Neuroanatomy Research at the Leading Edge

Neuroanatomy Research Advances

NEUROANATOMY RESEARCH AT THE LEADING EDGE

Additional books in this series can be found on Nova's website at:

https://www.novapublishers.com/catalog/index.php?cPath=23_29&seriesp=
Neuroanatomy+Research+at+the+Leading+Edge

Additional e-books in this series can be found on Nova's website at:

https://www.novapublishers.com/catalog/index.php?cPath=23_29&seriespe=
Neuroanatomy+Research+at+the+Leading+Edge

NEUROANATOMY RESEARCH AT THE LEADING EDGE

NEUROANATOMY RESEARCH ADVANCES

CIAN E. FLYNN
AND
BRANDON R. CALLAGHAN
EDITORS

Nova Biomedical
Nova Science Publishers, Inc.
New York

Copyright © 2010 by Nova Science Publishers, Inc.

All rights reserved. No part of this book may be reproduced, stored in a retrieval system or transmitted in any form or by any means: electronic, electrostatic, magnetic, tape, mechanical photocopying, recording or otherwise without the written permission of the Publisher.

For permission to use material from this book please contact us:
Telephone 631-231-7269; Fax 631-231-8175
Web Site: http://www.novapublishers.com

NOTICE TO THE READER

The Publisher has taken reasonable care in the preparation of this book, but makes no expressed or implied warranty of any kind and assumes no responsibility for any errors or omissions. No liability is assumed for incidental or consequential damages in connection with or arising out of information contained in this book. The Publisher shall not be liable for any special, consequential, or exemplary damages resulting, in whole or in part, from the readers' use of, or reliance upon, this material. Any parts of this book based on government reports are so indicated and copyright is claimed for those parts to the extent applicable to compilations of such works.

Independent verification should be sought for any data, advice or recommendations contained in this book. In addition, no responsibility is assumed by the publisher for any injury and/or damage to persons or property arising from any methods, products, instructions, ideas or otherwise contained in this publication.

This publication is designed to provide accurate and authoritative information with regard to the subject matter covered herein. It is sold with the clear understanding that the Publisher is not engaged in rendering legal or any other professional services. If legal or any other expert assistance is required, the services of a competent person should be sought. FROM A DECLARATION OF PARTICIPANTS JOINTLY ADOPTED BY A COMMITTEE OF THE AMERICAN BAR ASSOCIATION AND A COMMITTEE OF PUBLISHERS.

Library of Congress Cataloging-in-Publication Data

Neuroanatomy research advances / editors, Cian E. Flynn and Brandon R. Callaghan.
    p. ; cm.
 Includes bibliographical references and index.
 ISBN 978-1-60741-610-4 (hardcover)
 1. Neuroanatomy. 2. Headache--Pathophysiology. I. Flynn, Cian E. II. Callaghan, Brandon R.
 [DNLM: 1. Nervous System--anatomy & histology. 2. Brain--anatomy & histology. 3. Nerve Net--anatomy & histology. WL 101 N4924 2009]
 QM451.N38 2009
 611'.8--dc22
          2009030457

Published by Nova Science Publishers, Inc. ✦ *New York*

Contents

Preface   **vii**

Chapter I   Major Neuroanatomical and Neurochemical Substrates Involved in Primary Headaches   **1**
Mohtashem Samsam, Rafael Covenas, Raheleh Ahangari and Javier Yajeya Javier

Chapter II   Architectonic Studies: Past, Present and Future   **59**
Peiyan Wong and Jon H. Kaas

Chapter III   Correlation of Neurotrophin Expression and Survival-Promoting Capacities with Different Programmed Cell Death Periods in the Developing Murine Retina   **93**
Elvira Pyziak and Nicole Duenker

Chapter IV   Comparative Distribution of Orexin-like Immunoreactivity in the Brain of Vertebrates   **121**
Kristan G. Singletary, Christopher R. Hayworth and Yvon Delville

Chapter V   Visual Cortex: Crosstalk and Concomitant Communications between Extrastriate Visual Areas   **145**
Hiroyuki Nakamura and Kazuo Itoh

Chapter VI   Final Publications of Christfried Jakob: On the Frontal Lobe and the Limbic Region   **165**
Lazaros C. Triarhou

Chapter VII   The Human Olfactory System: An Anatomical and Cytoarchitectonic Study of the Anterior Olfactory Nucleus   **171**
Daniel Saiz Sánchez, Isabel Úbeda Bañón, Carlos de la Rosa Prieto, Lucía Argandoña Palacios, Susana García Muñozguren, Ricardo Insausti and Alino Martínez Marcos

Chapter VIII	Caudata (Amphibia) Brains and Telencephalon: Volumetric Organization and Hyperspatial Interpretations (CFA Projections) *Michel Thireau*	**183**
Chapter IX	Vagal Tone: Neuroanatomy, Function, and Application *Vladimir Miskovic and Louis A. Schmidt*	**197**
Chapter X	Quantitative Microscopic Analysis of Myelinated Nerve Fibers *Dimiter Prodanov, Hans K.P. Feirabend and Enrico Marani*	**207**
Index		**267**

Preface

Neuroanatomy is the study of the anatomical organization of the brain. Reciprocal communication between the brain and the cardiovascular system is important in sustaining neurobehavioral states that allow organisms to cope with their environment. Furthermore, in vertebrate animals, the routes that the myriad nerves take from the brain to the rest of the body, and the internal structure of the brain in particular, are both extremely elaborate. As a result, the study of neuroanatomy has developed into a discipline in itself, although it also represents a specialization within neuroscience. This book briefly covers the neuroanatomy of the vagal circuit, the functional significance of tonic cardiac vagal function and ways of quantifying this measure for research purposes. Also examined are the fiber composition and functional topography of peripheral nerves, and innovative methodologies that facilitate measurements of nerve fibers. This book contributes new insights to the controversial discussion about neurotrophin effects on different cell populations and at different time points in retinal programmed cell death (PCD). Other chapters in this book provide a comparative overview of the distribution of orexin cells and fibers across the brains of vertebrates in relation to function, the neuroanatomical structures and autonomic nerves involved in headaches and a reevaluation of the structure of the human anterior olfactory nucleus, with an updated description of this structure in the normal human.

Chapter I - Neuroanatomical structures involved in head pain are primarily the sensory distribution of four cranial nerves: the trigeminal—and to a lesser extent, facial, glossopharyngeal, and vagus—as well as the terminations of the upper three cervical nerves.

In addition, various pain sensitive cranial structures including the scalp and its blood supply, the head and neck muscles, intracranial and meningeal arteries, and dura mater including the venous sinuses are the major anatomical substrates of various types of headaches. Although brain tumors, different types of hemorrhage, hypertension, and meningitis may present as a headache, the migraine, cluster, and tension headaches are the three major types of primary headaches. Current opinion suggests a primary central nervous system activation may initiate a migraine. Several triggering factors such as disturbances of brain oxygenation and metabolism, alterations in the serotonin levels, low levels of brain tissue magnesium, altered transport of ions across the cell membrane, abnormal mitochondrial energy metabolism, and genetic abnormalities including mutations of the P/Q type calcium channel gene, Na^+/K^+ pump ATP1A2, or sodium channel Nav1.1 mutations have been linked to the pathogenesis of migraines. Patients with mutations in the calcium channel gene are more sensitive to environmental factors, which results in a wave of cortical spreading depression in the patient after the attack is initiated.

Moreover, several recent clinical and diagnostic studies indicate a dysfunction of the brainstem periaqueductal gray matter during migraine, or initiation of migraine by activation of the brainstem including the dorsal rostral and midline pons. Consistent with this, an active locus in the posterior hypothalamus has been implicated in cluster headache (CH). The headache phase involves the activation of the trigeminovascular system and possibly dilatation of the cranial blood vessels presumably mediated by the release of vasoactive substances and neuropeptides including the calcitonin gene-related peptide (CGRP). Increased serum CGRP levels were detected during migraine and CH. In addition, in CH, there is a release of parasympathetic peptide, vasoactive intestinal peptide. Currently, inhibiting the release of vasoactive substances and neuropeptides including the CGRP or nitric oxide, or blocking their receptors in the neuroanatomical substrates of head pain is a major focus in treatment of headaches.

Chapter II - The mammalian neocortex has a basic six-layered structure. Modifications to this fundamental design have lead to a diversity of structural and functional areas amongst mammals. Functional borders of certain cortical areas have shown good correspondence to anatomical borders identified by histological methods, the primary visual cortex of squirrels as an example (Kaas et al., 1972). This suggests a link between structure and function, an 'organology' of cortical areas where certain functions are localized in certain areas (Creutzfeldt, 1995). Perhaps through studying the fine anatomy of the neocortex, different functional areas can be identified by their differing fine anatomical structure. Architectonic studies attempt to better understand cortical morphology and parcellate the cortical sheet into distinct areas (Van Essen, 2004). This involves the use of staining methods to visualize various structural features. While architectonic studies came about as early as the 18th century, progress in this field has been hampered by technological limitations. In the past century, architectonic studies have acquired several tools that lead to great progress in the parcellation of the neocortex. This includes the availability of better microscopes, and staining methods that use antibodies with increased specificity and ligands that are able to show the distribution of their respective receptors. In the recent years, architectonic studies have taken on a more quantified, observer-independent approach to reduce variations from individual samples and subjectivity of different researchers. With improved functional imaging methods, there is a need for architectonic studies to come up with reliable spatial cortical maps that can be applied to functional imaging results. This will require the use of multiple approaches, observer-dependent and independent methods, and a battery of staining methods, including the histological, immunohistochemical and receptor-binding methods. In addition, continued efforts to develop better statistical methods for observer-independent methods, software to create spatial maps of the neocortical areas, and more sensitive, area-specific staining methods are necessary.

Chapter III - Programmed cell death (PCD) is a genuine developmental process of the nervous system, affecting not only projecting neurons but also proliferating neural precursors and newly postmitotic neuroblasts. It is widely accepted that during development neurotrophic factors control the survival of different neuronal cell types. In most survival studies published so far, enriched retinal ganglion cell cultures of dissociated cells were used, a system far from being physiological as the neurons lost cell-cell contacts. Besides, in the literature one finds contradictory reports on neurotrophin effects at different time points in retinal development: some studies observed that survival promoting effects of neurotrophins are limited to early neurons, others report effects restricted to differentiated neurons. Last but not least, a multitude of studies analysed survival-promoting effects of neurotrophins under pathological conditions, e.g. the survival of retinal ganglion cells after optic nerve lesion. However, the expression and effect of survival-promoting factors during developmental, naturally occurring PCD has not been investigated so far. In the study presented, the authors analyzed the cell types expressing neurotrophins and their receptors by immunocytochemical double labelling with cell type specific markers, correlated the expression profile of neurotrophins and their receptors with naturally occurring PCD periods of the developing retina and compared the survival-promoting capacity of neurotrophin signalling on different cell populations during early and late murine postnatal retinal PCD peaks using an *in vitro* culture system that retains the integrity of the retinal network. The authors found mRNA levels of the brain derived neurotrophic factor (BDNF) and neurotrophin-4 (NT4) receptor TrkB, insulin and ciliary neurotrophic factor (CNTF) receptors to be up-regulated during murine retinal development and their maximal expression to correlate with the main peaks of postnatal retinal PCD. BDNF, NT4 and insulin exhibited different survival promoting capacities during all postnatal retinal PCD phases affecting early, proliferating neurons as well as different populations of differentiated retinal cells. Although their receptors do not seem to be expressed on photoreceptors, these neurotrophins prevented apoptosis of both retinal ganglion and photoreceptor cells in organotypic murine retinal wholemount cultures. CNTF, by contrast, showed no short-term survival-promoting effect during murine retinal apoptosis, at least not after 24h culture *in vitro*. Thus, this chapter contributes new insights to the controversial discussion about neurotrophin effects on different cell populations and at different time points in retinal PCD.

Chapter IV - Orexin neuropeptides are highly conserved among vertebrates. This conservation extends to neuroanatomy and perhaps function. Orexin is thought to be involved in feeding, the sleep/wake cycle, stress and reproduction in mammals. However, its role in most vertebrates is unclear. In an effort to gain a better understanding of the function of orexin the authors compared orexin immunoreactive like (-lir) cell bodies and fiber distributions across tetrapods. The authors' studies support previous findings that orexin-lir neurons are concentrated in the vertebrate hypothalamus. In addition, there is a high degree of conservation of orexin-lir innervation across vertebrates.

While orexin cell bodies are located in the hypothalamus across vertebrates, there are slight differences in hypothalamic area. Discrepancies between species may be due to phylogenetic differences, and this could reflect diverging roles for the orexin system. It is interesting to note that in these vertebrates, aside from mammals, these orexin cell bodies are associated with neurosecretory areas and likely involved in homeostasis.

Examining orexin-lir fiber distribution can also help elucidate the function of orexins. Generally, there is moderate to dense orexin-lir innervation of the hypothalamus, midline thalamic areas, and ventral telencephalon. Overall similarities suggest that the orexin system is involved in general physiological or homeostatic roles, although slight differences could reflect a lineage relationship in vertebrate evolution and help to track phylogenies. As such, this short commentary will provide a comparative overview of the distribution of orexin cells and fibers across the brains of vertebrates in relation to function.

Chapter V - Extrastriate visual cortex has been divided into the dorsal and ventral stream visual areas. The dorsal stream visual areas are located in the occipito-parietal pathway directed to the superior temporal sulcus and inferior parietal lobule visual areas, underlying motion and spatial vision. These areas have been considered to receive visual information from magnocellular retinal ganglion cells through layer $4C\alpha$ and layer 4B of the primary visual area V1 (striate cortex), and then the cytochrome oxidase (CO)-rich thick stripes of the secondary visual area V2. On the other hand, the ventral stream visual areas are located in the occipito-temporal pathway directed to the inferior temporal cortex, underlying object vision. These areas have been considered to receive visual information from the parvocellular retinal ganglion cells through layer $4C\beta$ and layers 2-3 of V1, and then the CO-rich thin stripes and the CO-poor interstripe regions of V2. This parallel visual cortical information processing hypothesis is, however, too simple, and ignored abundant connections between the dorsal and the ventral stream visual areas (Nakamura et al., *Soc. Neurosci. Abstr., 18,* 294, 1992). In addition, recent analysis of the connections between V1 and V2 CO-modules provided a line of evidence against the dorsal versus ventral stream hypothesis (Sincich & Horton, *Science, 29,* 1734-1737, 2002; Nassi & Callaway, *J. Neurosci., 26,* 12789-12798, 2006), and thus the whole story of visual cortical information processing is now going to be reconstructed. The authors here describe the connections between the extrastriate visual areas based on the previous reports, and the authors' publications and unpublished data to construct a graph scheme of visual cortical network. The visual cortical network is hierarchically composed of several sets of visual areas and connections between them. Consider the areas as nodes and the connections as arcs, the network is a direct graph (Apollonio & Franciosa, *Descrete Math., 307,* 2598-2614, 2007). In this graph, functional groups of the areas and the connections are partial graphs. The partial graphs are dynamic in a sense that the nodes and arcs (the areas and connections) vary from time to time depending on what task or function is necessary. The dynamic partial graphs overlap each other to allow them common use of visual information.

Chapter VI - One of the foremost neuroanatomists of the twentieth century, Christfried (Christofredo) Jakob (1866–1956) left a legacy of over 30 monographs and 200 papers, now becoming appreciated in the English biomedical literature. Born in Germany, he was summoned in 1899 to Buenos Aires by the Argentinian psychiatric academia. He spent the rest of his professional life (save for a brief return to Germany between 1910–1912) in affiliation with the National Universities of La Plata and Buenos Aires. The writings of Jakob cover a wide spectrum of topics, from the pathology of neuropsychiatric disorders to the phylogeny, ontogeny and dynamics of the cerebral cortex and their mental corollaries, and ultimately some of the most fundamental neurophilosophical questions. Although in many respects his innovative ideas opened up new ways of thinking in brain and behavior research, they still remain largely unheeded, most likely owing to their exclusive appearance in German or Spanish. The present study revisits Jakob's last two formal publications, dating to 1949. These are entitled 'The task of the frontal lobe in connection with a synthetic quantification of its constitutive elements' and 'The neuronal quantification of the limbic region in its relation to the endogenous affective sphere' (co-authored with his pupils Eduardo A. Pedace and Andrés R. Copello, respectively), and represent the culmination of Jakob's thought, integrating morphofunctional concepts in his quest for understanding the neuroanatomical fundamentals of the human mind. Cognitive function and emotional processing are at the core of current neurobiological research, and Jakob's pioneering concepts remain worthy of consideration six decades later.

Chapter VII - The sense of smell is only poorly-developed in humans and neuroanatomical studies have therefore often neglected the olfactory system. Recent data have shown that the olfactory system is affected early in neurodegenerative conditions such as Alzheimer's and Parkinson's disease, where hyposmia appears before other symptoms. Such findings emphasize the importance of understanding olfactory system structure and function. The present work revisits the anatomic and cytoarchitectonic structure of the human olfactory system, with particular emphasis on poorly-characterized regions affected in neurodegenerative diseases such as the anterior olfactory nucleus. The anterior olfactory nucleus, the first relay in the olfactory pathway after the olfactory bulb, projects to the olfactory cortex as well as to the ipsi- and contralateral olfactory bulbs. Histologic studies have revealed that α-synuclein and tau proteins, markers of neurodegenerative diseases, accumulate in this nucleus in Parkinson's and Alzheimer's disease respectively. However, literature descriptions of the nucleus remain controversial, particularly regarding its extent and the classification of its different subdivisions. This study reevaluates the structure of the human anterior olfactory nucleus and provides an updated description of this structure in the normal human.

Chapter VIII - Studies on vertebrate brain evolution commonly use either qualitative or quantitative methods. The latter require cytological examination of tiny brains, to recognize various neurons populations and obtain their reliable volumetric data. Before the discovery of allometry, brain size was an obstacle to the interpretation of ratios.

Allometric analysis itself raises obstacles: a necessary use of an average rate for the calculation of indices and, moreover, a restriction to uni- or bi- dimensional comparisons.

With the use of Correspondence Factor Analysis (CFA), novel interpretations of the volumetric values of the different brain divisions are derived from a hyperspace in which the barycentric juxtaposition allows multidimensional comparisons (phi1phiN) between species and volumes projected on biplots.

Choosing to work on Caudata Order (newts and salamanders) allows us to understand the role of all the telencephalon neurons populations in a Vertebrate radiation, as well as the impact of neoteny on Caudata brain organization.

The main results obtained during the last ten years show that the brain of each species is taxonomically characteristic (= neurotaxonomy) under a general tendency to scale invariance (fractality).

Neurotaxonomy proposes support and possible arbitration in a wide variety of systematic questions (such as polymorphism and polytypy); and finally provide a key to understanding the brain and species hyperspaces links.

Chapter IX - Reciprocal communication between the brain and the cardiovascular system is important in sustaining neurobehavioral states that allow organisms to cope with their environment. The vagal circuit is one of the key brain cardio-regulatory circuits implicated in emotion regulation and stress responsiveness. Here the authors briefly cover the neuroanatomy of the vagal circuit, the functional significance of tonic cardiac vagal function, and ways of quantifying this measure for research purposes. The authors also illustrate the application of the vagal tone construct for research on stress vulnerability in clinical and nonclinical populations.

Chapter X - Better understanding of the structure and function of peripheral nerve fibers could facilitate the search of new treatments for demyelinating disorders and nerve regeneration and lead to further improvement of neural prostheses.

Availability of quantitative anatomic (morphometric) data is, therefore, crucial part of this process.

Due to the labor-intensiveness of the conventional morphometric protocols, extensive morphometric studies are still occasional. Therefore, many structures in the peripheral and central nervous systems are still poorly described quantitatively. In this chapter, the authors will give an account of the most important studies dealing with the fiber composition and topography of peripheral nerves and spinal roots.

The authors' research in this field was directed toward several objectives: to characterize better the (i) fiber composition and (ii) functional topography of peripheral nerves, and (iii) to device innovative methodologies that facilitate measurements of nerve fibers. Using the conventional morphometric approach, the authors have demonstrated that parametric population models could describe well the fiber composition of peripheral nerves. These models could be used for objective classification of the myelinated nerve fibers into $A\alpha$, $A\beta$, $A\gamma$ or $A\delta$ fiber classes. Anatomical and physiological criteria for such classification are derived for the rat. By means of nonparametric spatial statistics, it has been shown that some muscle representations are topographically organized along their course in the peripheral nerves. Presented results are discussed in the perspective of the development of nerve-electrode interfaces.

Finally, a comprehensive account is given on the new statistical approaches for fiber classification and spatial statistical analysis. Applicability of presented approaches is discussed for other PNS studies, for example in fiber regeneration and toxicology.

In: Neuroanatomy Research Advances
Editors: C. E. Flynn and B. R. Callaghan, pp.1-58

ISBN: 978-60741-610-4
©2010 Nova Science Publishers, Inc.

Chapter I

Major Neuroanatomical and Neurochemical Substrates Involved in Primary Headaches

Mohtashem Samsam[*,1,2], *Rafael Covenas*[3], *Raheleh Ahangari*[1] *and Javier Yajeya Javier*[3]

University of Central Florida, Burnett College of Biomedical Sciences and College of Medicine, Orlando, Florida, USA[1]
International University of Health Sciences (IUHS), St. Kitts, West Indies[2]
University of Salamanca, Institute of Neurosciences of Castilla y Leon (INCYL), Salamanca, Spain[3]

Abstract

Neuroanatomical structures involved in head pain are primarily the sensory distribution of four cranial nerves: the trigeminal—and to a lesser extent, facial, glossopharyngeal, and vagus—as well as the terminations of the upper three cervical nerves.

In addition, various pain sensitive cranial structures including the scalp and its blood supply, the head and neck muscles, intracranial and meningeal arteries, and dura mater including the venous sinuses are the major anatomical substrates of various types of headaches. Although brain tumors, different types of hemorrhage, hypertension, and meningitis may present as a headache, the migraine, cluster, and tension headaches are the three major types of primary headaches. Current opinion suggests a primary central nervous system activation may initiate a migraine. Several triggering factors such as disturbances of brain oxygenation and metabolism, alterations in the serotonin levels, low levels of brain tissue magnesium, altered transport of ions across the cell membrane,

---

[*]Correspondence should be sent: Mohtashem Samsam, MD, PhD, University of Central Florida, 4000 Central University Blvd., HPA-II, 320, Orlando, FL, 32816, USA, Phone: 407- 823 4810, Fax: 407- 823-3095, E-mail: msamsam@mail.ucf.edu

abnormal mitochondrial energy metabolism, and genetic abnormalities including mutations of the P/Q type calcium channel gene, Na^+/K^+ pump ATP1A2, or sodium channel Nav1.1 mutations have been linked to the pathogenesis of migraines. Patients with mutations in the calcium channel gene are more sensitive to environmental factors, which results in a wave of cortical spreading depression in the patient after the attack is initiated.

Moreover, several recent clinical and diagnostic studies indicate a dysfunction of the brainstem periaqueductal gray matter during migraine, or initiation of migraine by activation of the brainstem including the dorsal rostral and midline pons. Consistent with this, an active locus in the posterior hypothalamus has been implicated in cluster headache (CH). The headache phase involves the activation of the trigeminovascular system and possibly dilatation of the cranial blood vessels presumably mediated by the release of vasoactive substances and neuropeptides including the calcitonin gene-related peptide (CGRP). Increased serum CGRP levels were detected during migraine and CH. In addition, in CH, there is a release of parasympathetic peptide, vasoactive intestinal peptide. Currently, inhibiting the release of vasoactive substances and neuropeptides including the CGRP or nitric oxide, or blocking their receptors in the neuroanatomical substrates of head pain is a major focus in treatment of headaches.

Introduction

The neuroanatomical structures involved in headaches are mainly the trigeminal nerve [cranial nerves (CN) five, CNV], CNVII, CNIX, CNX, as well as the upper cervical nerves together with their target peripheral tissues including the skin, muscles, blood vessels, meninges, and other tissues. Autonomic nerves have also been implicated in headaches. Several neurotransmitter/ neuromodulator contents of these nerves mediate the transmission of pain. The trigeminal nerve has a major role in conducting the painful (nociceptive) information to the higher brain centers to register the pain. Central processes of the trigeminal primary sensory neurons reach the trigeminal nuclear complex in the brainstem. The ascending pathways include the fibers of the postsynaptic trigeminal sensory nuclei neurons, a major part of it originating in the caudal trigeminal nucleus and project to several supraspinal centers including the nucleus of the solitary tract, A5 cell group region/superior salivatory nucleus, the periaqueductal grey matter (PGA), the parabrachial nucleus, as well as the ventral posteromedial thalamic nuclei (Noseda et al., 2008). The painful information reaches the sensory cortical areas as well as other regions such as the limbic system for autonomic and affective responses to pain.

Several supraspinal centers with potential involvement in modulation of pain transmission have been identified. Among these multiple candidate efferent pathways with modulatory control of nociception, the well-known circuit includes the amygdala, PAG, dorsolateral pontomesencephalic tegmentum (DLPT) and rostroventromedial medulla (RVM) in the brainstem. This circuit controls both spinal and trigeminal dorsal horn pain transmission neurons via descending projections, and mediates both opioid and stimulation produced analgesia (Fields, 2000).

The descending antinociceptive system originates in the amygdaloid body and hypothalamus and project to the lower brainstem and spinal cord, via midbrain.

Descending modulation of pain is conducted mainly by the noradrenergic, serotonergic, and opioidergic systems. The midbrain PAG region sends excitatory projections to the neurons of the rostroventral medial medulla, the most important of which are the serotonergic neurons in the midline of the nucleus raphe magnus and also other serotonergic nuclei. Moreover, other descending inhibitory systems involved in antinociception in dorsal horn originate in the noradrenergic locus ceruleus and other brainstem nuclei (Jones, 1991; Basbaum and Jessel, 2000). In addition, two other medullary systems including the dorsal reticular nucleus and the caudal ventrolateral medulla are involved in the modulation of pain and function primarily as pronociceptive and antinociceptive centres, respectively (Millan, 2002). Both areas are connected with the spinal dorsal horn by closed reciprocal loops (Lima and Almedia, 2002; Tavares and Lima, 2007). The descending pain modulatory pathways function in both descending inhibition as well as the descending facilitation of pain. Neuroanatomical structures involved in the descending inhibition or facilitation of the pain are common (Millan, 2002). Recent clinical studies in primary headache patients, including the cluster headache and migraine, show activation of several regions including mainly the pons, midbrain, and hypothalamus among others (Cohen and Goadsby, 2006). These areas remain activated even after the resolution of headache following sumatriptan (an effective anti-migraine drug) treatment. This has led us to believe that the trigger of pain in migraine might be in the brainstem, and that a possible pathophysiology of migraine might be due to an abnormal central processing (Goadsby, 2007).

Within this chapter we review the neuroanatomical and neurochemical substrates of headache including the most important supraspinal structures with direct descending pathways to the dorsal horn and analyze the functional bases of some most recent clinical and imaging findings in primary headaches.

What is Pain?

Pain is an unpleasant sensory and emotional experience associated with actual or potential tissue damage or described in terms of such damage (Bonica, 1990). It is a complex sensory and psychological experience and is a common cause of suffering that may lead to disability and impairment of the quality of life and is a serious economic problem. Pain is highly individual and has a subjective nature which makes it difficult to define and to treat clinically. There are no painful stimuli that invariably elicit the perception of pain in all individuals (Basbaum and Jessell, 2000). Although many loci involved in pain have been identified, the exact pathomechanism of pain and especially headaches is still not clear.

Types of Pain

Pain can be acute or chronic. Acute pain is usually a persistent and sometimes a severe pain which might force the patient to seek medical attention. It is a protective and warning sign of a possible or actual damage. Chronic pain, however, is more complicated and may not be useful and makes the patients miserable. Chronic pain persists for a month beyond the usual course of an acute disease, or a reasonable time for an injury to heal, or is associated with a chronic pathologic process that causes continuous pain, or the pain recurs at intervals for months or years (Bonica, 1990). Pain can be subdivided into the nociceptive, neuropathic, and idiopathic (psychogenic) pains. Nociceptive pain is usually due to direct activation of the nociceptors in various tissues which develops in response to tissue injury and/ or inflammation. Neuropathic pain, however, bypasses the normal nociceptive pathway and is precipitated by direct injury to the peripheral or central nerves and often has a burning or electric sensation. The post herpetic neuralgia and phantom limb pain fall in this category (Bonica, 1990; Basbaum and Jessell, 2000). Idiopathic (psychologic) pain persists in the absence of an identified source of organic pain, or might be in excess of a documented organic lesion (Portenoy and Kanner, 1996).

Perception and Transmission of Pain

Pain is perceived by nociceptors, which are specialized sensory receptors distributed in various tissues. The transduction of painful stimuli is by these peripheral (free nerve) endings of the non-myelinated C fibers and thinly myelinated Aδ fibers. When superficial (e.g., skin) or deep (e.g., muscle) tissues are stimulated by a noxious stimulus, this activates the nociceptors, the peripheral endings of primary sensory neurons, whose cell bodies are located in the dorsal root ganglia or trigeminal ganglion. Their central axons terminate usually in the dorsal horn of the spinal cord or the trigeminal nucleus in the brainstem.

Different classes of nociceptors include the thermal, mechanical, polymodal, and silent nociceptors. Thermal nociceptors are activated by extreme temperature (> 45°C or < 5°C). The mechanical nociceptors show selective responses to strong pressure. Both are of Aδ fiber type. Polymodal nociceptors are small diameter non-myelinated C-fibers with a slow conduction velocity (1 m/s). These nociceptors respond to chemical, mechanical, and thermal (both hot and cold) stimuli and are therefore known as polymodal nociceptors. Silent nociceptors are usually found in the viscera and are not activated normally by noxious stimuli; however, their threshold is significantly reduced by inflammation and chemical insults (Basbaum and Jessell, 2000).

Central Relay of Nociceptive Afferents

Central axons of the pseudounipolar nociceptive neurons (afferents) reach predominantly the dorsal horn of the spinal cord or the brainstem medulla. Upon entering the dorsal horn of the spinal cord, fibers branch immediately and divide into ascending and descending branches which travel for one or two segments and form the posterolateral tract of Lissauer, that synapse with the cells in the outer part of the dorsal horn, in the substantia gelatinosa of Rolando. The trigeminal afferents terminate predominantly in the ipsilateral trigeminal nuclei in the brain stem (Carpenter, 1985; Snell, 2001).

The dorsal horn can be subdivided histologically into six distinct layers or laminae. The primary nociceptive afferent (central) fibers terminate on projection neurons in the dorsal horn of the spinal cord. The lamina I projection neurons receive direct input from myelinated (Aδ) nociceptive afferent fibers and indirect input from unmyelinated (C) fibers via stalk cell interneurons in lamina II. Neurons in lamina V are mainly of the wide dynamic-range type, which receive low-threshold input from the large-diameter myelinated Aβ fibers of mechanoreceptors as well as both direct and indirect inputs from nociceptive afferent Aδ and C fibers (Basbaum and Jessell, 2000). The *lateral spinothalamic tract in* the spinal cord transmits the pain and thermal stimuli to the higher brain centers. Its second-order neurons in the pathway originate in the dorsal horn of the spinal cord and cross obliquely to the opposite side, in the anterior gray and white commisures within one spinal segment and ascend in the contralateral white column as the lateral spinothalamic tract. It ascends through the brainstem as *spinal lemniscus* accompanied by anterior spinothalamic (for light/ crude touch and pressure) and the spinotectal tracts. Spinal lemniscus ascends in the posterior part of pons and the midbrain tegmentum. These fibers terminate predominantly in the ventral posterolateral nucleus of thalamus by synapsing on third-order neurons. These in turn ascend towards the sensory cerebral cortex (Carpenter, 1985; Snell, 2001).

The Anatomic Substrates of Head Pain

Nerve impulses conducting the head pain originate primarily in the peripheral sensory distribution of four cranial nerves including mainly the trigeminal nerve [cranial nerve (CN)V], and to a lesser extent CN VII (facial), CN IX (glossopharyngeal), and CN X (vagus) and also in terminations of the upper three cervical nerves (Feindel, 1960, Mayberg et al., 1984; Carpenter, 1985; Bonica, 1990; Liu et al., 2008). Intracranial vessels are the major structures involved in the intracranial pain. Even early studies by Wolff and associates suggested six basic mechanisms of headache that arise from intracranial sources. These include traction on the veins that pass to the venous sinuses from the surface of the brain, and displacement of the great venous sinuses, traction on the middle meningeal arteries, as well as the large arteries at the base of the brain and their branches, distension and dilatation of the intracranial arteries, inflammation in or about any of the pain sensitive structures of the head, and direct pressure by tumors (Wolff, 1943).

Headache from extracranial sources is mostly due to sustained contraction of muscles of the head and neck, tissue inflammation, distension of the extracranial arteries, and pain referred from diseases of the eye, sinuses, and teeth (Bonica, 1990). Since intracranial blood vessels are innervated by the sympathetic, parasympathetic and sensory nerves, we therefore review some major nerves implicated in headache as well as their neurotransmitter contents.

The Sensory Portion of the Trigeminal Nerve and the Corresponding Nuclei

Trigeminal nerve carries the major sensory innervation of the cranial structures. Most of the primary afferents of the trigeminal nerve [the cranial nerve five (CNV)] are composed of unipolar (pseudounipolar) neurons in the trigeminal (Gasserian) ganglion (TG) including their peripheral and central processes. The peripheral processes of the trigeminal nerve make up the ophthalmic (CNV/I), maxillary (CNV/II), and mandibular (CNV/III) nerves/ divisions, which are distributed in the head and face and innervate several tissues including the skin, vessels, muscles, dura mater, and deeper structures. The mandibular nerve contains the main motor innervation contributed by the CNV which originate in the motor nucleus of the trigeminal nerve in the pons. The central processes of the primary sensory neurons of the trigeminal ganglion make up the sensory root, which reaches the ventral surface of the pons. These central processes then pass through the spinal trigeminal tract and terminate in the trigeminal nuclear complex (TNC), composed of main sensory nucleus (MSN) and the spinal trigeminal nucleus (STN). The MSN is located in pons, while the STN is deep to the descending trigeminal tract and extends caudally as far as the second and third cervical segments. The spinal nucleus is further subdivided into three parts: subnucleus oralis, subnucleus interpolaris, and subnucleus caudalis (Olszewski, 1950; Kerr, 1970; Darian-Smith, 1973; Carpenter, 1985; Bonica, 1990).

The large A-beta fiber type neurons, whose cell bodies reside in the trigeminal (Gasserian) ganglion, transmit proprioceptive information from the anterior two-thirds of the head via the three major divisions of the trigeminal nerve. Their central processes synapse in the mesencephalic nucleus. The large myelinated mechanoreceptive and thermoreceptive low-threshold receptors/primary afferents pass centrally and divide into short ascending branches that terminate in the main sensory nucleus and long descending branches that pass through the trigeminal tract and give off collaterals to various parts of the underlying spinal nucleus to the main sensory nucleus and subnuclei oralis and interpolaris. The thermoceptive and nociceptive A-delta and C fibers descend in to terminate within the subnucleus caudalis (Bonica, 1990).

The descending fibers from the trigeminal primary afferents as well as the cranial nerves VII, IX, and X, make up the descending spinal tract, and their collaterals synapse with the second-order neurons in the spinal nucleus. The axons of second-order neurons cross to the opposite side to shape the ventral trigeminothalamic tract. However, some of the fibers from the main sensory nucleus and subnucleus oralis ascend ipsilaterally as the dorsal trigeminothalamic tract. Likewise, the fibers of the paleotrigeminothalamic tract cross to the opposite side, where some ascend to reach the ventral postero-medial (VPM) and the medial/intralaminar thalamic nuclei (MIT), however, other fibers pass into the reticular formation, where they synapse with ascending reticulothalamic fibers (Bonica, 1990). The trigeminal mesencephalic nucleus (TMN), however, is a collection of cell bodies of primary neurons, which instead of being localized in the trigeminal ganglion (TG) together with other somatic primary cell bodies have migrated into the mesencephalon (midbrain) and are known to be involved in proprioception through their peripheral fibers distributed in the head (Darian-Smith, 1973; Carpenter, 1985; Bonica, 1990). The central branches of these primary cells project to the motor nucleus of the CN V and make monosynaptic contact with somatomotor neurons to complete a two-neuron arc for the jaw-reflex, which is homologous with the spinal reflexes (Bonica, 1990).

Like many other areas of the nervous system, the trigeminal system has a somatotopic arrangement throughout the TG, the sensory root, the spinal tract and the spinal nucleus. The cutaneous distribution of the ophthalmic branch of the CNV innervates the tip and upper parts of the nose, upper parts of the face including the forehead and the scalp over the parietal bone. The maxillary branch innervates the skin of the lateral and lower parts of the nose, the cheeks, and the lateral parts of the forehead. The mandibular branch innervates the very lateral parts of the face including the area over the lower jaw and areas anterior and superior to the auricles (Bonica 1990; Wall and Melzack, 1994). The supratentorial dura mater is innervated by the branches of the trigeminal nerve, but the infratentorial part of the dura mater is innervated by the upper cervical spinal nerves as well as the vagus nerve (Feindel, 1960; Mayberg, 1984; Carpenter, 1985). There is also a somatotopic organization of the descending spinal trigeminal tract in the lower medulla oblungata. In a cross section of the human lower medulla, from posterior to the posterolateral and postero-anterior directions, the structures are distributed as the following: fasciculus gracilis is located posteriorly close to the midline; lateral to this, the fasciculus cuneatus, and more anterolaterally, the central processes of the cranial nerves (CN) seven (CNVII), CNIX, and CNX are located. Next to this wedge (in the cross section of the medulla oblongata), from posterior to anterior direction, the central processes of the mandibular, maxillary, and ophthalmic divisions terminate in the spinal trigeminal nucleus. In a rostrocaudal direction, Dejerine in 1914 described the somatotopic distribution of the trigeminal central terminals in CTN, responsible for the "onion peel" pattern of sensation in the face (Bonica, 1990).

We have also shown such somatotopic organization in the rat medulla by degenerative studies following sectioning the infraorbital and/or mandibular nerves and looked for the disappearance of neuropeptide contents of the trigeminal central terminals in caudal trigeminal nucleus (Knyihár Csillik et al., 1994).

Central processes of the trigeminal ganglion neurons terminate predominantly in the ipsilateral trigeminal nuclei and electrical stimulation of the trigeminal ganglion leads to depletion of neuropeptide contents of the central trigeminal terminals in the ipsilateral caudal trigeminal nucleus (CTN) (Samsam et al, 2000). However, a unilateral electrical stimulation of the trigeminal ganglion leads to a patchy depletion of neuropeptide immunoreactivity of the contralateral CTN in addition to their massive ipsilateral depletion (Samsam et al., 2001), indicating a possible bilateral termination of some trigeminal central fibers. Although, all these fibers may not be nociceptive, most of the trigeminal nociceptive fibers reach the CTN. This may have implication in bilateral perception of pain originating from one side in the periphery, but activating both sides central neurons in the brainstem. Contralateral depletions were not seen in all parts of the medulla, indicating that the degree and levels of termination of such contralateral central trigeminal terminals may not be the same in the entire trigeminal nucleus. Trigeminal nerve projections to the contralateral medullary and cervical dorsal horns were also reported by other groups (Pfaller and Arvidsson, 1988: Jacquin et al., 1990). This was in agreement with a study done by Hoskin and colleagues, stating that electrical stimulation of the middle meningeal artery of one side in the dura of monkey and cat increased the expression of C-fos in the ipsilateral and also contralateral trigeminocervical nucleus (Hoskin et al., 1999).

Neurotransmitters/ Neuromodulator Contents of the Trigeminal Ganglion

Several neuropeptides exist in the primary sensory neurons of the dorsal root ganglia (DRG) and the trigeminal ganglion (TG) neurons including their processes. Among these, excitatory amino acids such as glutamate and aspartate are found in large DRG neurons, and many other substances including several peptides are found in the DRG small neurons (Yaksh et al., 1980; Holzer, 1988; Bonica 1990). Glutamate is one of the main neurotransmitters of the TG neurons (Lazarov, 2002; Ramadan, 2003). Several neuropeptides such as substance P (SP), calcitonin gene-related peptide (CGRP) (Uddman et al., 1985; O'Connor and Van der Kooy, 1988) and neurokinin A (NKA), exist and co-exist together in a subpopulation of TG neurons and their processes (Edvinsson et al., 1987a; 1988; 1989; 1994; Uddman et al., 1985; Hardebo et al., 1989; Suzuki et al., 1989). Among several neuropeptides in the human TG, the CGRP and SP are the most abundant; the CGRP containing neurons make up about 40% of the cells, and 18% of the TG neurons express SP (Edinsson et al., 1989; McCulloch et al., 1986).

The neuronal processes of such neuropeptide containing sensory neurons are distributed in peripheral tissues such as in the skin and cornea, the cerebral blood vessels, as well as in parts of the central nervous system especially in the dorsal horn of the spinal cord and medulla. The CGRP containing nerve fibers innervate the cerebral arteries and pial arterioles on the cortex of brain and the dura mater (Edvinsson et al., 1987a; 1987b; 1994; Knyihar-Csillik et al., 1995; Fricke et al., 1997) including the human (Gulbenkian et al., 1995; 2001) as well. Both CGRP and SP are potent vasodilators and the CGRP effect has been reported to be ten to a thousand time stronger than SP in vasodilation (Edvinsson et al., 1972; 1987a; McCulloch et al., 1986; Jansen et al., 1991). The circulating CGRP was proposed to induce hyperaemia in certain pathological conditions (Brain et al., 1985). Several studies suggest that the headache phase of migraine is due to cranial vasodilation as well as to the activation and sensitization of the sensory nerves including the trigeminal nerve (Moskowitz 1984; Burstein et al., 2000; Villalón et al., 2002; Spierings, 2003; Silberstein, 2004). Trigeminal nerve and its target innervation, the cerebral vasculature, as well as the cerebral dura mater are involved in headaches (Wolff, 1943; Feindel, 1960; Moskowitz, 1984; Bonica, 1990).

Moreover, several neuropeptides including SP and CGRP found in the temporal and occipital tissues may be involved in extracranial pain (Uddman et al., 1986). Increased CGRP levels were found in the jugular blood of human subjects during migraine (Goadsby et al., 1988, 1990). Consistent with this, Gallai and associates found increased CGRP and NKA levels in human blood during migraine attacks (Gallai et al., 1995). In a series of studies we have also reported the depletion of CGRP-immunoreactivity in the peripheral and central trigeminal terminals (Knyihár-Csillik et al., 1994, 1995, 1996, 1997, 1998), as well as the CGRP, SP and NKA depletion centrally in the caudal trigeminal nucleus (CTN) (Samsam et al., 1996, 1999, 2000, 2001) following electrical stimulation of the rat TG.

Clinically however, efforts to find SP in the blood of migraine sufferers have failed (Goadsby et al., 1990, 2002; Friberg et al., 1994, Gallai et al., 1995; Alessandri et al., 2006), except to a recent article which shows increased plasma SP and CGRP levels and high angiotensin converting enzyme (ACE) activity in migraineurs during headache-free periods (Fusayasu et al., 2007).

Inhibiting the release of neuropeptides or blocking their receptors in the periphery (in order to block the neurogenic inflammation and vasodilation) and/or in the CNS, seems to be a reasonable strategy to alleviate the pain. In this respect, neurokinin (NK)-1 receptor antagonists such as RP67580 failed to inhibit or decrease the expression of c-fos and central trigeminal activity following electrical stimulation of the superior sagittal sinus, see the headache section of this chapter. Consistent with this, neither the neurokinin-1 (NK1) receptor antagonist RP67580 (0.23 or 2.3 mumol.kg-1, i.v.), nor the vasoactive intestinal peptide (VIP) antagonist (p-Cl-D-Phe6,Leu17)-VIP at 15 or 30 nmol.kg-1, i.v., had any effect on increased facial skin blood flow following electrical stimulation of the TG (Escott et al., 1995). Similarly, SP antagonists did not alleviate headache in clinical investigations (Diener, 1996; Goldstein et al., 1997), although this might be due to the poor bioavailability of this drug during such attacks.

All these indicated that SP may not have a major role in vasodilation in the peripheral trigeminal territory in human in primary headache. Therefore, CGRP remains a major neuropeptide in focus at the moment and indeed many efforts are made in recent years to block its release presynaptically and/ or inhibit its receptor(s) postsynaptically to treat migraine and possibly the cluster headaches, see Goadsby (2007), Linde (2006) and (Samsam et al., 2007a) for review.

Juluis and colleagues used an expression cloning strategy based on calcium influx and isolated the transient receptor potential vanilloid-1 (Trpv1) capsaicin receptor from sensory neurons. This receptor is a non-selective cation channel that is structurally related to members of the TRP family of ion channels. The Trpv1 receptor is also activated by increases in temperature (greater than $43^{\circ}C$) in the noxious range and functions as a transducer of painful thermal stimuli in vivo (Caterina et al., 1997). Capsaicin, the main pungent ingredient in 'hot' chilli peppers, elicits a sensation of burning pain by selectively activating sensory neurons that convey information about noxious stimuli to the central nervous system. Trpv1 receptors (at the mRNA and protein levels) are found in the sensory and TG of the rat and human (Szallasi et al., 1995; Caterina et al., 1997; Guo A et al., 1999; Hou et al., 2002). Indeed Trpv1 receptor is colocalized with a subpopulation of CGRP, SP, and NOS expressing TG neurons (Hou et al., 2002). This implicates the Trpv1 receptors in modulation of pain and transmitter release. For a comprehensive review on how neurons detect pain-producing stimuli of a thermal, mechanical or chemical nature and their signalling mechanisms, please see the (Julius and Basbaum, 2001).

In addition to the SP, NKA and CGRP, many other neuropeptides such as somatostatin (SST) and neurotensin (NT) and endorphins are also found in the trigeminal nerve. Cerebral blood vessels are innervated by nerve fibers containing neuropeptide Y (NPY), vasoactive intestinal polypeptide (VIP), peptide histidine isoleucine (PHI). Fibers containing other substances such as cholecystokinin (CCK), dynorphin B, galanin (Gal), gastrin releasing peptide and vasopressin, have also been reported to innervate the cerebral blood vessels (Uddman and Edvinson, 1989).

A comprehensive review on neurotransmitter/ neuromodulator contents of the TG and the mesencephalic trigeminal nucleus (MTN) indicates that in the TG, two subpopulations of primary sensory neurons, containing immunoreactive (IR) material, were identified: 1) numerous glutamate-, SP-, NKA-, CGRP-, CCK-, SST-, VIP- and Gal-IR ganglion cells showing a small and medium-sized somata, and 2) relatively less numerous larger-sized neuropeptide Y (NPY)- and peptide 19 (PEP 19)-IR trigeminal neurons. In addition, many nitric oxide synthase (NOS)- and parvalbumin (PV)-IR cells of all sizes as well as fewer, mostly large, calbindin D-28k (CB)-containing neurons were also seen. Most of the large ganglion cells were surrounded by SP-, CGRP-, SST-, CCK-, VIP-, NOS- and 5-HT-IR perisomatic networks. In the mesencephalic trigeminal nucleus (MTN) however, the main subpopulation of large-sized neurons were glutamatergic (Lazarov, 2002), but some neurons exhibit PV- or CB-immunostaining while certain small MTN neurons, most likely interneurons, were found to be GABAergic. The trigeminal primary proprioceptors have their cell bodies in the centrally located MTN within the brainstem and are a crucial component of the neural circuitry responsible for the generation and control of oromotor activities. The expression of classical neurotransmitters and their receptors in mesencephalic trigeminal neurons has been recently reviewed elsewhere (Lazarov, 2007). For a review of the major TG neuropeptides implicated in headache, please refer to Samsam et al., (2007b).

As mentioned above, the TG neurons express nitric oxide synthase (NOS) (Olesen et al., 1995; Lazarov 2002), and nitric oxide (NO) has also been implicated in pain and migraine (Olesen J et al., 1995; Thomsen and Olesen, 2001). Intravenous (i.v.) infusion of nitroglycerine (Iversen, 2001) and hα-CGRP (Lassen et al., 2002) in migraineurs can produce a migraine-like effect. Nitroglycerine induces the release of NO, a strong vasodilator, mediating the pain (Iversen, 2001). Nitric oxide is involved in the maintenance of the basal level of dural arterial blood flow as well as in the electrically evoked flow increases mediated by CGRP released from dural afferent fibres. The synergistic effect of NO and CGRP on the stimulated blood flow was postulated to be in part due to a NO mediated facilitation of the CGRP release (Messlinger et al., 2000), while prostaglandins are not significantly involved (Strecker et al., 2002). CGRP synthesis and release are coordinately stimulated by the vasodilator NO, a signaling mechanism occuring within the trigeminal ganglia neurons. Consistent with this, NO-synthase inhibitors antagonized neurogenic and CGRP induced dilation of dural meningeal vessels (Akerman et al., 2002). Although NO-dependent cyclic guanosine monophosphate (cGMP) signaling causes headache and migraine, the CGRP-dependent cyclic adenosine monophosphate (cAMP), was found to be more involved (Birk et al., 2006).

Moreover, the CGRP promoter activity was also found to be stimulated by NO donors and overexpression of inducible nitric oxide synthase (iNOS). Mechanisms involving the NO stimulation of the CGRP secretion were reported not to require cGMP or PI3-kinase signaling pathways, but rather, NO action required extracellular calcium and likely involved T-type calcium channels, and sumatriptan (an anti-migraine drug) greatly repressed NO stimulation of CGRP promoter activity and secretion (Bellamy et al., 2006).

In addition, CGRP is also co-expressed with brain-derived neurotrophic factor (BDNF) in a large subset of adult rat TG neurons, and recent evidence shows that CGRP potently enhances BDNF release from cultured trigeminal neurons, which implicates BDNF as a candidate mediator of trigeminal nociceptive plasticity (Buldyrev et al., 2006). The nerve growth factor (NGF) has also been implicated in pain (Basbaum and Woolf, 1999).

Female sex hormones are believed to regulate the synthesis and receptor expression of CGRP. The 17beta-estradiol enhanced neurogenic vasodilatation, suggesting an increase in the release of CGRP from the perivascular nerves. This may be one of the mechanisms through which 17beta-estradiol exacerbates migraine in women (Gupta et al., 2007a). Several recent evidence indicates estrogens involvement in migraine (Gupta et al., 2007b; Varga et al., 2006; Pardutz et al., 2007).

Cholecystokinin peptides mediate several functions both in the CNS and in the gastrointestinal tract where they act as neurotransmitters and regulate digestive functions. CCK peptides induce neurogenic vasodilation both in cerebral and mesenteric vessels. This effect is mediated by NO and seems to be presynaptic, regulating both cerebral and splanchnic blood flow (Ruíz-Gayo et al., 2006). Pituitary adenylate cyclase-activating peptide (PACAP) has also been reported in the sensory innervation of intracranial vessels originating from the TG (Edvinsson, 2001; Edvinsson and Uddman, 2005). Opiate, such as dynorphin B containing nerve fibers are found surrounding the brain blood vessels (Moskowitz et al., 1986). Endomorphins such as endomorphin-2, which are endogenous peptides with potent analgesic activity, have been observed in primary sensory afferent fibers, which might serve as endogenous ligands for pre and post synaptic mu receptors to modulate pain perception (Martin-Schild et al., 1998). Met-Enk is present in primary afferent fibers and TG (Yaksh et al., 1988; Zhang et al., 1994; Saria et al., 1997). Met-Enk containing neurons and terminals are present in several CNS regions including the mesencephalon and spinal cord, and Met-Enk may be released from such terminals upon somatic stimulation (Yaksh and Elde, 1981). Increased levels of Met-Enk (Mosnaim et al., 1985, 1986) and β- endorphin levels have been detected in the plasma of migraine patients (see Edvinsson, 2006 for review).

Increase (Yaksh and Elde, 1981; Cesselin et al., 1985) or decrease (Cesselin et al., 1985; Bourgoin et al., 1988), of Met-Enk out flow into the cerebrospinal fluid (CSF) were reported in different experimental pain conditions. These variations might depend on the type of nociception (acute, chronic, local or general) (Langemark et al., 1995). Increased plasma (Nakamura and Yoshino, 1990; Negri et al., 1993) and synovial tissue (Suzuki et al., 1992; Shiga et al., 1993) levels of Met-Enk have also been reported during pain.

Opiates decrease the duration of the action potential of the nociceptors and consequently decreasing the Ca^{++} influx, which leads to a decrease in neurotransmitter release from primary afferents. In addition, opiates hyperpolarize the postsynaptic neurons in the dorsal horn by activating the K^+ conductance (Basbaum and Jessell, 2000). Somatostatin (SST) is involved in hypothalamic regulation of metabolic, neuroendocrine and autonomic functions, as well as modulation of nociceptive information in the spinal trigeminal nucleus and spinal cord of the rat (Dalsgaard et al., 1984). SST (Ositelu et al., 1987; Kai-Kai, 1989; Alvarez and Priestley, 1990a; Del Fiacco and Quarta, 1994; Zhao et al., 1998), and neurotensin (NT) were also found in the TG of the rat (Alvarez and Priestly, 1990b; Zhao et al., 1998) and human (Del Fiacco and Quarta, 1994), as well as in the brainstem trigeminal nucleus (Massari et al., 1983). Somatostatin-IR fibers in layer II of the CTN originate mainly from primary trigeminal afferents, whereas, layer I SST-IR fibers belong mostly to the interneurons of layer I and II of the CTN (Alvarez and Priestley, 1990b). Moreover, electrical stimulation of the TG leads to a depletion (and release) of SST in the ipsilateral CTN (Samsam et al., 2002). Somatostatin (Gazelius et al., 1981) and opiates inhibit the release of SP from sensory neurons and relieve pain and autonomic symptoms of cluster headache (Sicuteri et al., 1984, 1986) and migraine attacks (Kapicioglu et al., 1997). The i.v. administration of a synthetic octapeptide analogue of SST (SMS 201-995) blocked plasma protein extravasation (and neurogenic inflammation) within the rat or guinea pig dura mater following electrical stimulation of the TG or capsaicin administration (Matsubara et al., 1992). This indicates that peripheral tissues may be the target of Octreotide action in pain relief. However, Octreotide failed to suppress C-fos-IR of rat CTN or pain behaviours following intracisternal capsaicin administration (Kemper et al., 2000), which might possibly be due to its poor penetration to the brain (Kitazawa et al., 1998; Schmidt et al., 1998).

Serotonin has long been implicated in the pathogenesis of migraine (Edvinsson L et al., 1983; Moskowitz MA, 1984), stroke and vasospasm. Edvinsson and colleagues showed the presence of a central serotonergic innervation of pial arteries and arterioles in the rat, possibly originating from both median and dorsal raphé nucle (Edvinsson L et al., 1983). Systemic serotonin levels have also been associated with migraine headaches (Hamel, 1999). Serotonin (5-HT) is a monoamine neurotransmitter synthesized in serotonergic neurons in the CNS and enterochromaffin cells in the gastrointestinal tract, and is a vasoconstrictor which controls the cerebral blood flow (McBean DE et al., 1990), see (Zhang et al., 2007) for review. Several serotonin (5-HT$1_{B/D}$) receptor agonists known as triptan family of drugs are currently being used to treat migraine.

Autonomic Nerves Innervating the Intracranial Vessels and their Major Neurotransmitter Contents

In addition to the trigeminal and upper cervical nerves, the intracranial vessels are also innervated by the sympathetic and parasympathetic nerve fibers.

Moreover, the preganglionic sympathetic and parasympathetic (in sacral segments) neurons in the intermediolateral gray column of the spinal cord receive descending modulatory inputs from higher brain centers to control the autonomic output. These are mainly the serotonergic, noradrenergic and peptidergic fibers (Bowker, 1983, Millan, 1999).

Sympathetic Nerves

The cerebrovascular system (the extra- as well as intracerebral vessels) receives a well-developed innervation by the adrenergic fibers originating in the superior cervical sympathetic ganglion (Nielsen and Owman, 1967; Nelson and Rennels, 1970; Betz 1972, Edvinsson et al., 1975; Owman et al., 1978), as well as the inferior cervical ganglion and the stellate ganglion (Arbab et al., 1988). The stellate fibres innervate the vertebral arteries towards the basilar artery and its branches (Arbab MA et al., 1988).

The sympathetic nerves of superior cervical ganglion origin contain noradrenalin (NA), neuropeptide Y (NPY), and adenosine triphosphate (ATP) (Edvinsson et al., 1983;

Gulbenkian et al., 2001). Moreover, the NPY is colocalized with NA in sympathetic nerves (Edvinsson et al., 1984), and are involved in vasoconstriction and the regulation of the cerebral blood flow (Edvinsson and Uddman, 2005). In addition, there are other sources of noradrenergic fibers from locus Ceruleus (LC) and hypothalamus to small pial vessels for control of local blood flow (Duverger et al., 1987; Lou et al., 1987).

Parasympathetic Nerves

The parasympathetic nerve fibers innervating the intracranial blood vessels originate mainly from neurons in the otic and sphenopalatine ganglia and their major neurotransmitters include the acetylcholine (Ach), VIP, pituitary adenylate cyclase activating peptide (PACAP), and nitric oxide (NO) (Motavkin and Dovbish 1971; Edvinsson et al., 1972; 1989; Larsson et al., 1976; Hara et al., 1985; Suzuki et al., 1988; 1990; Uddman et al., 1993; Goadsby et al., 1996; Uddman et al., 1999). The VIP, PACAP, and NO have been shown to dilate the isolated cerebral arteries (Jansen-Olesen et al., 1994; Goadsby et al., 1996; Uddman et al., 1993), while Ach can induce both constriction and relaxation of isolated cerebral arteries (Lee, 1980) and that atropine can not block the vasodilation in these preparations (Lee, 1982). This might be due to the effect of additional neurotransmitters/ neuromodulators involved during vasodilation, and/ or the ability of Ach to inhibit prejunctionally the autonomic nerves neurotransmitter release (Lee, 2000). For further reading on the autonomic nerves involvement in headache, please refer to the review by Edvinsson and Uddman (2005) whose studies in the last four decades significantly increased our understanding in this field.

The Ascending Spinal Tracts Involved in Transmission of Pain

The noxious information received by the primary sensory neurons is then transmitted by the spinal and medullary dorsal horn postsynaptic (secondary) neurons projecting to several supraspinal centers including the thalamus, hypothalamus, nucleus tractus solitarius (NTS), the parabrachial nucleus (PBN), the PAG, and amygdale, and other areas. The third-order neurons from the thalamus project to the sensory cortex and limbic structures to register the pain. The axons of nociceptive-specific and wide dynamic range neurons originating from various dorsal horn laminae make up the five major ascending pathways that carry the nociceptive information from the spinal cord to the brain. These include the spinothalamic, spinoreticular, spinomesencephalic, cervicothalamic, and spinohypothalamic tracts (Basbaum and Jessell, 2000).

The spinomesencephalic tract is believed to mediate the affective component of pain. This pathway ascends in the anterolateral quadrant of the spinal cord to the mesencephalic reticular formation and periaqueductal gray matter, and via the spinoparabrachial tract, it projects to the parabrachial nuclei. Neurons of the parabrachial nuclei project to the amygdaloid nucleus of the limbic system involved in emotions (Basbaum and Jessell, 2000). In mammals, two main ascending pathways encoding the sensory discriminative and affective aspects of pain are the spinothalamic and spinoparabrachial tracts respectively (Millan 1999, 2002).

In a similar way several functional ascending tracts convey sensory trigeminal information from the head and face to the higher brain centers. These include the ventral and dorsal trigeminothalamic tracts, the neotrigeminothalamic tract as well as the paleotrigeminothalamic system. Most of the former three tracts terminate predominantly in the ventroposteromedial thalamic nucleus (VPM) in a somatotopic organization and from there the third-order neurons reach mainly the sensory cortex of the brain. The ventral trigeminothalamic tract (also called the ventral trigeminal lemniscus) fibers carry the touch, pressure, and proprioceptive information by means of neurons whose cell bodies are located in the main sensory nucleus, and in the subnucleus oralis, as well as in the mesencephalic nucleus. The axons of most of these neurons cross the midline in pons and ascend as ventral trigeminal lemniscus close to the medial and spinal lemnisci. The dorsal trigeminothalamic tract is made up by the axons from the ipsilateral trigeminal main sensory nucleus which ascends in close relationship with the ipsilateral medial lemniscus to the thalamus. However, axons from the caudal trigeminal nucleus (CTN) neurons which carry the thermal and nociceptive (pain) impulses as well as the touch and pressure sensations also join the ventral trigeminothalamic tract and reach the thalamus and the sensory cortex. A group of these long fiber tracts known as the neotrigeminothalamic tract, projects directly to the VPM and the posteromedial thalamic nuclei. In addition, the axons of some other neurons originating in the CTN which are not somatotopically organized (nonlemniscal), ascend on both sides as the paleotrigeminothalamic tract to the brainstem reticular formation, synapsing on the reticulothalamic fibers that project to the periaqueductal gray (PAG), the hypothalamus, the nucleus submedius, and the medial and intralaminar thalamic nuclei to synapse on neurons of these structures which send inputs to the limbic forebrain centers and with diffuse projections to many other parts of the brain (Carpenter 1985, Bonica, 1990).

The Supraspinal Centers Involved in Modulation of Pain

Several regions in the brain are involved in the processing of the nociceptive information including the affective component of the pain. The supraspinal systems involved in processing the nociceptive information include the thalamus, the hypothalamus, the limbic system, and the cerebral cortex. In addition, brain structures involved in pain sensation have considerable interaction with the autonomic control system. The insular and anterior cingulate cortices, amygdala, hypothalamus, periaqueductal grey, parabrachial nucleus, nucleus of the solitary tract, ventrolateral medulla and raphe nuclei receive converging nociceptive and visceral inputs from the spinal and trigeminal dorsal horns and initiate arousal, affective, autonomic, motor and pain modulatory responses to painful stimuli, see (Benarroch, 2006) for review. Pain was originally suggested to have three major dimensions including the sensory-discriminative (such as identification of the sensory stimulus in terms of space, time, intensity and submodalities such as mechanical, thermal, and chemical stimuli), motivational-affective (mechanisms leading to escape and other forms of aversive behavior), and cognitive-evaluative dimentions (Melzack and Wall, 1965; Bonica, 1990). As mentioned earlier, two major ascending pathways carrying the sensory discriminative and affective aspects of pain in mammals are the spinothalamic and spinoparabrachial tracts respectively (Millan 1999, 2002). The sensory inputs to the thalamus and parabrachial nuclei are coming from the projection neurons of dorsal horn laminae. These in turn relay such information to the cortical and amygdalar regions for perception of painful stimulus. Among several thalamic nuclei that are involved in the processing of nociceptive information, the lateral nuclear group (composed of ventroposterior medial nucleus, the ventroposterior lateral, and posterior nucleus) and the medial nuclear group (composed of central lateral nucleus and the intralaminar complex) are the most important ones (Basbaum and Jessel, 2000). Several earlier studies reviewed by Bonica support the idea that the ventrobasal thalamus and the somatosensory cortex receive inputs from the rapidly conducting lateral ascending pathways, have anatomic and physiologic characteristics that permit processing of sensory discriminative information, whereas the neural areas comprising the medial ascending pathways (the reticular formation, hypothalamus, medial thalamus, and limbic systems) are involved in motivational and affective features of pain (Bonica, 1991). The fast pain impulses mainly travel to the ventral posterolateral nucleus of the thalamus directly, and then reach the cerebral cortex (Snell, 2001). The lateral thalamus seems to mediate the information about the location of an injury, information usually conveyed to consciousness as acute pain (Basbaum and Jessel 2000). The majority of slow pain fibers in the lateral spinothalamic tract end up in the reticular formation which then activates many parts of the nervous system. The post-central gyrus, the cingulate gyrus of the limbic system and the insular gyrus (Craig et al., 1994a, 1994b, and 1996) are the sites concerned with the reception and interpretation of the nociceptive information. Hypothalamus is involved in co-ordinating the sensory and autonomic information. It receives sensory information from dorsal horn through major ascending pathways. The hypothalamus is extensively interlinked with the nucleus tractus solitarius (NTS), the periaqueductal gray (PAG) matter and rostral ventromedial medulla (RVM), together with the corticolimbic structures (Millan, 1999), see below. Activation of the hypothalamic and limbic forebrain systems mediate the supraspinal autonomic reflex responses concerned with ventilation, circulation, and neuroendocrine function, and the motivational drive and unpleasant affect that trigger the organism to action (Bonica, 1990). Electrical stimulation of the limbic structures including the hippocampus, fornix, or amygdala or posterior medial hypothalamus in awake animals provoked escape or other mixed behavioural responses to stop the stimulation, but stimulation of the lateral hypothalamus has been used as a reward in behavioral training (Olds and Olds, 1963). The affective dimension of pain is made up of feelings of unpleasantness and emotions associated with future implications, termed secondary affect. Experimental and clinical studies show serial interactions between pain sensation intensity, pain unpleasantness, and secondary affect. Spinal pathways to limbic structures and medial thalamic nuclei provide direct inputs to brain areas involved in affect (Price, 2000). Another source is from spinal pathways to somatosensory thalamic and cortical areas and then through a cortico-limbic pathway. The latter integrates nociceptive input with contextual information and memory to provide cognitive mediation of pain affect. Both direct and cortico-limbic pathways converge on the same anterior cingulate cortical and subcortical structures whose function establishes the emotional valence and response priorities (Price, 2000).

Descending Pathways Involved in Modulation of Pain

There are several descending pathways that are involved in the modulation of the neuronal activity of the ascending pathways and can have an inhibitory or facilitatory effect on the pain sensation. The existence of a specific system modulating the pain was proposed in 1965 when Melzack and Wall (1965) explained the gate-control theory of pain. The anatomical regions involved in the inhibition or facilitation of pain overleap often. These differences in the inhibitory or facilitatory modulations are mainly due to the receptor subtypes and different intracellular signalling mechanisms. Descending pathways can modulate nociception through several interaction sites in the spinal and dorsal medullary horns including the presynaptic interactions with the primary afferent terminals, and/or projections to the postsynaptic secondary neurons, and/or projections on local interneurons, or interactions with other descending pathways. Moreover, the descending modulatory pathways make synaptic connections with the preganglionic sympathetic and parasympathetic (in sacral segments) neurons in the intermediolateral gray column of the spinal cord, to control the autonomic output as well as descending projections to the ventral horn motor neurons to mediate responses to pain such as reflex escape (Bowker et al., 1983; Willis and Westlund, 1997; Millan, 1999, 2002; Hokfelt et al., 2000).

Several centers with potential for modulating pain transmission have been identified. Among these multiple candidate efferent pathways with modulatory control of nociception, the most completely described pain modulating circuit includes the amygdala, the periaqueductal gray (PAG) matter, dorsolateral pontomesencephalic tegmentum (DLPT) and rostral ventromedial medulla (RVM) in the brainstem. This circuit controls both spinal and trigeminal dorsal horn pain transmission neurons via descending projections, and mediates both opioid and stimulation produced analgesia (Fields, 2000). It is due to many different neurotransmitter contents of this circuit that it can modulate bi-directional control of pain through "On" cells that facilitate and "Off" cells that inhibit dorsal horn nociceptive neurons. There is evidence that this circuit contributes to analgesia in humans and may be activated by acute stress or the expectation of relief. Conversely, through the facilitating effect of "On" cells, this circuit is theoretically capable of generating or enhancing perceived pain intensity, which may provide a physiological mechanism for the pain enhancing actions of mood, attention and expectation (Fields, 2000).

The descending antinociceptive system originates in the amygdaloid body and hypothalamus and project to the lower brainstem and spinal cord, via the PAG and RVM. The PAG coordinates the activity of the descending antinociceptive pathway (Reynolds, 1969; Mayer et al., 1971; Liebeskind et al., 1973; Yaksh et al., 1976; Basbaum and Field, 1979; Behbehani and Fields, 1979; Reichling et al., 1988; Reichling and Basbaum, 1990). Such modulation is exerted mainly by the noradrenergic, serotonergic, and opioidergic systems. The midbrain PAG region has excitatory projections to the RVM neurons, the most important of which are the serotonergic neurons in the midline of the nucleus raphe magnus and also other serotonergic nuclei. The other descending inhibitory systems involved in antinociception in dorsal horn originate in the noradrenergic locus ceruleus and other brainstem nuclei (Jones, 1991; Basbaum and Jessel, 2000).

Two other medullary systems involved in the modulation of pain transmission include the dorsal reticular nucleus and the caudal ventrolateral medulla, which function primarily as pronociceptive and antinociceptive centres, respectively. Both areas are connected with the spinal dorsal horn by closed reciprocal loops (Lima and Almedia, 2002; Tavares and Lima, 2007).

Neuroanatomical structures involved in the descending inhibition or facilitation of the pain are common and overleap with each other (Fields et al., 1991; Urban et al., 1999a,b,c; Basbaum and Jessel, 2000). Descending pathways reach the spinal cord through the dorsolateral and ventrolateral funiculi which are differentially involved in descending inhibition and facilitation. The dorsolateral funiculus seems to carry the descending inhibition via noradrenergic and serotonergic fibers to the dorsal horn, whereas the ventrolateral funiculus is involved in the mechanism of descending facilitation (Zhuo and Gebhart, 1997; Watkins et al., 1998; Wei and Dubner, 1998). A detailed review of the structures involved in the modulation of pain as well as the major descending pathways which monosynaptically innervate the spinal cord together with their known neurotransmitter contents, written by Millan is a comprehensive source of further reading in this area (Millan MJ, 2002). Here we review some of the most important supraspinal structures with direct descending pathways to the dorsal horn to provide neuroanatomical and functional bases to some most recent clinical and imaging findings in primary headaches discussed in this chapter.

Hypothalamus

Stimulation of the anterior hypothalamus suppresses the pain by descending inhibitory control that originates from neurons in pressor regions of the anterior hypothalamus and is highly selective for nociceptive inputs to Class 2 neurons in the dorsal horn (Workman and Lumb, 1997). The hypothalamic nuclei including the medial preoptic, and major part of lateral hypothalamus elicit antinociception presumably through glutamatergic projections to the periaqueductal grey (PAG) and rostroventromedial medulla (RVM) including the raphe magnus nucleus (Murphy et al., 1999, Jiang and Behbehani, 2001; Aimone et al., 1988, Behbehani et al., 1988; Cechetto and Saper, 1988; Holden and Naleway, 2001). Several other hypothalamic nuclei including the paraventricular, the arcuate nucleus, tuberomammillary nucleus, and the posterior periventricular nucleus give direct projections to the dorsal horn and other regions of the spinal cord (Cechetto and Saper, 1988) with defined neurotransmitters. Direct hypothalamic-trigeminal connections have also been found (Malik and Burstein, 1998), and hypothalamus is known to modulate autonomic and nociceptive responses including the trigeminovascular nociceptive pathways (Bartsch T et al., 2004). Hypothalamus is believed to be involved in central disinhibition of the trigeminal-autonomic reflex in these syndromes (May and Goadsby, 1999a; Benjamin L et al., 2004). Goadsby and associates injected the somatostatin (SST)-antagonist "cyclo-somatostatin" into the posterior hypothalamus of the rat and observed reduced A- and C-fibre responses to dural stimulation, leading to decreased spontaneous activity. Responses to facial thermal stimulation were also decreased. Their study indicates that blockade of somatostatin receptors in the posterior hypothalamus has an anti-nociceptive effect on dural and facial input, probably mediated via

GABAergic mechanisms. Therefore, posterior hypothalamus may play a role in the pathophysiology of primary headache disorders, such as migraine or cluster headache (Bartsch et al., 2005). The posterior hypothalamus activation has been reported in paroxysmal hemicrania (PH), cluster headache (CH), short-lasting unilateral neuralgiform headache with conjunctival injection and tearing (SUNCT) as well as in hemicrania continua (HC), and is believed to be a major cranial autonomic feature associated with primary headaches, see the headache sections. Also in this respect, deep brain stimulation of the posterior hypothalamus was beneficial in intractable pain of CH and SUNCT (Leone et al., 2004; 2005a,b). Stereotactic lesions of the ergotropic portion of the posterior hypothalamus {posteromedial (Sano triangle) hypothalamotomy} normalize the violent, aggressive, restless behaviours in human (Sano and Mayanagi, 1988). However, another report indicates that stimulation of the Sano triangle in the posteromedial hypothalamic region during the neurosurgical procedure to reach the subthalamic nuclei to treat a patient suffering from Parkinson's disease, developed acute transient aggressive behavior during intraoperative electrical test stimulation (Bejjani et al., 2002). Similar abnormal behavior is seen in more than 90% of the CH attacks (Bahra et al., 2002). Obviously, it is clear that hypothalamus is an important center in at least CH. As we will see in the cluster headache section, the area activated in headache is the posterior hypothalamus, seen by functional imaging studies (May et al., 1999c; Matharu and Cohen, 2006), and deep brain stimulation of the posterior hypothalamus, rather than the anterior hypothalamus was effective in intractable pain of CH. These findings give rise to questions that hypothalamic activation as a direct perpetrator of the painful attacks, and may indicate the hypothalamic activation during these headache attacks to be an association rather than a direct effect (Cohen and Goadsby, 2006). Although the modulatory effects of hypothalamus, as well as the central sensitization, activating the supranuclear centers should also be considered.

Parabrachial Nucleus

Parabrachial nucleus (PBN), in the dorsolateral pontomesencephalic tegmentum of the brainstem is regarded as an important locus for the processing and integration of the sensory and autonomic information from oral, gastrointestinal, and postabsorptive receptor sites and plays an important role in the regulation of the cardiovascular system, and respiration as well as regulating food intake (Bertrand and Hugelin, 1971; Mraovitch et al., 1982; Halsell and Travers, 1997; Baird et al., 2001). It is involved in emotional and cognitive aspects of pain and receives direct nociceptive information from spinal and medullary dorsal horns as well as those coming from the viscera. Different parts of the PBN send several projections to the nucleus tractus solitarius (NTS), the RVM, as well as the medullary and spinal dorsal horns. The caudal trigeminal nucleus neurons project to the parabrachial nucleus, as well as other regions including the commissural subnucleus of the solitary tract, A5 cell group region/superior salivatory nucleus, lateral periaqueductal grey matter, inferior colliculus, as well as the ventroposteromedial thalamic nuclei. Histological investigations revealed immunoreactivity for 5HT1(D) and CGRP. This implicated these central areas as being possible targets of triptan family and/or drug inhibiting the CGRP action (Noseda et al.,

2008), see the headache section of this chapter. Injection of horseradish peroxidase into the right lateral parabrachial region, retrogradely labeled laminae I, II and III neurons of the medullary dorsal horn bilaterally, with an ipsilateral predominance, indicating that neurons in the medullary dorsal horn and spinal cord project directly to the lateral parabrachial region (Wang et al., 2001). Anterograde and retrograde transport methods revealed descending projections from the parabrachial nucleus (PB) to the trigeminal sensory nuclear complex (TSNC) and spinal dorsal horn (SpDH). The ventrolateral PB, including Kölliker-Fuse nucleus (KF), send axons terminating mainly in the ventrolateral parts of rostral trigeminal nuclei of the principalis, oralis, and interpolaris, as well as in the inner lamina II of the medullary (nucleus caudalis) and spinal dorsal horn. These descending projections are bilateral, but with an ipsilateral dominance. Moreover, TSNC received a more dominant ipsilateral projection from PB nucleus than spinal dorsal horn. The cells of origin of the descending tracts from the PB nucleus are believed to be located mainly in KF, but TSNC was reported to receive fewer projections from the KF than spinal dorsal horn. The TSNC receives a considerable projection from the medial subnucleus of PB and the ventral parts of the lateral subnuclei of PB, such as the central lateral subnucleus and lateral crescent area (Yoshida et al., 1997). The PB stimulation exerts inhibitory influences on the spontaneous activity and responses evoked by nonnociceptive and nociceptive skin and deep afferent inputs in trigeminal subnucleus caudalis neurons (Chiang et al., 1994). Endomorphin-2 (EM2) is colocalized with SP and CGRP in the nucleus of the solitary tract (NTS) and with SP, CGRP and mu opioid receptor (MOR) in the parabrachial nucleus, implicating them in the regulation of pain (Greenwell et al., 2007). The exact function of these CGRP or SP containing neurons in PB and NTS is not clear, although they are known to be excitatory neurotransmitter/ neuromodulator in spinal and medullary dorsal horns. The anti-nociceptive effect of morphin is well known (Basbaum and Jessel, 2000), and release of endogenous morphin from trigeminal afferents in the caudal trigeminal nucleus together with other excitatory neurotransmitters was proposed to block their further release and help in antinociception (Samsam et al., 2002).

Nucleus Tractus Solitarius

The nucleus tractus solitarius (NTS) is located in the medulla and lower pons, and modulates processing of sensory information. It receives visceral sensations and taste from cranial nerves (CN) seven CNVII, CNIX, and CNX (Iversen et al., 2000; Gamboa-Esteves et al., 2001a), as well as monosynaptic projections from dorsal horn neurons receiving sensory afferent inputs. Such projections may represent pathways through which NTS neurons are influenced by nociceptive and non-nociceptive information from the dorsal horn and thereby can co-ordinate the appropriate autonomic response, including adjustments in cardiorespiratory reflex output (Gamboa-Esteves et al., 2001b). The NTS is interconnected to PBN and coordinates the sensory and autonomic information and has reciprocal interconnections with the hypothalamus, the limbic system as well as the cerebral cortex, and sends efferents to the PAG, the nucleus raphe magnus (NRM), as well as the spinal cord

(Mtui et al, 1993; Tavares and Lima, 1994; Wiertelak et al., 1997; Pan et al., 1999; Iversen, 2000; Millan 2002; Komisaruk and Whipple, 2005).

Electrical stimulation of the NTS causes pronounced analgesia (Lewis et al., 1987; Aicher and Randich, 1990). This analgesia appears to involve opioids and is pharmacologically dissociable from the hemodynamic changes elicited by NTS stimulation. Therefore, the NTS might serve as a neural substrate for inter-relationships between stress, cardiovascular function, alterations in respiration, and pain sensitivity (Lewis et al., 1987). In contrast, other studies indicate the NTS involvement in facilitation of pain, and suggest that neural structures have the capacity for opposed actions, in that both the NTS and NRM underlie hyperalgesia as well as analgesia (Randich and Gebhart, 1992; Wiertelak et al., 1997).

Rostroventromedial Medulla

The Rostroventromedial medulla (RVM) is one of the sites that is involved in both inhibition and facilitation of pain. Such dual functions play an important role in the modulation of nociception in painful conditions due to tissue inflammation and injury (Li et al., 1998; Wei et al., 1999; Fields, 2000; Porreca et al., 2001; Millan 2002; Hjornevik et al., 2008; Randich et al., 2008). The RVM is composed of several nuclei including the nucleus raphe magnus (NRM) located medially, with a large number of serotonergic neurons, the nucleus reticularis gigantocellularis, located more dorsally and/or laterally, the nucleus gigantocellularis pars alpha, and the nucleus reticularis paragigantocellularis lateralis with many direct descending inputs to the dorsal horn laminae (Basbaum and Fields, 1984; Carpenter 1984; Fields et al., 1991; Urban and Gebhart, 1999). The RVM is primarily under the influence of the supraspinal structure involved in the processing of painful information by receiving inputs from the PAG, PBN, the NTS and others, although the RVM may also receive direct sensory inputs as well (Fields et al., 1991; Millan, 2002). The amygdala, PAG, dorsolateral pontomesencephalic tegmentum (DLPT) and RVM form one of the most important efferent circuits for pain modulation in the brainstem.

As mentioned earlier, this circuit controls both spinal and trigeminal dorsal horn pain transmission neurons via descending projections, and mediates both opioid and stimulation produced analgesia (Fields, 2000). This modulates bi-directional control of pain through "On" cells that facilitate and "Off" cells that inhibit dorsal horn nociceptive neurons or conversely, through the facilitating effect of "On" cells, this circuit is theoretically capable of generating or enhancing perceived pain intensity, which may provide a physiological mechanism for the pain enhancing actions of mood, attention and expectation (Fields, 2000).

Dorsal Reticular Nucleus of the Medulla

Dorsal reticular (DRt) nucleus is located in the reticular formation medial to the spinal trigeminal nucleus, pars caudalis, lateral to the NTS, ventral to the cuneate nucleus and dorsal to the ventral reticular nucleus (Tavares and Lima, 1994; 2007). The DRt nucleus is possibly implicated in the modulation of the ascending nociceptive transmission involved in the motivational-affective dimension of pain, as well as the endogenous supraspinal pain control system centered in the periaqueductal gray matter-rostral ventromedial medulla-spinal cord circuitry; and the motor reactions associated with pain (Leite-Almeida, 2006). Dorsal reticular nucleus has been reported to have both descending facilitatory (Almeida 1993) and inhibitory (Bouhassira, 1992; Gall, 2000) effects. Several studies indicate a pronociceptive function of the DRt nucleus since it facilitates the nociception by enhancing the response capacity of dorsal horn neurons to noxious stimulation. Stimulation of the DRt nucleus induces hyperalgesia (Almeida et al., 1993; 1996; 1999; Dugast et al., 2003), whereas its lesioning decreases the inflammatory pain revealed by a decrease in the c-fos expression in the spinal cord (Almeida et al., 1999; 2002).

The pronociceptive action of the DRt nucleus is mediated by direct excitatory descending fibres to the superficial and deep laminae of the spinal dorsal horn, and the reciprocal connections from the spinal dorsal horn back to the DRt nucleus, establishing a spinal dorsal horn- DRt nucleus- spinal dorsal horn loop (Almeida et al., 1993; Tavares and Lima, 1994; Almeida 1999; Tavares and Lima 2007). The GABAergic spinal neurons have been suggested to buffer and counteract the amplifying effect of the reverberative spinal dorsal horn- DRt nucleus- spinal dorsal horn loop (Tavares and Lima, 2007).

On the other hand, DRt nucleus is believed to have neurons responsible for supraspinally mediated diffuse noxious inhibitory controls, which is activated by tissue damage and can induce analgesis (Bouhassira et al., 1992). Consistent with this, unilateral quinolinic acid-induced lesions of the DRt nucleus significantly reduced the inhibitions produced by heterotopic noxious stimuli (supraspinally mediated diffuse noxious inhibitory controls) of the C-fibre-evoked responses of the convergent neurons (Bouhassira et al., 1992).

Periaqueductal Grey Matter

The midbrain periaqueductal gray (PAG), has been known to be involved in pain and analgesia, fear and anxiety, vocalization, lordosis and cardiovascular control (Reynolds, 1969; Behbehani MM 1995). The major intrinsic circuit within the PAG is a tonically-active GABAergic network and that inhibition of this network is an important mechanism for activation of outputs of the PAG (Behbehani 1995). The PAG matter coordinates the activity of the descending antinociceptive pathway (Mayer et al., 1971; Liebeskind et al., 1973; Yaksh et al., 1976; Basbaum and Fields, 1979; Behbehani and Fields, 1979; Reichling et al., 1988; Reichling and Basbaum, 1990; Fields et al., 1991). It receives direct and indirect nociceptive fibers from the dorsal horn (Hylden 1986; Millan 1999). Descending modulation of pain is exerted mainly by the noradrenergic, serotonergic, and opioidergic systems. The midbrain PAG region has excitatory projections to the neurons of the rostroventral medial medulla, the most important of which are the serotonergic neurons in the midline of the nucleus raphe magnus (NRM) and also other serotonergic nuclei. The NRM contains serotonergic neurons that project to the spinal cord via the dorsal part of the lateral funiculus and inhibits the dorsal horn neurons via direct and indirect (through enkephalinergic interneurons) connections. The other descending inhibitory systems involved in antinociception in dorsal horn originate in the noradrenergic locus ceruleus and other brainstem nuclei. The local- circuit endogenous opoid -containing interneurons in the superficial dorsal horn of the spinal cord which are activated by such brainstem serotoninergic and noradrenergic neurons, inhibit the presynaptic release of neurotransmitters from primary sensory central terminals as well as inhibit the postsynaptic neurons (Basbaum and Jessell, 2000). The PAG is involved in the control of emotion including the anxiety and fear by its reciprocal interconnections with the hypothalamus, the parabrachial nucleus, the nucleus tractus solitarius, and several corticolimbic regions such as the frontal cortex and amygdale, see (Millan 2002) for review. There are evidences that PAG neurons project directly to the trigeminal nucleus as well as the dorsal horn. The CCK-substance P cell group in the PAG project to the spinal cord dorsal horn (Skirboll et al., 1983), and many serotonergic PAG neurons project axons simultaneously to both the trigeminal sensory complex and forebrain regions, which may have a possible role in the limbic or affective-motivational aspect of the pain (Li et al., 1993). Consistent with this, evoked trigeminal neuronal activity in the spinal cord was reversibly inhibited by stimulation of the PAG (Knight and Goadsby, 2001). Several other studies by Goadsby and colleagues indicate the involvement of PAG in descending inhibition of pain in the trigeminal system (Knight, et al., 2002; 2003). However, there are studies reporting the activation of the brainstem red nucleus and substantia nigra before the occipital signals elevation in visually-triggered migraine (Welch et al., 1998; Cao et al., 2002) as well as other types of headache patients (Welch et al., 2002), indicating the brainstem structures might be involved in the initiation of migraine attack. Using high resolution MRI, increased iron concentration/accumulation in multiple deep nuclei including the PAG has been detected in repeated migraine attacks which was proposed to serve as a possible generator of migraine attacks due to dysfunction of PAG matter (Welch et al., 2002). It remains unclear whether iron accumulation in the antinociceptive network has a causative role in the development of (chronic) migraine headache (Kruit et al., 2008). Neurotensin (NT) and SP as well as opioid peptides induced antinociception when administered locally in the rat PAG (Clineschmidt et al., 1982; Behbehani and Pert, 1984; Al-Rodhan et al., 1991; Gioia and Bianchi, 1991; Behbehani, 1992).

Neurotensin however, has a bipolar (facilitatory and inhibitory) effect on pain modulation: facilitation predominates at low (picomolar) doses of NT injected into the rostroventral medial medulla (RVM), whereas higher doses (nanomolar) produce antinociception, presumably by a receptor selective action (Smith et al., 1997). It is known that NT containing neurons of the PAG project to RVM (Beitz, 1982) and inhibit the pain transmission (Clineschmidt et al., 1979; Kalivas et al., 1982; Fang et al., 1987; Behbehani, 1992), however, its concentration might be an important factor. Therefore, NT concentration in different circumstances might be involved in nociception or antinociception.

In the following sections of this chapter we will introduce different proposed pathophysiology of major types of primary headaches, while focusing more on the recent basic and clinical research, as well as the alterations in functional neuroanatomy, and neurochemical changes in primary headaches.

Three main types of primary headaches include the tension type headache, cluster headaches and migraine headaches.

Tension Type Headache

Tension-type headache (TTH) is the most common form of the primary headaches (Jensen and Olesen, 2000). It is a diffuse, dull, aching, band-like headache, which becomes worse on touching the scalp and aggravated by noise; it is associated by tension. It has both chronic and episodic forms and commonly co-exists with depression. The duration of pain may be from many hours to days, and the frequency of pain could be daily or infrequent, it may get worse towards the end of the day and may persist over many years (Lindsay and Bone, 2004). The mechanism of pain is believed to be muscular, and increased tenderness of peripheral myofacial tissue has been suggested. Recent studies using suprathreshold single and repetitive (2 Hz) electrical stimulation of muscle and skin in cephalic (temporal and trapezius) and extracephalic (anterior tibial) regions between patients with chronic TTH and healthy subjects provides evidence for generalized increased pain sensitivity in chronic TTH and suggests that pain processing in the central nervous system is abnormal in this disorder (Ashina et al.,, 2006). Limited studies revealed a normal level of neuropeptides such as CRRP in the cerebrospinal fluid (CSF) of tension headache patients (Bach et al., 1994). The plasma levels of CGRP, VIP, SP, and NPY measured in the peripheral (antecubital veins) or cranial (jugular vein) circulation were also unultered in patients with chronic tension- type headaches (Ashina et al., 1999; 2000b). Experimentally, the plasma CGRP levels did not change during and after infusion of the nitroglycerine in chronic tension headache patients (Ashina et al, 2000a). However, Ashina's study shows interictal plasma CGRP was increased in eight patients with a pulsating pain quality and suggests that headaches with symptoms that fulfill International Headache Society criteria for tension-type headache may be pathophysiologically related to migraine, if the headache has a pulsating quality (Ashina et al., 2000b). The CGRP receptor anatagonists may be helpful in treatment of a subpopulation of the TTH patients.

Treatment of TTh includes the reassurance and attempts to reduce stress and analgesic over-use. Traditionally, tricyclic antidepressants have been used. For acute treatment, the most common interventions involve the use of simple analgesics and anti-inflammatory medications, often taken by the patient without a prescription. For preventive treatment, amitriptyline is the best-studied drug, but nortriptyline, mirtazapine, tizanidine, the selective serotonin reuptake inhibitors, and other medications are also suggested (Bigal, 2008). Advances in the nonpharmacologic, complementary and alternative approaches to TTH treatment, including psychological therapies, acupuncture, and physical treatments (Sun-Edelstein, 2008) as well as the current pharmacologic strategies in the treatment of TTH patients has been recently reviewed (Bigal, 2008) else where.

Cluster Headaches

Cluster headache (CH), is a severe unilateral pain around one eye, associated with conjunctival injection, lacrimation, rhinorrhea, and occationaly a transient Horner's syndrome. The duration of pain is usually for 10 minutes to 2 hours, and its frequency is once or many times per day, often wakening from sleep at night. Clusters of attacks are separated by weeks or even months (Lindsay and Bone, 2004). Cluster headache is the most frequent trigeminal autonomic cephalalgia (TAC) with characteristic association of headache and loco-regional signs and symptoms of facial parasympathetic involvement (Goadsby, 1994; 1997). The apparent features of circadian rhythmicity of attacks and circannual periodicity of cluster period, together with the neuroendocrine abnormalities, are suggestive of a neurochronobiological disorder with a central-diencephalic pathogenetic involvement, confirmed by direct evidence in functional neuroimaging studies of posterior hypothalamic activation during cluster attack, the paroxysmal hemicrania (PH), as well as the short-lasting unilateral neuralgiform headache with conjunctival injection and tearing (SUNCT). The CH, PH, and SUNCT have been grouped as the trigeminal autonomic cephalalgia (TACs) in the second edition of International Headache Society (IHS) classification (Olsen, 2004). Goadsby and colleagues used voxel-based morphometry, an objective and automated method of analyzing changes in the brain structure, to study the structure of the brain of patients with cluster headache. They found a co-localization of structural changes and alterations in local brain activity with positron emission tomography (PET) in the same area of the brain in the same patients, and concluded that this periodic headache is associated with a hitherto unrecognized brain abnormality in the hypothalamic region (May, 1999b). A later study using PET in spontaneous or nitroglycerine (NTG) induced cluster headache, there was an activation of the ipsilateral posterior inferior hypothalamic gray, as well as other regions of the brain including the contralateral ventroposterior thalamus, the anterior cingulate cortex, the ipsilateral basal ganglia, the right anterior frontal lobe, and both insulae, while in patients out of the bout who experienced only a mild NTG headache, activation of the hypothalamic gray matter was not seen (May et al., 2000). Consistent with these, several functional MRI (fMRI) studies indicate activation of the ipsilateral inferior posterior hypothalamus (May et al., 1999a), or activation of the bilateral hypothalamus (Sprenger et al., 2005) in SUNCT. Significant activation of the contralateral posterior hypothalamus has also been reported in PH, which is a severe, strictly unilateral headache that lasts 2 to 30 minutes, occurs more than five times daily, and is associated with trigeminal autonomic symptoms, which is responsive to indomethacin (Matharu and Cohen, 2006). In addition, contralateral ventral midbrain, which extended over the red nucleus and the substantia nigra were also activated in the latter study. Consistent with hypothalamic neuronal dysfunction in patients with CH, the photon MR spectroscopy (1H-MRS) in 26 patients with CH revealed a reduced hypothalamic N-acetylaspartate/creatine level (Lodi et al., 2006; Wang et al., 2006).

Neuropeptide level alterations have also been detected in CH patients. The CGRP and VIP levels increase in the cranial venous blood in patients with episodic cluster headaches while no changes were seen in NPY or SP levels (Goadsby and Edvinsson, 1994). Increase in plasma calcitonin gene-related peptide from the extracerebral circulation was detected during nitroglycerine-induced cluster headache attack (Fanciullacci, 1995). Significant increase in serum levels of both CGRP and VIP with no change in NPY or SP was detected in blood withdrawn from external jugular vein of patients during the cluster headache. Oxygen or sumatriptan (subcutaneous injection) aborted the pain and normalized the CGRP levels. Consistent with these, earlier studies using electrical stimulation of the superior sagittal sinus in cat by activating the trigeminovascular system showed increased CGRP and VIP levels in the external jugular vein, indicating the VIP response is mediated via a brainstem reflex involving the superior salivatory nucleus (Zagami A.S., et al., 1990). The increased CGRP and VIP levels is believed to be due to activation of a brainstem reflex, with trigeminal nerve being the afferent limb and cranial parasympathetic outflow component of the facial nerve (CNVII) serves as the efferent limb (Edvinsson, 2001; Edvinsson and Uddman, 2005; Edvinsson, 2006). The headache-eliciting effect of the parasympathetic neurotransmitter, VIP and its effect on cerebral arteries and brain haemodynamics in man were recently studied. Infusion of VIP caused a decrease in the blood velocity in the middle cerebral artery without affecting regional cerebral blood flow. In spite of a marked vasodilator effect in the extracranial vessels and increased plasma VIP, healthy subjects developed only a very mild headache (Hansen et al., 2006). Significant increase in blood VIP levels have also been detected during chronic paroxysmal hemicrania (CPH) attack which was normalized with indomethacin treatment (Goadsby and Edvinsson, 1996b). It was postulated that CPH is characterized by activation of both sensory and parasympathetic cranial fibers, and that CPH pathophysiology may resemble that of cluster headache (Edvinsson, 2006).

Several treatment strategies including surgical procedures are currently applied to treat cluster headaches. Ergotamine and sumatriptan, oxygen inhalation, locally applied anesthetic agents, and prednisolone are used to treat CH. For prevention and prophylactic treatment, the methysergide, calcium channel blockers, or lithium bicarbonate are being used (Lindsay and Bone, 2004). The Hypothalamic deep brain stimulation (DBS) is an efficacious and safe procedure to relieve otherwise intractable chronic CH and SUNCT (Leone et al., 2005b).

Although the outcomes are encouraging, the invasive nature of the technique and the occurrence of rare but major adverse events have suggested a safer peripheral approach with occipital nerve stimulation (Proietti Cecchini et al., 2008).

Migraine Headache

Migraine is a complex, disabling disorder of the brain that manifests itself as attacks of often severe, throbbing head pain with sensory sensitivity to light, sound and head movement (Goadsby, 2007). According to the International Headache Society (HIS), migraine is a repeated episodic headache of 4- 72 hrs duration characterized by any two of (unilateral, throbbing, worsened by movement, moderate or severe) or any one of (nausea and/or vomiting, photophobia and phonophobia) features (Olsen, 2004). It affects about 15% of the population (Lipton, 2001) and is one of the most costly neurological disorders. According to the world health organization, the mental and neurological disorders collectively account for 30.8% of all years of healthy life lost to disability, whilst migraine, one amongst these, alone accounts for 1.4% and is in the top 20 causes of disability worldwide (Leonardi, 2005). Considering a complete picture of the socioeconomic effect of headaches, as well as the effect on the life of the person, the partner and children, and on the possible impact even when headache-free including a fear of the next attack (Stovner et al., 2008), one may get even more reliable data about the impact of primary headaches on the society . International Classification of Headache Disorders (ICHD) adopted by the IHS is one of the main sources of diagnostic criteria for various types of headaches (Olsen, Headache Classification Subcommittee of the International Headache Society, 2004).

There are two recognizable types of migraine headaches: a) migraine without aura (common migraine), and b) migraine with aura (classic migraine). Migraine occurs more in women and the female/male ratio is 3/1 for both types of migraine headaches (Breslau and Rasmussen, 2001). These headaches may be accompanied by nausea, vomiting, hypersensitivity to light (photophobia), and hypersensitivity to sound (phonophobia), and may be aggravated by physical activity. The majority of migraine headaches fall in this category. However, before the headache starts, approximately 19-30% of migraine patients (Rasmussen and Olesen, 1992; Gérardy et al., 2008) experience some neurological symptoms which are mainly visual including the flashing lights, fortifications, scotomas, as well as sensory, and motor disturbances, collectively called aura which occur about 20-40 minutes before the headache. Traditionally (Blau, 1980), based on the clinical symptoms there are five phases of a complete migraine which includes the prodrome, aura, headache, headache termination, and postdrome, however, all five phases may not occur in patients, see Linde M (2006) for review. Migraine is manifested by 3 major phases, the trigger, aura, and the headache phases.

The Pathomechanism and Trigger for Migraine

The migraine attack is a complex neurobiological and neurovascular process (Tfelt-Hansen et al., 2008). The exact pathomechanism of migraine is not known, however, several factors especially in the last 2-3 decades have been implicated in the pathogenesis of migraine. These include dysfunction in the wall of the cerebral blood vessels or disorders of flow, possibly related to abnormal vessel contractility, platelet disturbance or due to circulating vasoactive substances (including the neuropeptides), or disturbance of brain oxygenation and metabolism (Moskowitz, 1984). Several other triggering factors such as alterations in serotonin (5-HT) levels, low levels of brain tissue magnesium, altered transport of ions across the cell membrane, abnormal mitochondrial energy metabolism and reduction of mitochondrial phosphorylation potential, and inheritance have also been implicated in the pathogenesis of migraine (Schoenen et al., 1994; Hamel, 1999; Arommaa et al., 1999; Knight et al., 2002; Boska et al., 2002; Kors et al., 2004; Sandor et al., 2005; Zhang et al., 2007). However, basic investigations revealed an involvement of the brainstem structures in migraine pathophysiology (Lance et al., 1983; Goadsby, 1991), and that the migraine attack itself might start in the brainstem. Consistent with this, several evidence in recent years indicate the trigger phase of migraine is initiated by neuronal hyperexcitability and activation of the brain including the brainstem (and perhaps not the cortical structures), which continues and is unaffected even after relief of the headache by sumatriptan (a potent antimigraine drug) treatment (Weiller, 1995; Goadsby et al., 2002; Spierings, 2003; Denuelle et al., 2007). A dysfunction of the brainstem PAG was seen in several patients during migraine (Welch et al., 2001). Several positron emission tomographic (PET) studies indicate that migraine with or without aura is initiated with activation of the brainstem (Weiller et al., 1995), the dorsal rostral pons (Bahra et al., 2001; Matharu et al., 2004), the dorsal midline pons (Géraud et al., 2005) or the dorsal pons (Afridi et al., 2005), see (Cohen and Goadsby, 2006) for review). PET studies in migraine patients without aura revealed higher regional cerebral blood flow (rCBF) in the contralateral brainstem (Weiller et al., 1995) and dorsal pons (Bahra et al.,

2001) during an attack compared with the headache-free state. There was activation of other places such as anterolateral cingulated cortex, as well as the visual and auditory association cortices, and these activations were abolished by administration of sumatriptan, but the brainstem activation still persisted (Weiller et al., 1995). Another PET study indicates similar persistent activation of the brainstem and hypothalamus persisted even after headache relief by sumatriptan (Géraud et al., 2005). As indicated earlier, the PAG is involved in antinociception and PAG has inhibitory effect on the nociceptive response to trigeminal stimulation (Knight and Goadsby, 2001; Knight et al., 2005). Consistent with this, blockade of P/Q type voltage gated calcium channels in the PAG facilitated the trigeminal nociception (Knight et al., 2002). Therefore, a newer view to migraine considers it to be a sensory dysmodulation, a system failure of normal sensory processing (Goadsby, 2007).

Moreover, a number of genetic abnormalities including mutations of the P/Q type calcium channel gene (Ophoff et al., 1996, 2001), and Na^+/K^+ pump ATP1A2 (De Fusco M et al., 2003; Vanmolkot et al., 2003) or sodium channel Nav1.1 mutations (Dichgans et al., 2005) have been linked to the pathogenesis of familial hemiplegic migraine (Goadsby et al., 2002; Kors et al., 2004; Wessman et al., 2004) which are accompanied by aura. These mutations make patients more susceptible to migraine attacks (van den Maagdenberg et al., 2004). Several factors such as alcohol, odors or foods, weather changes and estrogen depletion are believed to trigger the migraine (Smetana, 2000; Kelman, 2007).

The migraine aura, which may follow the trigger phase is observed in less than 30% (Rasmussen and Olesen, 1992; Gérardy et al., 2008) of migraine patients, possibly involves cortical spreading depression (CSD), which is described as a wave of transient intense spike activity that starts in the occipital cortex and spreads rostrally with a speed of 2-6mm/min, possibly leading to a long lasting neuronal inhibition (Lauritzen et al., 1983; Lauritzen, 2001; Goadsby et al., 2002). The CSD is followed by a characteristic regional decrease in cerebral blood flow (oligemia) (Lauritzen, 2001; Gorji, 2001; Sanchez del Rio and Reuter, 2004; Tfelt-Hansen et al., 2008), although other theories were proposed, see (Spierings, 2004) for review. Specific symptoms experienced by a number of migraine patients during aura include mainly the visual disturbances such as flashing lights, zigzags (fortifications), scotomas, and other symptoms that may last for less than an hour before the onset of headache.

The CSD is considered to be the basis for migraine aura. The characteristic form and development of sensory disturbances during migraine auras is neurally driven and involves a disturbance of the cerebral cortex (Lauritzen, 1994), the CSD of Leão described in 1944. Several neurological disorders including the migraine have been linked to different channelopathies. The CACNA-1a (the alpha(1) subunit of neuronal Ca(v)2.1 Ca(2+) channels) knock-in mouse model of migraine has shown an increased susceptibility to CSD (van den Maagdenberg et al., 2004). There seems to be a link between the channelopathies and migraine aura in familial hemiplegic migraine (FHM), see (Goadsby, 2004) and (Goadsby and Kullmann, 2005) for review. Mutations of the P/Q type calcium channel gene (CACNA1A) (Ophoff et al., 1996, 2001), knwon as FHM-I which comprise about 50% of the FHM cases leads to an enhanced glutamate release. Mutations in Na^+/K^+ pump ATP1A2 (De Fusco et al., 2003; Vanmolkot et al., 2003) linked to chromosome 1q23, known as FHM-II, comprise about 20% of the FHM and results to a smaller electrochemical gradient for sodium (Na^+), leading to a reduction/ inactivation of astrocytic glutamate transporters which results in accumulation of synaptic glutamate. This in turn, may have other consequences. Astrocyte involvement in CSD has also been proposed (Linde, 2006). Astroglia usually monitor extracellular glutamate and maintain it at low levels, metabolize glutamate, or release it back into the extracellular space. Glutamate in turn, can induce an increase in astroglial cell volume with a resulting decrease of the extracellular space, and thereby alter the concentration of extracellular substances. Failed astroglial functions may result into neuronal dysfunction (Hansson et al., 2000). Consistent with this, the glial spike theory proposes the spreading depression (SD) to be a slowly propagating, regenerative event in the neuroglial compartment. By altering the neuronal microenvironment, this glial spike helps trigger and coordinate the neuronal depolarization of SD (Leibowitz , 1992). The glial spike is facilitated by neuronally released agents acting at the neuroglial plasma membrane. The conduction velocity-determining propagation mechanism of SD is further proposed to be a wave of intracellular Ca(2+)-induced Ca2+ release (cytocal wave) that travels through the glial compartment of the nervous tissue (Leibowitz, 1992). The wave of SD was shown to be a propagating wave in the astroglial gap-junction coupled network facilitated (increased) by glutamate (Blomstrand et al., 1999). Sodium channel Nav1.1 (SCN1A) mutations (Dichgans et al., 2005) have been linked to the pathogenesis of FHM-III, which facilitates repetitive high frequency discharges leading to a possible increase in synaptic glutamate release. The synaptic build-up of glutamate and perhaps other neurotransmitters would sensitize the surrounding neuronal structures and renders the individual more susceptible to migraine attack. A recent study analyzing 12 ion transport genes from several European populations indicates common variants of moderate effect size in ion transport genes do not play a major role in susceptibility to common migraine within these European populations, although there is some evidence for epistatic interaction between potassium and calcium channel genes (KCNB2 and CACNB2), but multiple rare variants or trans-regulatory elements of these genes were not ruled out (Nyholt, 2008). Increasing knowledge of the pathomechanism of migraine including the synaptic alterations in CSD sheds lights into the effective treatment of migraine including the possibility of gene therapy. In addition, a number of patients with right to left cardiac shunts have been found to suffer from a high incidence of migraine headaches which are significantly reduced after the correction of the problem (Wilmshurst and Nightingale, 2001; Azarbal et al., 2005; Tsimikas, 2005). The right to left shunting of blood in a patent foramen ovale (PFO) could serve as a conduit for chemicals that would exert a trigger effect on hyper excitable neurons leading to the development of migraine. Although some studies indicate a higher prevalence of migraine, especially migraine with aura, in patients with PFO, and there was an improvement in their symptoms after percutaneous closure of the PFO (Del Sette et al. 1998, Anzola et al., 1999; 2008; Wilmshurst et al., 2000; Schwerzmann, 2005; Luermans, 2008; Hasan, 2008), other studies actually question the causal relationship between PFO and migraine (Rundek et al., 2008; Jesurum et al., 2008).

The headache phase of migraine, seems to be probably due to the cranial vasodilation as well as to the activation and sensitization of the sensory nerves, mainly the trigeminal nerve (Moskowitz, 1984; Bonica, 1990; Burstein et al., 2000; Villalón et al., 2002; Spierings, 2003; Silberstein, 2004), although there is evidence that migraine pain could be started without initial dilatation of the middle cerebral artery (Kruuse et al., 2003), see below. Headache follows most of the migraine attacks and is experienced commonly in the frontotemporal region. Since the parenchyma of the brain itself is insensitive to pain, blood vessels as well as the cerebral sinuses, meninges and their innervations including their neuropeptide contents have been implicated in generation and conduction of pain.

Moskowitz in 1984, proposed the trigeminovascular theory, as a possible base to explain the pathomechanism of migraine headaches. Although growing evidence indicates that the trigeminovascular theory is not the trigger for migraine, however, many agree that the trigeminal nerve and its innervation of the cranial vessels are involved in the pain phase of migraine. According to the trigeminovascular theory, a trigger for headache (such as injury to the blood vessel wall) is accompanied by local production and synthesis or transport of molecules from circulation, which are nociceptive (e.g., 5-HT, histamine, bradykinin, prostaglandins). These substances lower threshold or depolarize sensory nerve fibers by binding to specific receptors on these fibers. Depolarization is accompanied by local release of neurotransmitters (such as substance P) from axonal varicosities and by orthodromic (convey the information to the brainstem and higher brain centers to register the pain) and antidromic conduction. Antidromic conduction is depolarization-induced substance P (SP) release into the blood vessel wall. Released SP increases vascular permeability and dilates cerebral blood vessels, leading to a headache. SP at high concentrations degranulates mast cells leading to release of other vasoactive substances such as histamine which all together enhance the vasodilation and build up a local inflammation (Moskowitz, 1984). Since this process leads to inflammation which is mediated by neural activity, it therefore, is referred to as neurogenic inflammation. However, this view has changed over years and the trigger for migraine is believed to be primarily in the brain including the brainstem (Goadsby et al., 2002). First of all SP has not been detected in the blood of migraine patients (Goadsby et al., 1990; 2002; Gallai et al., 1995; Alessandri et al., 2006). Moreover, SP receptor (neurokinin-1) antagonists failed to alleviate the pain of migraine patients (Diener, 1996; Goldstein et al., 1997; May and Goadsby 2001), therefore, there is a doubt about the inflammation and plasma protein extravasation in human meningeal vessels during migraine (Peroutka, 2005), and the neurogenic vasodilatation mediated by CGRP via the direct (i.e., endothelium-independent) relaxation of the vascular smooth muscle seems to be involved in the pain of migraine (Peroutka, 2005), rather than the plasma protein extravasation. A similar view was also indicated elsewhere (Goadsby, 2007). Many In vivo models have been used to induce a migraine like attack experimentally, in order to study and explain the possible pathomechanism of migraine headaches. These include the constriction of carotid arteriovenous anastomoses in pigs, electrical stimulation of the TG or the superior sagittal sinus in rats and chemical stimulation of the sensory nerve fibers with capsaicin, vasodilator substances such as prostaglandin E1, nitroglycerine, histamine, or CGRP, which have been used in human to induce a vascular type of headache. Finally, several in vitro models have also been developed; many of these models have been recently reviewed by Saxena and associates (Arulmani et al., 2006).

Electrical stimulation of the rat TG promotes extravasation of albumin from plasma within the postcapillary venules in the receptive field of the trigeminal nerve (e.g.: dura), presumably mediated by release of neuropeptides (Markowitz, 1987). A unilateral electrical stimulation (5 Hz, 5ms, 0.1- 1 mA) of the rat TG for 5 min, led to an increased CGRP-immunoreactivity and significant swelling (3- 4 times the normal size) and enlargement of the ipsilateral perivascular club-like nerve terminals in the dura mater (Knyihár-Csillik et al., 1995). The CGRP and SP innervations of the dura are robust and the patterns of distribution of these neuropeptides are essentially the same. The majority of the fibers are perivascular and innervate branches of the anterior and middle meningeal arteries and the superior sagittal and transverse sinuses; other CGRP/SP fibers appear end "free" within the dural connective tissue (Keller, and Marfurt, 1991).

Following a 30 min electrical stimulation (5 Hz, 5ms, 0.1- 1 mA) of the rat TG, the club-like perivascular nerve terminals and enlarged varicosities were found corroded and collapsed due to disintegration or bursting of the terminals and of the en passant beads (Knyihár-Csillik et al., 1995). These changes seem to be due to the release of their neuropeptide content into the blood vessels or into the tissue. CGRP levels increased in the superior sagittal sinus of the rat following electrical stimulation of the TG and this increase was attenuated when the rats (Buzzi et al., 1991) or cats (Goadsby and Edvinsson, 1993) were treated with dihydroergotamine and/or sumatriptan (a serotonin receptor 1D and B (5-HT$_{1D/B}$) agonist, anti-migraine drug) prior to electrical stimulation. Consistent with this, in 7 of 8 migraine patients responding to subcutaneous administration of sumatriptan, elevated CGRP levels were normalized and the headache was relieved (Goadsby and Edvinsson, 1993). Moreover, intravenous administration of sumatriptan, prior to electrical stimulation of the TG, prevented disintegration of the perivascular terminals and induced accumulation of CGRP in terminals and preterminal portions of peripheral sensory axons in dura mater (Knyihár-Csillik et al., 1997) by an agonistic action at 5-HT$_{1D}$ receptors.

Consistent with this, electrical stimulation of the dural surface (10-20 V, 5-10 Hz, 10-30 min) also caused a release of CGRP from trigeminal afferents innervating the dura mater, thereby causing vasodilation and increasing the meningeal blood flow. These effects were dose dependently inhibited by topical application of the CGRP antagonist hCGRP8-37 (Messlinger et al., 1995).

As indicated earlier, nitric oxide (NO) is also a very important molecule in the regulation of cerebral and extra cerebral cranial blood flow and arterial diameters and therefore is involved in nociceptive processing. Inhibition of NO production or blockade of steps in the NO-cGMP pathway or scavenging of NO have been proposed in treatment of migraine and other headaches (Olesen, 2008).

Examining the central transmission of pain, several experiments revealed that electrical stimulation of the TG releases CGRP (Knyihár-Csillik et al., 1998; Samsam et al., 1999) and SP as well as NKA (Samsam et al., 1996; 1999; 2000) from the central terminals in the ipsilateral caudal trigeminal nucleus (CTN) as well as some pathy depletion (release) of CGRP, SP and NKA from the contralateral CTN (Samsam et al., 2001). Such depletion is significant in CTN in the lower medulla, where majority of the central terminals of the dull pain conveying afferents of the TG neurons terminate.

This is accompanied by an increase in the expression of early gene, the c-fos oncoprotein in the CTN, indicating the release of excitatory neurotransmitters from central trigeminal terminals located in the CTN (Knyihár-Csillik et al., 1997).

We also noticed a co-release of CGRP, SP, and NKA from the trigeminal central neurons in the medulla oblongata (Samsam et al., 2000), indicating a possible co-transmittory or co-modulatory role of these neuropeptides in transmission of pain in the trigeminal nerve territory.

Substance P (Otsuka and Konishi, 1976; Lembeck and Gamse, 1977; Woolf and Wiesenfeld-Hallin, 1986; Oku et al., 1987) and NKA (Saria et al., 1985; Gamse and Saria, 1986) act as excitatory transmitters which may activate the neuronal network in the ipsilateral CTN in medulla and higher brain centers to record the painful stimulus. In this regard, noxious stimuli including the electrical stimulation of the TG, increases the expression of the early activating gene, the c-fos oncoprotein in medulla (Nozaki et al., 1992; Kaube et al., 1993; Knyihár-Csillik et al., 1997). CGRP has been reported to enhance the action of SP when these peptides are co-administered in the CNS (Wiesenfeld-Halin et al., 1984; Goodman and Iversen, 1986). Substance P causes a dose dependent characteristic caudally directed biting and scratching response in mice and rats when administered in the spinal cord (Hylden and Wilcox, 1981; Piercey et al., 1981; Seybold et al., 1982) which lasts only for a few minutes. CGRP (20 µg) alone, did not cause such an effect, but when administered with SP (CGRP 20µg, SP 10µg) the duration of the behavioural response was increased (Wiesenfeld-Halin et al., 1984; Goodman, and Iversen, 1986). The CGRP was proposed to inhibit an enzyme involved in SP degradation (Greves et al., 1985). Therefore, central release of CGRP might possibly be also correlated with the intensity and/or duration of painful stimuli in such animal experiments.

However, the strong excitatory activity of the glutamate released from the trigeminal central terminals can not be ignored. Glutamate has been implicated in cortical spreading depression, trigeminovascular activation and central sensitization (Basbaum and Woolf, 1999; Yaksh, 1999; Ramadan, 2003). Consistent with these, Memantine and MK-801, selective NMDA receptor antagonists partially reduced capsaicin induced c-fos expression (Mitsikostas et al., 1998).

Sumatriptan was reported to decrease the expression of c-fos in the rat medulla oblongata (Hoskin et al., 1996), but it failed to reduce c-fos activity in the rat CTN (Knyihár-Csillik et al., 1997) in our experiments. There are evidences showing activation of the brainstem during migraine attacks (Bahra et al., 2001) and that sumatriptan relieved the headache but brainstem activation persisted. Indeed in our studies, electrical stimulation of trigeminal ganglion in rat increased c-fos expression in the CTN and intravenous administration of sumatriptan prior to the attack failed to decrease c-fos activity in the CTN (Knyihár-Csillik et al., 1997). There are reports however, indicating a poor penetration of sumatriptan through the blood brain barrier (Goadsby and Knight, 1997; Goadsby, 1997a; 1997b), since other triptans as well as dihydroergotamine are able to inhibit the activation of CTN in animals undergoing superior sagittal or dural stimulation (Goadsby, and Boes, 2001; Donaldson et al., 2002; Lambert et al., 2002).

Consistent with this, expression of Fos-like immunoreactivity (Fos-LI) in the trigeminal nucleus following electrical stimulation of the TG in guinea-pig, was inhibited by each of the following drugs, the NK1 receptor antagonist GR205171, or N-methyl-D-aspartate receptor antagonist (MK-801) (Clyton et al., 1997). Since both SP and glutamate are released centrally following experimental activation of the trigeminovascular system, each may be significant neurotransmitter/ neuromodulator involved in the activation of the CTN neuronal cells (Clayton et al., 1997). Intravenously administered CGRP receptor antagonists alpha-CGRP-

(8-37) and BIBN4096BS inhibit the trigeminocervical complex evoked activity following electrical stimulation of the superior sugittal sinus of the cat or local activation by exposure to glutamate and α-CGRP (Storer et al., 2004). These results sugget that the non-presynaptic CGRP receptors in the trigeminocervical complex can be inhibited by CGRP receptor blockade and that a CGRP receptor antagonist would be effective in the acute treatment of migraine and cluster headache (Storer et al., 2004).

Consistently, the CGRP-antagonist BIBN4096BS lowered the activity of neurons with meningeal input in the rat CTN (Fischer et al., 2005). Electrical stimulation of the CTN which leads to a pronounced increase of facial blood flow, was also blocked by 0.3 mg/kg, i.v. injection of BIBN4096BS (Just et al., 2005).

Therefore, a combined peripheral (on target tissues) and central action of CGRP antagonists in the trigeminal nucleus makes these drugs potential candidates for treatment of migraine, especially in patients with cardiovascular disease, where triptans might have some limitations due to their vasoconstrictive activity on 5-HT 1B/D receptors on coronary arteries, or in patients with second rebound attack, see (Arulmani et al., 2006; Linde, 2006) for review.

Since CGRP is also co-expressed with brain-derived neurotrophic factor (BDNF) in a large subset of adult rat TG neurons, neurotrophic factors can possibly mediate the trigeminal nociceptive plasticity (Buldyrev et al., 2006). Neurotrophins (of NGF family including the BDNF and NT3-5) are a family of structurally related proteins that regulate the survival, differentiation and maintenance of function of different populations of peripheral and central neurons through different high affinity tyrosine kinase ($TrK_{(A-C)}$) and p75 (the low affinity neurotrophin) receptors. They are also essential for modulating activity-dependent neuronal plasticity.Very low concentrations of BDNF can excite hippocampal neurons, as well as the cortex and the cerebellum. The BDNF and neurotrophin-4/5 depolarized neurons just as rapidly as the neurotransmitter glutamate, even at a more than thousand-fold lower concentration; Neurotrophin-3 produced much smaller responses, and nerve growth factor was ineffective (Kafitz et a.l, 1999). The neurotrophin-induced depolarization seems to be due to the activation of a sodium ion conductance which was reversibly blocked by K-252a, a protein kinase blocker which prefers Trk receptors. Therefore, a very rapid excitatory action of neurotrophins, places them among the most potent endogenous neuro-excitants in the mammalian central nervous system described so far (Kafitz et a.l, 1999) and can have an effect on overall activity of the trigeminal nociceptive transmission.

There are evidences that the nerve growth factor (NGF) levels increase during inflammation and that NGF binds to TrkA receptors expressed on nociceptors. The NGF-TrkA complex is then transported retrogradely to the cell body, where it increases the transcription of neuropeptides such as SP and ion channels (Basbaum, and Woolf, 1999). Controling the BDNF and/or NGF release should open some areas of interest in the treatment of migraine. For a comprehensive review on the role of various neurochemical substances involved in headache, please see (Samsam et al., 2007a; 2007b).

Even if vascular involvement may not be the origin of migraine, the pain phase has been linked to the dilatation of the cranial blood vessels, including the arteriovenous anastomotic shunts. There are studies that indicate activation of the trigeminal system leads to dilatation of cranial blood vessels, including arteriovenous anastomotic shunts, causing the headache (De Vries et al., 1999; Villalón et al., 2002). In contrast to this, there are studies showing that the pain phase is independent of the vasodilation. Although distension of the intracranial blood vessels is painful, there are evidences that migraine pain may already start during cerebral hypoperfusion which seems to drive changes in the vessel calibre (Nichols et al., 1990; Olesen et al., 1990; May et al., 2001; Kruuse et al., 2003). In fact, there is evidence that migraine pain could be started without initial dilatation of the middle cerebral artery (Kruuse et al., 2003).

Conclusion

Several structures including the trigeminal nerve [cranial nerve five (CNV)], especially its ophthalmic branch, the CNVII, CNIX, CNX, and the upper cervical nerves, as well as the autonomic nervous system together with their target innervations in the periphery including the skin, muscle, and the intracranial and extracranial vessels are involved in the sensory and autonomic processing of the nociceptive information from the head. Trigeminal nerve is the major system that conveys the noxious stimuli to its brainstem and spinal nuclei terminating on central neurons. These trigeminal nuclei neurons in turn make up the ascending tracts that project to several supraspinal centers and reach the thalamus and sensory cortex to register the pain.

Several neurotransmitter/ neuromodulator contents of the above-mentioned nerves including the neuropeptides such as CGRP, SP, NKA, VIP, the nitric oxide (NO), and some others with vasoactive properties have been implicated in vasodilation of the cranial vessels which is believed to be responsible for the pain phase of headache. However, accumulating evidence shows a strong relation between headache and the CGRP release from the trigeminovascular system. In addition, NO, a vasodilator which may act synergistically with CGRP, is an important molecule in the regulation of cerebral and extra cerebral blood flow in the head and is therefore involved in pain processing. Substances inhibiting the CGRP and/ or NO production and/or release, or blocking their receptors, are potential drugs for the treatment of migraine and other types of headaches. Some of these are already in use or are in early clinical development (Olesen, 2008). In cluster headache, the VIP content of the parasympathetic nerves has been linked to the facial vasomotor system (Edvinsson and Uddman, 2005). Central release of several of such neuropeptides alone or together with other neurotransmitters/ neuromodulators, in the trigeminal nucleus act on their appropriate receptors and activate the pain processing pathways in the central nervous system (CNS). The supraspinal centers involved in the processing of nociceptive information include various brainstem nuclei, the thalamus, cerebral cortex, the hypothalamus, and the limbic system. In addition, brain structures involved in pain sensation have considerable interaction with the autonomic control system. The ventrolateral medulla and raphe nuclei, parabrachial nucleus, nucleus of the tractus solitarius, the periaqueductal grey (PAG) matter, amygdala, hypothalamus, the insula and anterior cingulate cortex, receive converging nociceptive and visceral inputs from the spinal and trigeminal dorsal horns and are believed to be involved in the arousal, affective, autonomic, motor and pain modulatory responses to painful stimuli (Benarroch, 2006). Several centers with potential for modulating pain transmission have been also discussed in this chapter. The best known pain modulating circuit includes the amygdala, periaqueductal gray (PAG), dorsolateral pontomesencephalic tegmentum (DLPT) and rostroventromedial medulla (RVM) in the brainstem. This circuit controls both spinal and trigeminal dorsal horn pain transmission neurons via descending projections, and mediates both opioid and stimulation produced analgesia (Fields, 2000). The well-known inhibitory descending modulation of pain is exerted mainly by the noradrenergic, serotonergic, and opioidergic systems. The midbrain PAG region has excitatory projections to the neurons of the rostroventral medial medulla, the most important of which are the serotonergic neurons in the midline of the nucleus raphe magnus and also other serotonergic nuclei. The other descending inhibitory systems involved in antinociception in the dorsal horn, originate in the noradrenergic locus ceruleus and other brainstem nuclei (Basbaum and Jessel, 2000).

However, the neuroanatomical structures involved in the descending inhibition or facilitation of pain are common and overleap with each other. Descending pathways reach the spinal cord through the dorsolateral and ventrolateral funiculi which are differentially involved in descending inhibition and facilitation. The dorsolateral funiculus seems to carry the descending inhibition via noradrenergic and serotonergic fibers to the dorsal horn, whereas the ventrolateral funiculus is involved in the mechanism of descending facilitation (Millan, 2002). Basic investigations indicated the involvement of brainstem in migraine pathophysiology (Lance et al., 1983; Goadsby, 1991), and that the migraine attack itself might start in the brain stem. Consistent with this, increased activity in a number of such supraspinal centers for control and modulation of pain has been observed in the brainstem and brain during headache (Cohen and Goadsby, 2006). Several studies in recent years propose that the trigger for migraine might be the neuronal hyperexcitability and activation of the brainstem which continues and is unaffected even after relief of the headache by sumatriptan (a potent antimigraine drug) treatment (Weiller, 1995; Goadsby et al., 2002; Spierings, 2003; Denuelle et al., 2007), or it might be due to a dysfunction of the brainstem PAG matter during migraine (Welch et al., 2001). Several positron emission tomographic studies indicate that migraine with or without aura is initiated with activation and higher regional cerebral blood flow (rCBF) of the dorsal midbrain including the PAG, and dorsal pons close to the locus ceruleus in spontaneous migraine (Weiller et al., 1995), the dorsal rostral pons (Bahra et al., 2001; Matharu et al., 2004), the dorsal midline pons (Géraud et al., 2005) or the dorsal pons (Afridi et al., 2005) during an attack compared with the headache-free state. Activation of other places such as anterolateral cingulated cortex, as well as the visual and auditory association cortices were abolished by administration of sumatriptan, but the brain stem activation still persisted (Weiller et al., 1995). Another PET study indicates similar persistent activation of the brainstem and hypothalamus even after headache relief by sumatriptan (Géraud et al., 2005) in migraine patients. Consistent with these, several functional MRI (fMRI) studies indicate activation of the ipsilateral inferior posterior hypothalamus (May et al., 1999a), or activation of the bilateral hypothalamus (Sprenger et al., 2005) in short-lasting unilateral neuralgiform headache with conjunctival injection and tearing (SUNCT). The posterior hypothalamus activation has been reported in paroxysmal hemicrania (PH), cluster headache (CH), and SUNCT, as well as hemicrania continua (HC), and is proposed to play a important role in the pathophysiology of primary headache disorders, such as migraine or cluster headache, or SUNCT (May, 1999b, c; May et al., 2000; Bartsch et al., 2005). Significant activation of the contralateral posterior hypothalamus has also been reported in paroxysmal hemicrania. Posterior hypothalamus is believed to be a major cranial autonomic feature associated with primary headaches. Also in this respect, deep brain stimulation of the posterior hypothalamus was beneficial in intractable pain of CH and SUNCT (Leone et al., 2004; 2005a,b) patients. Involvement of the posterior hypothalamus in CH seen by functional imaging studies, and that the deep brain stimulation of the posterior hypothalamus rather than the anterior hypothalamus was effective in intractable CH patients, give rise to questions about hypothalamic activation as a direct perpetrator of the painful attacks, and may indicate the hypothalamic activation during these headache attacks to be an association rather than a direct effect (Cohen and Goadsby, 2006). Due to the overleap of several supraspinal centers discussed in this chapter which are involved in both facilitation and inhibition of pain, the complexity of the system and the limitation in technology, it is difficult to precisely know whether activation of these areas are the cause or the effect, and to know what exactly is going on in these areas during regional increase in cerebral blood flow. However, there is strong evidence to associate activation of the brain and brainstem with the attacks, and to believe in the existence of an imbalance between the nociceptive modulating nuclei during headache. Therefore, migraine at the moment might be considered to be a sensory dysmodulation, a system failure of normal sensory processing (Goadsby, 2007).

In addition, the peripheral and central sensitizations that refer to heightened state of pain should also be considered. Central sensitization involves an increase in the excitability of medullary dorsal horn (subnucleus caudalis) and spinal dorsal horn neurons due to several conditions including the neuronal depolarization; removal of the voltage-dependent magnesium block of the N-methyl-D-aspartate (NMDA) receptor; release of calcium from intracellular stores; phosphorylation of the NMDA, alpha amino-3-hydroxy-5-methyl-4-isoxazole-propionate (AMPA), and neurokinin (NK) 1 receptors via activation of protein kineses; a change in the neuron's excitability; and an increase in synaptic strength have been implicated in trigeminal nociceptive pathways, and several neurotransmitters/ neuromodulators are involved (Basbaum and Woolf, 1999; Yaksh 1999; Dubner and Ren, 2004).

References

Afridi, SK; Giffin, NJ; Kaube, H; Friston, KJ; Ward, NS; Frackowiak, RS; Goadsby, PJ. A positron emission tomographic study in spontaneous migraine. *Arch Neurol*, 2005 62, 1270-1275.

Aicher, SA; Randich, A. Antinociception and cardiovascular responses produced by electrical stimulation in the nucleus tractus solitarius, nucleus reticularis ventralis, and the caudal medulla. *Pain*, 1990 42, 103-119.

Aimone, LD; Bauer, CA; Gebhart, GF. Brain-stem relays mediating stimulation-produced antinociception from the lateral hypothalamus in the rat. *J Neurosci*, 1988 8, 2652-2663.

Akerman, S; Williamson, DJ; Kaube, H; Goadsby, PJ. Nitric oxide synthase inhibitors can antagonize neurogenic and calcitonin gene-related peptide induced dilation of dural meningeal vessels. *Br J Pharmacol*, 2002 137, 62-68.

Alessandri, M; Massanti, L; Geppetti, P; Bellucci, G; Cipriani, M; Fanciullacci, M. Plasma changes of calcitonin gene-related peptide and substance P in patients with dialysis headache. *Cephalalgia*, 2006 26, 1287-1293.

Almeida, A; Tavares, I; Lima, D; Coimbra, A. Descending projections from the medullary dorsal reticular nucleus make synaptic contacts with spinal cord lamina I cells projecting to that nucleus: an electron microscopic tracer study in the rat. *Neuroscience*, 1993 55, 1093-106.

Almeida, A; Tjølsen, A; Lima, D; Coimbra, A; Hole, K. The medullary dorsal reticular nucleus facilitates acute nociception in the rat. *Brain Res Bull*, 1996 39, 7-15.

Almeida, A; Størkson, R; Lima, D; Hole, K; Tjølsen, A. The medullary dorsal reticular nucleus facilitates pain behaviour induced by formalin in the rat. *Eur J Neurosci*, 1999 11, 110-122.

Almeida, A; Cobos, A; Tavares, I; Lima, D. Brain afferents to the medullary dorsal reticular nucleus: a retrograde and anterograde tracing study in the rat. *Eur J Neurosci*, 2002 16, 81-95.

Alvarez, FJ; Priestly, JV. Anatomy of somatostatin-immunoreactive fibers and cell bodies in the rat trigeminal subnucleus caudalis. *Neuroscience*, 1990a 38, 343-357.

Al-Rodhan, NR; Richelson, E; Gilbert, JA; McCormick, DJ; Kanba, KS; Pfenning, MA; Nelson, A; Larson, EW; Yaksh, TL. Structure-antinociceptive activity of neurotensin and some novel analogues in the periaqueductal gray region of the brainstem. *Brain Res*, 1991 557, 227-235.

Alvarez, FJ; Priestly, JV. Ultrastructure of somatostatin-immunoreactive nerve terminals in laminae I and II of the rat trigeminal subnucleus caudalis. *Neuroscience*, 1990b 38, 359-371.

Anzola, GP; Magoni, M; Guindani, M; Rozzini, L; Dalla Volta, G. Potential source of cerebral embolism in migraine with aura: a transcranial Doppler study. *Neurology*, 1999 52, 1622-1625.

Anzola, GP; Meneghetti, G; Zanferrari, C; Adami, A; Dinia, L; Del Sette, M. SAM Study Group. Is migraine associated with right-to-left shunt a separate disease? Results of the SAM study. *Cephalalgia*, 2008 28, 360-366.

Arbab, MA; Wiklund, L; Delgado, T; Svendgaard, NA. Stellate ganglion innervation of the vertebro-basilar arterial system demonstrated in the rat with anterograde and retrograde WGA-HRP tracing. *Brain Res*, 1988 445, 175-180.

Arommaa, M; Rautava, P; Sillanpaa, M; Helenius, H; ojanlatva, A. Familial occurrence of headache. *Cephalalgia*, 1999 25, 49-52.

Arulmani, U; Gupta, S; Massen Van Den Brink, A; Centurion, D; Villalon, CM; Saxena, PR. Experimental migraine models and their relevance in migraine therapy. *Cephalalgia*, 2006 26, 642-659.

Ashina, M; Bendtsen, L; Jensen, R; Ekman, R; Olesen, J. Plasma levels of substance P, neuropeptide Y and vasoactive intestinal polypeptide in patients with chronic tension-type headache. *Pain*, 1999 83, 541-547.

Ashina, M; Bendtsen, L; Jensen, R; Sakai, F; Olesen, J. Possible mechanisms of glyceryl-trinitrate-induced immediate headache in patients with chronic tension-type headache. *Cephalalgia*, 2000a 20, 919-924.

Ashina, M; Bendtsen, L; Jensen, R; Schifter, S; Jansen-Olesen, I; Olesen, J. Plasma levels of calcitonin gene-related peptide in chronic tension-type headache. *Neurology*, 2000b 55, 1335-1340.

Ashina, S; Bendtsen, L; Ashina, M; Magerl, W; Jensen, R. Generalized hyperalgesia in patients with chronic tension-type headache. *Cephalalgia*, 2006 26, 940-948.

Azarbal, B; Tobis, J; Suh, W; Chan, V; Dao, C; Gaster, R. Association of interatrial shunts and migraine headaches: impact of transcatheter closure. *J Am Coll Cardiol*, 2005 45, 489- 492.

Bach, FW; Langemark, M; Ekman, R; Rehfeld, JF; Schifter, S; Olesen, J. Effect of sulpiride or paroxetine on cerebrospinal fluid neuropeptide concentrations in patients with chronic tension-type headache. *Neuropeptides*, 1994 27, 129-136.

Bahra, A; Matharu, MS; Buchel, C; Frackowiak, RS; Goadsby, PJ. Brainstem activation specific to migraine headache. *Lancet*, 2001 357, 1016-1017.

Bahra, A; May, A; Goadsby, PJ. Cluster headache: a prospective clinical study with diagnostic implications. *Neurology*, 2002 58, 354-361.

Baird, JP; Travers, SP; Travers, JB. Integration of gastric distension and gustatory responses in the parabrachial nucleus. *Am J Physiol Regul Integr Comp Physiol*, 2001 281, R1581-593.

Baird, JP; Travers, JB; Travers, SP. Parametric analysis of gastric distension responses in the parabrachial nucleus. *Am J Physiol Regul Integr Comp Physiol*, 2001 281, R1568-R1580.

Bartsch, T; Levy, MJ; Knight, YE; Goadsby, PJ. Differential modulation of nociceptive dural input to (hypocretin) orexin A and B receptor activation in the posterior hypothalamic area. *Pain*, 2004 109, 367-378.

Bartsch, T; Levy, MJ; Knight, YE; Goadsby, PJ. Inhibition of nociceptive dural input in the trigeminal nucleus caudalis by somatostatin receptor blockade in the posterior hypothalamus. *Pain*, 2005 117, 30-39.

Basbaum, A; Field, H. The origin of descending pathways in the dorsolateral funiculus of the spinal cord of the cat and rat: further studies on the anatomy of pain modulation, *J. Comp. Neurol*, 1979 187, 513- 532.

Basbaum, AI; Fields, HL. Endogenous pain control systems: brainstem spinal pathways and endorphin circuitry. *Annu Rev Neurosci*, 1984 7, 309-338.

Basbaum, A I; Woolf, CJ. Pain. *Current Biology*, 1999 9, R429- R431.

Basbaum, AI. Jessell, TM. The Perception of Pain. In: Kandel ER, Schwartz JH, Jessell TM editors. *Principles of Neural Science*, 4th edition. New York: McGraw Hill; 2000; 473-491

Behbehani, M; Fields, H. Evidence that an excitatory connection between the periaqueductal gray and nucleus raphe magnus mediates stimulation produced analgesia. *Brain Res*, 1979 170, 85- 93.

Behbehani, M; Pert, A. A mechanism for analgesic effect of neurotensin as revealed by behavioural and electro-physiological techniques. *Brain Res*, 1984 324, 35-42.

Behbehani, MM; Park, MR; Clement, ME. Interactions between the lateral hypothalamus and the periaqueductal gray. *J Neurosci*, 1988 8, 2780-2787.

Behbehani, M M. Physiological mechanisms of the analgesic effect of neurotensin. *Ann N Y Acad Sci*, 1992 668, 253-265.

Behbehani, MM. Functional characteristics of the midbrain periaqueductal gray. *Prog Neurobiol*, 1995 46, 575-605.

Beitz, AJ. The organization of afferent projections to midbrain periaqueductal region of the rat. *Neuroscience*, 1982 7, 135-159.

Bejjani, BP; Houeto, JL; Hariz, M; Yelnik, J; Mesnage, V; Bonnet, AM; Pidoux, B; Dormont, D; Cornu, P; Agid, Y. Aggressive behavior induced by intraoperative stimulation in the triangle of Sano. *Neurology*, 2002 59, 1425-1427.

Bellamy, J; Bowen, EJ; Russo, AF; Durham, PL. Nitric oxide regulation of calcitonin gene-related peptide gene expression in rat trigeminal ganglia neurons. *Eur J Neurosci*, 2006 23, 2057-2066.

Benarroch, EE. Pain-autonomic interactions. *Neurol Sci*, 2006 27, Suppl 2:S130-133.

Benjamin, L; Levy, MJ; Lasalandra, MP; Knight, YE; Akerman, S; Classey, JD; Goadsby, PJ. Hypothalamic activation after stimulation of the superior sagittal sinus in the cat: a Fos study. *Neurobiol Dis*, 2004 16, 500-505.

Bertrand, F; Hugelin, A. Respiratory synchronizing function of nucleus parabrachialis medialis: pneumotaxic mechanisms. J Neurophysiol, 1971 34, 189-207.

Betz, E. Cerebral blood flow: its measurement and regulation. *Physiol Rev*, 1972 52, 595-630.

Bigal, ME; Rapoport, AM; Hargreaves, R. Advances in the pharmacologic treatment of tension-type headache. *Curr Pain Headache Rep*, 2008 12, 442-446.

Birk, S; Kruuse, C; Petersen, KA; Tfelt-Hansen, P; Olesen, J. The headache-inducing effect of cilostazol in human volunteers. *Cephalalgia*, 2006 26, 1304-1309.

Blau, JN. Migraine prodromes separated from the aura: complete migraine. *Br Med J*, 1980 281, 658-660.

Blomstrand, F; Khatibi, S; Muyderman, H; Hansson, E; Olsson, T; Rönnbäck, L. 5-Hydroxytryptamine and glutamate modulate velocity and extent of intercellular calcium signalling in hippocampal astroglial cells in primary cultures. *Neuroscience*, 1999 88, 1241-1253.

Bonica, JJ. *Management of Pain*. Second edition. Volume I and II. Philadelphia: Lea & Febiger; 1990.

Boska, M; Welch, K; Barker, P; Nelson, J; Schultz, L. Contrasts in cortical magnesium, phospholipid and energy metabolism between migraine syndromes. *Neurology*, 2002 58, 1227-1233.

Bouhassira, D; Villanueva, L; Bing, Z; le Bars, D. Involvement of the subnucleus reticularis dorsalis in diffuse noxious inhibitory controls in the rat. *Brain Res*, 1992 595, 353-357.

Bourgoin, S; Le Bars, D; Clot, AM; Hamon, M; Cesselin, F. Spontaneous and evoked release of methionine-enkephalin-like material from the spinal cord of arthritic rats in vivo. *Pain*, 1988 32, 107-114.

Bowker, RM; Westlund, KN; Sullivan, MC; Wilber, JF; Coulter, JD. Descending serotonergic, peptidergic and cholinergic pathways from the raphe nuclei: a multiple transmitter complex. *Brain Res*, 1983 288, 33-48.

Brain, SD; Williams, TJ; Tippins, JR; Morris, HR; MacIntyre, I. Calcitonin gene-related peptide is a potent vasodilator. *Nature*, 1985 313, 54-56.

Breslau, N; Rasmussen, BK. The impact of migraine: Epidemiology, risk factors, and co-morbidities. *Neurology*, 2001 56, (6 Suppl 1):S4-12.

Buldyrev, I; Tanner, NM; Hsieh, HY; Dodd, EG; Nguyen, LT; Balkowiec, A. Calcitonin gene-related peptide enhances release of native brain-derived neurotrophic factor from trigeminal ganglion neurons. *J Neurochem*, 2006 99, 1338-1350.

Burstein, R; Yarnitsky, D; Goor-Aryeh, I; Ransil, BJ; Bajwa, ZH. An association between migraine and cutaneous allodynia. *Ann Neurol*, 2000 47, 614-624.

Buzzi, MG; Carter, WB; Shimizu, T; Heath III, H; Moskowitz, MA. Dihydroergotamine and Sumatriptan attenuate levels of CGRP in plasma in rat superior sagittal sinus during electrical stimulation of the trigeminal ganglion. *Neuropharmacol*, 1991 30, 1193-1200.

Cao, Y; Aurora, SK; Nagesh, V; Patel, SC; Welch, KM. Functional MRI-BOLD of brainstem structures during visually triggered migraine. *Neurology*, 2002 59, 72-78.

Carpenter, MB. *Core Text of Neuroanatomy*. Third edition. Baltimore: Williams & Wilkins; 1985.

Caterina, MJ; Schumacher, MA; Tominaga, M; Rosen, TA; Levine, JD; Julius, D. The capsaicin receptor: a heat-activated ion channel in the pain pathway. *Nature*, 1997 389, 816-824.

Cechetto, DF; Saper, CB. Neurochemical organization of the hypothalamic projection to the spinal cord in the rat. *J Comp Neurol*, 1988 272, 579-604.

Cesselin, F; Le Bars, D; Bourgoin, S; Artaud, F; Gozlan, H; Clot, A M; Besson, J M; Hamon, M. Spontaneous and evoked release of methionine-enkephalin-like material from the rat spinal cord in vivo. *Brain Res*, 1985 339, 305-313.

Chiang, CY; Hu, JW; Sessle, BJ. Parabrachial area and nucleus raphe magnus-induced modulation of nociceptive and nonnociceptive trigeminal subnucleus caudalis neurons activated by cutaneous or deep inputs. *J Neurophysiol*, 1994 71, 2430-2445.

Clayton, JS; Gaskin, PJ; Beattie, DT. Attenuation of fos-like immunoreactivity in the trigeminal nucleus caudalis following trigeminovascular activation in the anaesthetised guinea pig. *Brain Res*, 1997 775, 74-80.

Clineschmidt, B V; McGuffin, J C; Bunting, PB. Neurotensin: antinociceptive action in rodents. *Eur J Pharmacol*, 1979 54, 129-139.

Clineschmidt, B V; Martin, GE; Veber, DF. Antinociceptive effects of neurotensin and neurotensin-related peptides. *Ann NY Acad Sci*, 1982 400, 283-306.

Coffield, JA; Bowen, KK; Miletic, V. Retrograde tracing of projections between the nucleus submedius, the ventrolateral orbital cortex, and the midbrain in the rat. *J Comp Neurol*, 1992 321, 488-499.

Cohen, AS; Goadsby, PJ. Functional neuroimaging of primary headache disorders. *Expert Rev Neurother*, 2006 6, 1159-1171.

Craig, AD; Bushnell, MC; Zhang, ET; Blomqvist, A. A thalamic nucleus specific for pain and temperature sensation. *Nature*, 1994a 372, 770-773.

Craig, AD; Bushnell, MC. The thermal grill illusion: unmasking the burn of cold pain. *Science*, 1994b 265, 252-255.

Craig, AD; Reiman, EM; Evans, A; Bushnell, MC. Functional imaging of an illusion of pain. *Nature*, 1996 384, 258-260.

Dalsgaard, CJ; Vincent, SR; Hökfelt, T; Wiesenfeld-hallin, Z; Gustafsson, L; Elde, R; Dockray, GJ. Effects of cysteamine on pain behaviour and on somatostatin and substance P-like immunoreactivity in the substantia gelatinosa of the rat. *Eur J Pharmacol*, 1984 104, 295-301.

Darian-Smith, I. The trigeminal system. In: Iggo, A. (editor), *Handbook of sensory physiology*. New York: Springer-Verlag; 1973; 271- 314.

De Fusco, M; Marconi, R; Silvestri, L; Atorino, L; Rampoldi, L; Morgante, L; Ballabio, A; Aridon, P; Casari, G. Haploinsufficiency of ATP1A2 encoding the Na+/K+ pump alpha2 subunit associated with familial hemiplegic migraine type 2. *Nat Genet*, 2003 33, 192-196.

Del Fiacco, M; Quarta, M. Somatostatin, galanin and peptide histidine isoleucine in the newborn and adult human trigeminal ganglion and spinal nucleus: immunohistochemistry, neuronal morphometry and co-localization with substance P. *J Chem Neuroanat*, 1994 7, 171-184.

Del Sette, M; Angeli, S; Leandri, M; Ferriero, G; Bruzzone, GL; Finocchi, C; Gandolfo, C. Migraine with aura and right-to-left shunt on transcranial Doppler: a case-control study. *Cerebrovasc Dis*, 1998 8, 327-330.

Denuelle, M; Fabre, N; Payoux, P; Chollet, F; Geraud, G. Hypothalamic activation in spontaneous migraine attacks. *Headache*, 2007 47, 1418-1426

De Vries, P; Villalon, CM; Saxena, PR. Pharmacological aspects of experimental headache models in relation to acute antimigraine therapy. *Eur J Pharmacol*, 1999 375, 61-74.

Dichgans, M; Freilinger, T; Eckstein, G; Babini, E; Lorenz-Depiereux, B; Biskup, S; Ferrari, MD; Herzog, J; van den Maagdenberg, AM; Pusch, M; Strom, TM. Mutation in the neuronal voltage-gated sodium channel SCN1A in familial hemiplegic migraine. *Lancet*, 2005 366, 371-377.

Diener, HC. Substance-P antagonist RPR100893-201 is not effective in human migraine attacks. In: Olesen J, Tfelt-Hansen P, editors. *Proceedings of the 6th International Headache Seminar*. New York: Lippincott-Raven; 1996.

Donaldson, C; Boers, PM; Hoskin, KL; Zagami, AS; Lambert, GA. The role of 5-HT1B and 5-HT1D receptors in the selective inhibitory effect of naratriptan on trigeminovascular neurons. *Neuropharmacology*, 2002 42, 374-385.

Dubner, R; Ren, K. Brainstem mechanisms of persistent pain following injury. *J Orofac Pain*, 2004 18, 299-305.

Dugast, C; Almeida, A; Lima, D. The medullary dorsal reticular nucleus enhances the responsiveness of spinal nociceptive neurons to peripheral stimulation in the rat. *Eur J Neurosci*, 2003 18, 580-588

Duverger, D; Edvinsson, L; MacKenzie, ET; Oblin, A; Rouquier, L; Scatton, B; Zivkovic B. Concentrations of putative neurovascular transmitters in major cerebral arteries and small pial vessels of various species. *J Cereb Blood Flow Metab*, 1987 7, 497-501.

Edvinsson, L. Sensory nerves in man and their role in primary headaches. *Cephalalgia*, 2001 21, 761-764.

Edvinsson, L. Neuronal signal substances as biomarkers of migraine. *Headache*, 2006 46, 1088-1094.

Edvinsson, L; Nielsen, KC; Owman, C; Sporrong, B. Cholinergic mechanisms in pial vessels. Histochemistry, electron microscopy and pharmacology. *Z Zellforsch Mikrosk Anat*, 1972 134, 311-325.

Edvinsson, L; Aubineau, P; Owman, C; Sercombe, R; Seylaz, J. Sympathetic innervation of cerebral arteries: prejunctional supersensitivity to norepinephrine after sympathectomy or cocaine treatment. *Stroke*, 1975 6, 525-330.

Edvinsson, L; Falck, B; Owman, C. Possibilities for a cholinergic action on smooth musculature and on sympathetic axons in brain vessels mediated by muscarinic and nicotinic receptors. *J Pharmacol Exp Ther*, 1977 200, 117-126.

Edvinsson, L; Degueurce, A; Duverger, D; MacKenzie, ET; Scatton, B. Central serotonergic nerves project to the pial vessels of the brain. *Nature*, 1983 306, 55-57.

Edvinsson, L; Emson, P; McCulloch, J; Tatemoto, K; Uddman, R. Neuropeptide Y: cerebrovascular innervation and vasomotor effects in the cat. *Neurosci Lett*, 1983 43, 79-84.

Edvinsson, L; Emson, P; McCulloch, J; Tatemoto, K; Uddman, R. Neuropeptide Y: immunocytochemical localization to and effect upon feline pial arteries and veins in vitro and in situ. *Acta Physiol Scand*, 1984 122, 155-163.

Edvinsson, L; Ekman, R; Jansen, I; McCulloch, J; Uddman, R. Calcitonin gene-related peptide and cerebral blood vessels: distribution and vasomotor effects. *J Cereb Blood Flow Metab*, 1987a 7, 720-728.

Edvinsson, L; Ekman, R; Jansen, I; Ottosson, A; Uddman, R. Peptide-containing nerve fibers in human cerebral arteries: immunocytochemistry, radioimmunoassay, and in vitro pharmacology. *Ann Neurol*, 1987b 21, 431-437.

Edvinsson, L; Brodin, E; Jansen, I; Uddman, R. Neurokinin A in cerebral vessels: characterization, localization and effects in vitro, *Regul Pept*, 1988 20, 181- 197.

Edvinsson, L; Hara, H; Uddman, R. Retrograde tracing of nerve fibers to the rat middle cerebral artery with true blue: colocalization with different peptides. *J Cereb Blood Flow Metab*, 1989 9, 212-218.

Edvinsson, L; Jansen, I; Cunha e Sa, M; Gulbenkian, S. Demonstration of neuropeptide containing nerves and vasomotor responses to perivascular peptides in human cerebral arteries. *Cephalalgia*, 1994 14, 88-96.

Edvinsson, L; Uddman, R. Neurobiology of primary headaches. *Brain Res Rev*, 2005 48, 438-456.

Escott, KJ; Beattie, DT; Connor, HE; Brain, SD. Trigeminal ganglion stimulation increases facial skin blood flow in the rat: a major role for calcitonin gene-related peptide. *Brain Res*, 1995 669, 93-99.

Fanciullacci, M; Alessandri, M; Figini, M; Geppetti, P; Michelacci, S. Increase in plasma calcitonin gene-related peptide from the extracerebral circulation during nitroglycerin-induced cluster headache attack. *Pain*, 1995 60, 119-123.

Fang, F; Morean, J L; Fields, H L. Dose dependent antinociceptive action of neurotensin microinjected into the rostroventromedial medulla of the rat. *Brain Res*, 1987 420, 171-174.

Feindel, W; Penfield, W; McNaughton, F. The tentorial nerves and localization of intracranial pain in man. *Neurology*, 1960 10, 555-563.

Fields, HL; Heinricher, MM; Mason, P. Neurotransmitters in nociceptive modulatory circuits. *Annu Rev Neurosci*, 1991 14, 219-245.

Fields, HL. Pain modulation: expectation, opioid analgesia and virtual pain. *Prog Brain Res*, 2000 122, 245-253.

Fischer, MJ; Koulchitsky, S; Messlinger, K. The nonpeptide calcitonin gene-related peptide receptor antagonist BIBN4096BS lowers the activity of neurons with meningeal input in the rat spinal trigeminal nucleus. *J Neurosci*, 2005 25, 5877-5883.

Friberg, L; Olesen, J; Olsen, TS; Karle, A; Ekman, R; Fahrenkrug, J. Absence of vasoactive peptide release from brain to cerebral circulation during onset of migraine with aura. *Cephalalgia*, 1994 14, 47- 54.

Fricke, B; von Düring, M; Andres, KH. Topography and immunocytochemical characterization of nerve fibers in the leptomeningeal compartments of the rat. A light- and electron-microscopical study. *Cell Tissue Res*, 1997 287, 11-22.

Fusayasu, E; Kowa, H; Takeshima, T; Nakaso, K; Nakashima, K. Increased plasma substance P and CGRP levels, and high ACE activity in migraineurs during headache-free periods. *Pain*, 2007 128, 209-214.

Gall, O; Villanueva, L; Bouhassira, D; Le Bars, D. Spatial encoding properties of subnucleus reticularis dorsalis neurons in the rat medulla. *Brain Res*, 2000 873, 131-134.

Gallai, V; Sarchielli, P; Flofidi, A; Francceschini, M; Codini, M; Trequattrini, A;

Palumbo, R. Vasoactive peptide levels in the plasma of young migraine patients with and without aura assessed both interictally and ictally. *Cephalalgia*, 1995 15, 384- 390.

Gamboa-Esteves, FO; Lima, D; Batten, TF. Neurochemistry of superficial spinal neurones projecting to nucleus of the solitary tract that express c-fos on chemical somatic and visceral nociceptive input in the rat. *Metab Brain Dis*, 2001a 16, 151-164.

Gamboa-Esteves, FO; Tavares, I; Almeida, A; Batten, TF; McWilliam, PN; Lima, D. Projection sites of superficial and deep spinal dorsal horn cells in the nucleus tractus solitarii of the rat. *Brain Res*, 2001b 921, 195-205.

Gamse, R; Saria, A. Nociceptive behavior after intrathecal injection of substance P, neurokinin A and calcitonin gene-related peptide in mice. *Neurosci Lett*, 1986 70, 143-147.

Gazelius, B; Brodin, E; Olgart, L; Panopoulos, P. Evidence that substance P is a mediator of antidromic vasodilatation using somatostatin as a release inhibitor. *Acta Physiol Scand*, 1981 113, 155-159.

Géraud, G; Denuelle, M; Fabre, N; Payoux, P; Chollet, F. Positron emission tomographic studies of migraine. *Rev Neurol* (Paris), 2005 161, 666-670.

Gérardy, PY; Fumal, A; Schoenen, J. Epidemiology and economic repercussion of headache: an inquiery among the administrative and technical personnel of the Liège University. *Rev Med Liege*, 2008 63, 310-314.

Gioia, M; Bianchi, R. Ultrastructure of substance P immunoreactive elements in the periaqueductal gray mater of the rat. *Peptides*, 1991 12, 1235-1238.

Goadsby, PJ; Edvinsson, L; Ekman, R. Release of vasoactive peptides in the extracerebral circulation of humans and the cat during activation of the trigeminovascular system. *Ann. Neurol*, 1988 23, 193- 196.

Goadsby, PJ; Edvinsson, L; Ekman, R. Vasoactive peptide release in the extracerebral circulation of human during migraine headache. *Ann. Neurol*, 1990 28, 183- 187.

Goadsby, PJ; Zagami, AS; Lambert, GA. Neural processing of craniovascular pain: a synthesis of the central structures involved in migraine. *Headache*, 1991 31, 365-371.

Goadsby, PJ; Edvinsson, L. The trigeminovascular system and migraine: studies characterizing cerebrovascular and neuropeptide changes seen in humans and cats. *Ann Neurol*, 1993 33, 48-56.

Goadsby, PJ; Edvinsson, L. Human in vivo evidence for trigeminovascular activation in cluster headache. Neuropeptide changes and effects of acute attacks therapies. *Brain*, 1994 117, 427-434.

Goadsby, PJ; Uddman, R; Edvinsson, L. Cerebral vasodilatation in the cat involves nitric oxide from parasympathetic nerves. *Brain Res*, 1996 707, 110-118.

Goadsby, PJ. Is a central action of acute antimigraine drugs essential? *Cephalalgia*, 1997a 17, 10-11.

Goadsby, PJ. Current concepts of the pathophysiology of migraine. *Neurol Clin*, 1997b 15, 27-42.

Goadsby, PJ; Lipton, RB. A review of paroxysmal hemicranias, SUNCT syndrome and other short-lasting headaches with autonomic feature, including new cases. *Brain*, 1997 120, 193-209.

Goadsby, PJ; Knight, Y. Inhibition of trigeminal neurones after intravenous administration of naratriptan through an action at 5-hydroxy-tryptamine (5-HT(1B/1D)) receptors. *Br J Pharmacol*, 1997 122, 918-922.

Goadsby, PJ; Boes, CJ. Zolmitriptan: differences from sumatriptan. *Curr Med Res Opin*, 2001 17, S46-50.

Goadsby, PJ; Lipton, RB; Ferrari, MD. Migraine--current understanding and treatment. *N Engl J Med*, 2002 346, 257-270.

Goadsby, PJ. Migraine aura: a knockin mouse with a knockout message. *Neuron*, 2004 41, 679-780.

Goadsby, PJ. Kullmann, DM. Another migraine gene. *Lancet*, 2005 366, 345-6.

Goadsby, PJ. Recent advances in understanding migraine mechanisms, molecules and therapeutics. *Trends Mol Med*, 2007 13, 39-44.

Goldstein, DJ; Wang, O; Saper, JR; Stoltz, R; Silberstein, SD; Mathew, NT. Ineffectiveness of neurokinin-1 antagonist in acute migraine: a crossover study. *Cephalalgia*, 1997 17, 785-790.

Gonzalez-Rey, E; Varela, N; Chorny, A; Delgado, M. Therapeutical approaches of vasoactive intestinal peptide as a pleiotropic immunomodulator. *Curr Pharm Des*, 2007 13, 1113-1139.

Goodman, EC; Iversen, LL. Calcitonin gene-related peptide: Novel neuropeptide. *Life Sci*, 1986 38, 2169-2178.

Gorji, A. Spreading depression: a review of the clinical relevance. *Brain Res Brain Res Rev*, 2001 38, 33-60.

Greenwell, TN; Martin-Schild, S; Inglis, FM; Zadina, JE. Colocalization and shared distribution of endomorphins with substance P, calcitonin gene-related peptide, gamma-aminobutyric acid, and the mu opioid receptor. *J Comp Neurol*, 2007 503, 319-333.

Greves, LE; Nyberg, F; Terenius, L; Hökfelt, T. Calcitonin gene-related peptide is a potent inhibitor of substance P degradation. *Eur J Pharmacol*, 1985 115, 309-311.

Gulbenkian, S; Barroso, CP; Cunha e Sá, M; Edvinsson, L. The peptidergic innervation of human coronary and cerebral vessels. *Ital J Anat Embryol*, 1995 100 Suppl 1, 317-327.

Gulbenkian, S; Uddman, R; Edvinsson, L. Neuronal messengers in the human cerebral circulation. *Peptides*, 2001 22, 995-1007.

Guo, A; Vulchanova, L; Wang, J; Li, X; Elde, R. Immunocytochemical localization of the vanilloid receptor 1 (VR1): relationship to neuropeptides, the P2X3 purinoceptor and IB4 binding sites. *Eur J Neurosci*, 1999 11, 946-958.

Gupta, S; Mehrotra, S; Villalon, C; De Vries, R; Garrelds, I; Saxena, P; Vandenbrink, AM. Effects of female sex hormones on responses to CGRP, acetylcholine, and 5-HT in rat isolated arteries. *Headache*, 2007a 47, 564-575.

Gupta, S; Mehrotra, S; Villalon, CM; Perusquia, M; Saxena, PR; MaassenVanDenBrink, A. Potential role of female sex hormones in the pathophysiology of migraine. *Pharmacol Ther*, 2007b 113, 321-340.

Halsell, CB; Travers, SP. Anterior and posterior oral cavity responsive neurons are differentially distributed among parabrachial subnuclei in rat. *J Neurophysiol*, 1997 78, 920-938.

Hamel, E. The biology of serotonin receptors: focus on migraine pathophysiology and treatment. *Can J Neurol Sci*, 1999 26 Suppl 3, S2-6.

Hansson, E; Muyderman, H; Leonova, J; Allansson, L; Sinclair, J; Blomstrand, F; Thorlin, T; Nilsson, M; Rönnbäck, L. Astroglia and glutamate in physiology and pathology: aspects on glutamate transport, glutamate-induced cell swelling and gap-junction communication. *Neurochem Int*, 2000 37, 317-329.

Hara, H; Hamill, GS; Jacobowitz, DM. Origin of cholinergic nerves to the rat major cerebral arteries: coexistence with vasoactive intestinal polypeptide. *Brain Res Bull*, 1985 14, 179-188.

Hardebo, JE; Suzuki, N; Owman, C. Origins of substance P- and calcitonin gene-related peptide-containing nerves in the internal carotid artery of rat. *Neurosci Lett*, 1989 101, 39-45.

Hasan, MY. Migraine and patent foramen ovale: exploring the association and a possible treatment option. *J Pak Med Assoc.*, 2008 58, 453-455.

Helliwell, RJ; McLatchie, LM; Clarke, M; Winter, J Bevan, S; McIntyre, P. Capsaicin sensitivity is associated with the expression of the vanilloid (capsaicin) receptor (VR1) mRNA in adult rat sensory ganglia. *Neurosci Lett*, 1998 250, 177-180.

Hjornevik, T; Jacobsen, LM; Qu, H; Bjaalie, JG; Gjerstad, J; Willoch, F. Metabolic plasticity in the supraspinal pain modulating circuitry after noxious stimulus-induced spinal cord LTP. *Pain*, 2008 140, 456-464.

Hökfelt, T; Arvidsson, U; Cullheim, S; Millhorn, D; Nicholas, AP; Pieribone, V; Seroogy, K; Ulfhake, B. Multiple messengers in descending serotonin neurons: localization and functional implications. *J Chem Neuroanat*, 2000 18, 75-86.

Holden, JE; Naleway, E. Microinjection of carbachol in the lateral hypothalamus produces opposing actions on nociception mediated by alpha(1)- and alpha(2)-adrenoceptors. *Brain Res*, 2001 911, 27-36.

Holzer, P. Local effector functions of capsaicin-sensitive sensory nerve endings: involvement of tachykinins, calcitonin gene-related peptide and other neuropeptides. *Neuroscience*, 1988 24, 739-768.

Hoskin, KL; Kaube, H; Goadsby, PJ. Sumatriptan can inhibit trigeminal afferents by an exclusively neural mechanism. *Brain*, 1996 119, 1419-1428.

Hoskin, KL; Zagami, AS; Goadsby, PJ. Stimulation of the middle meningeal artery leads to Fos expression in the trigeminocervical nucleus: a comparative study of monkey and cat. *J. Anat*, 1999 194, 579- 588.

Hou, M; Uddman, R; Tajti, J; Kanje, M; Edvinsson, L. Capsaicin receptor immunoreactivity in the human trigeminal ganglion. *Neurosci Lett*, 2002 330, 223-226.

Hylden, J L; Wilcox, G L. Intrathecal substance P elicits a caudally-directed biting and scratching behaviour in mice. *Brain Res*, 1981 217, 212-215.

Hylden, JL; Hayashi, H; Dubner, R; Bennett, GJ. Physiology and morphology of the lamina I spinomesencephalic projection. *J Comp Neurol*, 1986 247, 505-515.

Iversen, S. Iversen, L. Saper, CB. The Autonomic Nervous System and the Hypothalamus. In: Kandel ER, Schwartz JH, Jessell TM, editors. *Principles of Neural Science*: 4th edition, New York: McGraw Hill; 2000; 973.

Iversen, HK. Human migraine models. *Cephalalgia*, 2001 21, 781-785.

Jacquin, FM; Nicolas, L; Rhoades, WR. Trigeminal projections to contralateral dorsal horn: central extent, peripheral origins, and plasticity. *Somatosens. Mot. Res*, 1990 7, 153- 183.

Jansen, I; Alafaci, C; McCulloch, J; Uddman, R; Edvinsson, L. Tachykinins (substance P, neurokinin A, neuropeptide K, and neurokinin B) in the cerebral circulation: vasomotor responses in vitro and in situ. *J Cereb Blood Flow Metab*, 1991 11, 567-575.

Jansen-Olesen, I; Goadsby, PJ; Uddman, R; Edvinsson, L. Vasoactive intestinal peptide (VIP) like peptides in the cerebral circulation of the cat. *J Auton Nerv Syst*, 1994 49 Suppl:S97-103.

Jensen, R; Olesen, J. Tension-type headache: an update on mechanisms and treatment. *Curr Opin Neurol*, 2000 13, 285-289.

Jesurum, JT; Fuller, CJ; Kim, CJ; Krabill, KA; Spencer, MP; Olsen, JV; Likosky, WH; Reisman, M. Frequency of migraine headache relief following patent foramen ovale "closure" despite residual right-to-left shunt. *Am J Cardiol*, 2008 102, 916-620

Jiang, M; Behbehani, MM. Physiological characteristics of the projection pathway from the medial preoptic to the nucleus raphe magnus of the rat and its modulation by the periaqueductal gray. *Pain*, 2001 94, 139-147.

Jones, SL. Descending noradrenergic influences on pain. *Prog Brain Res*, 1991 88, 381-394.

Julius, D; Basbaum, AI. Molecular mechanisms of nociception. *Nature*, 2001 413, 203-310.

Just, S; Arndt, K; Doods, H. The role of CGRP and nicotinic receptors in centrally evoked facial blood flow changes. *Neurosci Lett*, 2005 381, 120-124.

Kafitz, KW; Rose, CR; Thoenen, H; Konnerth, A. Neurotrophin-evoked rapid excitation through TrkB receptors. *Nature*, 1999 401, 918-921.

Kai-Kai, MA. Cytochemistry of the trigeminal and dorsal root ganglia and spinal cord of the rat. *Comp Biochem Physiol A*, 1989 93, 183-193.

Kalivas, PW; Jennes, L; Nemeroff, CB; Prange, A J. Neurotensin: topographical distribution of brain sites involved in hypothermia and antinociception. *J Comp Neurol*, 1982 210, 225-238.

Kapicioglu, S; Gokce, E; Kapicioglu, Z; Ovali, E. Treatment of migraine attacks with a long-acting somatostatin analogue (Octreotide. SMS 201-995). *Cephalalgia*, 1997 17, 27-30.

Kaube, H; Keay, K A; Hoskin, K L; Bandler, R; Goadsby, P J. Expression of C-fos like immunoreactivity in the caudal medulla and upper cervical spinal cord following stimulation of the superior sagittal sinus in cat. *Brain Res*, 1993 629, 95-102.

Keller, JT; Marfurt, CF Peptidergic and serotoninergic innervation of the rat dura mater. *J Comp Neurol*, 1991 309, 515-534.

Kelman, L. The triggers or precipitants of the acute migraine attack. *Cephalalgia*, 2007 27, 394-402.

Kemper, RH; Jeuring, M; Meijler, WJ; Korf, J; Ter Horst, GJ. Intracisternal octreotide does not ameliorate orthodromic trigeminovascular nociception. *Cephalalgia*, 2000 20, 114-121.

Kerr, FWL. Fine structure and functional characteristics of the primary trigeminal neurons. In: Hassler, R. and Walker A.E. (Ed.), *Trigeminal neuralgia*. Stuttgart: Georg Thieme Verlag, 1970; 180- 190.

Kitazawa, T; Terasaki, T; Suzuki, H; Kakee, A; Sugiyama, Y. Efflux of taurocholic acid across the blood-brain barrier: interaction with cyclic peptides. *J Pharmacol Exp Ther*, 1998 286, 890-895.

Knight, YE; Goadsby, PJ. The periaqueductal grey matter modulates trigeminovascular input: a role in migraine? *Neuroscience*, 2001 106, 793-800.

Knight, YE; Bartsch, T; Kaube, H; Goadsby, PJ. P/Q-type calcium-channel blockade in the periaqueductal gray facilitates trigeminal nociception: a functional genetic link for migraine? *J Neurosci*, 2002 22, RC213.

Knight, YE; Bartsch, T; Goadsby, PJ. Trigeminal antinociception induced by bicuculline in the periaqueductal gray (PAG) is not affected by PAG P/Q-type calcium channel blockade in rat. *Neurosci Lett*, 2003 336, 113-116.

Knight, YE; Classey, JD; Lasalandra, MP; Akerman, S; Kowacs, F; Hoskin, KL; Goadsby, PJ. Patterns of fos expression in the rostral medulla and caudal pons evoked by noxious craniovascular stimulation and periaqueductal gray stimulation in the cat. *Brain Res*, 2005 1045, 1-11.

Knyihar-Csillik, E; Tajti, J; Samsam, M; Vécsei, L. Central representation of CGRP-positive trigeminal neurons in the medulla oblongata of the albino rat. *European Headache Federation, The 2nd international conference on Headache*, Liege, Belgium, 1994, Abstract p 41.

Knyihár-Csillik, E; Tajti, J; Samsam, M; Sáry, G; Vécsei, L. Electrical stimulation of the Gasserian ganglion induces structural alterations of calcitonin gene-related peptide-immunoreactive perivascular sensory nerve terminals in the rat cerebral dura mater: a possible model of migraine headache. *Neurosci Lett*, 1995 184, 189-192.

Knyihár-Csillik, E; Samsam, M; Tajti, J; Sáry, Gy; Buzas, P; Vécsei, L. Anatomical basis of Headache: changes in the intracellular equilibrium of a pain-related neuropeptide in an experimental migraine model. *Ann Anat*, 1996 178, p 220.

Knyihár Csillik, E; Tajti, J; Samsam, M; Sáry, G; Buzás, P; Vécsei, L. Effect of a serotonin agonist (Sumatriptan) on the peptidergic innervation of the rat cerebral dura mater and on the expression of c-fos in the caudal trigeminal nucleus in an experimental migraine model. *J Neurosci Res*, 1997 48, 449- 464.

Knyihár Csillik, E; Tajti, J; Samsam, M; Sáry, G; Buzás, P; Vécsei, L. Depletion of calcitonin gene-related peptide from the caudal trigeminal nucleus of the rat after electrical stimulation of the Gasserian ganglion. *Exp Brain Res*, 1998 118, 111-114.

Komisaruk, BR; Whipple, B. Functional MRI of the brain during orgasm in women. *Annu Rev Sex Res*, 2005 16, 62-86.

Kors, EE; Vanmolkot, KR; Haan, J; Frants, RR; van den Maagdenberg, AM; Ferrari, MD. Recent findings in headache genetics. *Curr Opin Neurol*, 2004 17, 283-288

Kruuse, C; Thomsen, L; Birk, S; Oleesen, J. Migraine can be induced by sildenafil without changes in middle cerebral artery diameter. *Brain*, 2003 126, 241-247.

Lambert, GA; Boers, PM; Hoskin, KL; Donaldson, C; Zagami, AS. Suppression by eletriptan of the activation of trigeminovascular sensory neurons by glyceryl trinitrate. *Brain Res*, 2002 953, 181-188.

Lance, JW; Lambert, GA; Goadsby, PJ; Duckworth, JW. Brainstem influences on the cephalic circulation: experimental data from cat and monkey of relevance to the mechanism of migraine. *Headache*, 1983 23, 258-265.

Langemark, M; Bach, F W; Ekman, R; Olesen, J. Increased cerebrospinal fluid Met-enkephalin immunoreactivity in patients with chronic tension-type headache. *Pain*, 1995 63, 103-107.

Larsson, LI; Edvinsson, L; Fahrenkrug, J; Håkanson, R; Owman, C; Schaffalitzky de Muckadell, O; Sundler, F. Immunohistochemical localization of a vasodilatory polypeptide (VIP) in cerebrovascular nerves. *Brain Res*, 1976 113, 400-404.

Lassen, LH; Haderslev, PA; Jacobsen, VB; Iversen, HK; Sperling, B; Olesen, J. CGRP may play a causative role in migraine. *Cephalalgia*, 2002 22, 54-61.

Lauritzen, M; Olsen, T; Lassen, N; Paulson, O. Regulation of regional cerebral blood flow during and between migraine attacks. *Ann Neurol*, 1983 14, 569-572.

Lauritzen, M. Pathophysiology of the migraine aura. The spreading depression theory. *Brain*, 1994 117, 199-210.

Lauritzen, M. Cortical spreading depression in migraine. *Cephalalgia*, 2001 21, 757-760.

Lazarov, NE. Comparative analysis of the chemical neuroanatomy of the mammalian trigeminal ganglion and mesencephalic trigeminal nucleus. *Prog Neurobiol*, 2002 66, 19-59.

Lazarov, NE. Neurobiology of orofacial proprioception. *Brain Res Rev,* 2007 56, 362-383.

Lee, TJ. Direct evidence against acetylcholine as the dilator transmitter in the cat cerebral artery. *Eur J Pharmacol*, 1980 68, 393-394

Lee, TJ. Cholinergic mechanism in the large cat cerebral artery. *Circ Res*, 1982 50, 870-879.

Lee, TJ. Nitric oxide and the cerebral vascular function. *J Biomed Sci*, 2000 7, 16-26.

Leibowitz, DH. The glial spike theory. I. On an active role of neuroglia in spreading depression and migraine. *Proc Biol Sci*, 1992 250,287-295.

Leite-Almeida, H; Valle-Fernandes, A; Almeida, A. Brain projections from the medullary dorsal reticular nucleus: an anterograde and retrograde tracing study in the rat. *Neuroscience*, 2006 140, 577-595.

Lembeck, F; Gamse, R. Lack of algesia effect of substance P on paravascular pain receptors. *Naunyn Schmiedebergs Arch Pharmacol*, 1977 29, 295-303.

Leonardi, M; Steiner, TJ; Scher, AT; Lipton, RB. The global burden of migraine: measuring disability in headache disorders with WHO's Classification of Functioning, Disability and Health (ICF). *J Headache Pain*, 2005 6, 429-240.

Leone, M; Franzini, A; Broggi, G; May, A; Bussone, G. Long-term follow-up of bilateral hypothalamic stimulation for intractable cluster headache. *Brain*, 2004 127, 2259-2264.

Leone, M; Franzini, A; D'Andrea, G; Broggi, G; Casucci, G; Bussone, G. Deep brain stimulation to relieve drug-resistant SUNCT. *Ann Neurol*, 2005a 57, 924-927.

Leone, M; Franzini, A; Felisati, G; Mea, E; Curone, M; Tullo, V; Broggi, G; Bussone, G. Deep brain stimulation and cluster headache. *Neurol Sci*, 2005b Suppl 2, s138-139.

Lewis, JW; Baldrighi, G; Akil, H. A possible interface between autonomic function and pain control: opioid analgesia and the nucleus tractus solitarius. *Brain Res*, 1987 424, 65-70.

Li, YQ; Takada, M; Matsuzaki, S; Shinonaga, Y; Mizuno, N. Identification of periaqueductal gray and dorsal raphe nucleus neurons projecting to both the trigeminal sensory complex and forebrain structures: a fluorescent retrograde double-labeling study in the rat. *Brain Res,* 1993 623, 267-277.

Li, HS; Monhemius, R; Simpson, BA; Roberts, MH. Supraspinal inhibition of nociceptive dorsal horn neurones in the anaesthetized rat: tonic or dynamic? *J Physiol*, 1998 506, 459-469.

Liebeskind, JC; Guilbaud, G; Besson, JM; Oliveras, JL. Analgesia from electrical stimulation of the periaqueductal gray matter in the cat: behavioral observations and inhibitory effects on spinal cord interneurons. *Brain Res*, 1973 50, 441-446.

Linde, M. Migraine: a review and future directions for treatment. *Acta Neurol Scand*, 2006 114, 71-83.

Lipton, RB; Stewart, WF; Diamond, S; Diamond, ML; Reed, M. Prevalence and burden of migraine in the United States: data from the American Migraine Study II. *Headache*, 2001 41, 646-657.

Lima, D; Almeida, A. The medullary dorsal reticular nucleus as a pronociceptive centre of the pain control system. *Prog Neurobiol*, 2002 66, 81-108.

Lindsay, KW. Bone, I. Headache. In: Lindsay KW, Bone I, editors. *Neurology and Neurosugery*, 4th edithion. Philadelphia: Churchill Livingstone; 2004; 67- 72.

Liu, Y; Broman, J; Edvinsson, L. Central projections of the sensory innervation of the rat middle meningeal artery. *Brain Res*, 2008 1208, 103-110.

Lodi, R; Pierangeli, G; Tonon, C; Cevoli, S; Testa, C; Bivona, G; Magnifico, F; Cortelli, P; Montagna, P; Barbiroli, B.Study of hypothalamic metabolism in cluster headache by proton MR spectroscopy. *Neurology*, 2006 66, 1264-1266.

Lou, HC; Edvinsson, L; MacKenzie, ET. The concept of coupling blood flow to brain function: revision required? *Ann Neurol*, 1987 22, 289-297.

Luermans, JG; Post, MC; Temmerman, F; Thijs, V; Schonewille, WJ; Plokker, HW; Suttorp, MJ; Budts, WI. Closure of a patent foramen ovale is associated with a decrease in prevalence of migraine: a prospective observational study. *Acta Cardiol*, 2008 63, 571-7.

Malick, A; Burstein, R. Cells of origin of the trigeminohypothalamic tract in the rat. *J Comp Neurol*, 1998 400, 125-144.

Markowitz, S; Saito, K; Moskowitz, M.A. Neurogenically mediated leakage of plasma protein occurs from blood vessels in dura mater but not brain. *J Neurosci*, 1987 7, 4129-4136.

Martin-Schild, S; Gerall, A A; Kastin, A J; Zadina, J E. Endomorphin-2 is an endogenous opioid in primary sensory afferent fibers. *Peptides*, 1998 19, 1783-1789.

Massari, VJ; Tizabi, Y; Park, CH; Moody, TW; Halke, CJ; O′Donohue, TL. Distribution and origin of bombesin, substance P and somatostatin in cat spinal cord. *Peptides*, 1983 4, 673-681.

Matharu, MS; Bartsch, T; Ward, N; Frackwiak, RS; Weiner, R; Goadsby, PJ. Central neuromodulation in chronic migraine patients with suboccipital stimulators: a PET study. *Brain*, 2004 127, 220-230.

Matharu, MS; Cohen, AS; Frackowiak, RS; Goadsby, PJ. Posterior hypothalamic activation in paroxysmal hemicrania. *Ann Neurol*, 2006 59, 535-545.

Matsubara, T; Moskowitz, MA; Huang, Z. UK-14,304, R(-)-alpha-methyl-histamine and SMS201-995 block plasma protein leakage within dura mater by prejunctional mechanism. *Eur J Pharmacol*, 1992 224, 145-150.

May, A; Bahra, A; Büchel, C; Frackowiak, RS; Goadsby, PJ. Hypothalamic activation in cluster headache attacks.*Lancet*. 1998 352, 275-578.

May, A; Goadsby, PJ. The trigeminovascular system in humans: pathophysiologic implications for primary headache syndromes of the neural influences on the cerebral circulation. *J Cereb Blood Flow Metab*, 1999a 19, 115-127.

May, A; Ashburner, J; Büchel, C; McGonigle, DJ; Friston, KJ; Frackowiak, RS; Goadsby, PJ. Correlation between structural and functional changes in brain in an idiopathic headache syndrome. *Nat Med*, 1999b 5, 836-838.

May, A; Bahra, A; Büchel, C; Turner, R; Goadsby, PJ. Functional magnetic resonance imaging in spontaneous attacks of SUNCT: short-lasting neuralgiform headache with conjunctival injection and tearing. *Ann Neurol*, 1999c 46, 791-794.

May, A; Bahra, A; Büchel, C; Frackowiak, RS; Goadsby, PJ. PET and MRA findings in cluster headache and MRA in experimental pain. *Neurology*, 2000 55, 1328-1335.

May, A; Goadsby, PJ. Substance P receptor antagonists in the therapy of migraine. *Expert Opin Investig Drugs*, 2001 10, 673-678.

May, A; Buchel, C; Turner, R; Goadsby, PJ. Magnetic resonance angiography in facial and other pain: neurovascular mechanisms of trigeminal sensation. *J Cereb Blood Flow Metab*, 2001 21, 1171-1176.

Mayberg, MR; Zervas, NT; Moskowitz, MA. Trigeminal projections to supratentorial pial and dural blood vessels in cats demonstrated by horseradish peroxidase histochemistry. *J Comp Neurol*, 1984 223, 46-56.

Mayer, DJ; Wolfle, TL; Akil, H; Carder, B; Liebeskind, JC. Analgesia from electrical stimulation in the brainstem of the rat. *Science*, 1971 174, 1351- 1354.

McBean, DE; Sharkey, J; Ritchie, IM; Kelly, PA. Evidence for a possible role for serotonergic systems in the control of cerebral blood flow. *Brain Res*, 1990 537, 307-310.

McCulloch, J; Uddman, R; Kingman, TA; Edvinsson, L. Calcitonin gene-related peptide: functional role in cerebrovascular regulation. *Proc Natl Acad Sci U S A,* 1986 83, 5731-5735.

Melzack, R; Wall, PD. Pain mechanisms: A new theory. *Science*, 1965 150, 971- 979.

Messlinger, K; Hanesch, U; Kurosawa, M; Pawlak, M; Schmidt, RF. Calcitonin gene related peptide released from dural nerve fibers mediates increase of meningeal blood flow in the rat. *Can J Physiol Pharmacol*, 1995 73, 1020-1024.

Messlinger, K; Suzuki, A; Pawlak, M; Zehnter, A; Schmidt, RF. Involvement of nitric oxide in the modulation of dural arterial blood flow in the rat. *Br J Pharmacol*, 2000 129, 1397-1404.

Millan, MJ. The induction of pain: an integrative review. *Prog Neurobiol*, 1999 57, 1-164.

Millan, MJ. Descending control of pain. *Prog Neurobiol*, 2002 66, 355-474.

Mitsikostas, DD; Sanchez del Rio, M; Waeber, C; Moskowitz, MA; Cutrer, FM. The NMDA receptor antagonist MK-801 reduces capsaicin-induced c-fos expression within rat trigeminal nucleus caudalis. *Pain*, 1998 76, 239-248.

Moskowitz, MA. The neurobiology of vascular head pain. *Ann Neurol*, 1984 16, 157-168.

Moskowitz, M A; Brezina, L R; Kuo, C. Dynorphin B-containing perivascular axons and sensory neurotransmitter mechanisms in brain blood vessels. *Cephalalgia*, 1986 6, 81-86.

Mosnaim, AD; Wolf, ME;; Chevesich, J; Callaghan, OH; Diamond, S. Plasma methionine enkephalin levels. A biological marker for migraine? *Headache*, 1985 25, 259-261.

Mosnaim, AD; Chevesich, J; Wolf, ME; Freitag, FG; Diamond, S. Plasma methionine enkephalin. Increased levels during a migraine episode. *Headache*, 1986 26, 278-281.

Motavkin, PA; Dovbish, TV. Histochemical characteristics of acetylcholinesterase of the nerves innervating the brain vessels. *Acta Morphol Acad Sci Hung*, 1971 19, 159-173.

Mraovitch, S; Kumada, M; Reis, DJ. Role of the nucleus parabrachialis in cardiovascular regulation in cat. *Brain Res*, 1982 232, 57-75.

Mtui, EP; Anwar, M; Gomez, R; Reis, DJ; Ruggiero, DA. Projections from the nucleus tractus solitarii to the spinal cord. *J Comp Neurol*, 1993 337, 231-252.

Murphy, AZ; Rizvi, TA; Ennis, M; Shipley, MT. The organization of preoptic-medullary circuits in the male rat: evidence for interconnectivity of neural structures involved in reproductive behavior, antinociception and cardiovascular regulation. *Neuroscience*, 1999 91, 1103-1116.

Nakamura, H; Yoshino, S. Opioid peptides in RA: modulation of immunologic mechanisms and mental states. *Arerugi*, 1990 39, 110-117.

Negri, M; Lomanto, D; Tonnarini, G; Bernardinis, G B; d'Alessandro, M; Mariani, P; Speranza, V. Plasma opioid levels during extracorporeal gallstone lithotripsy. *Am J Gastroentrol*, 1993 88, 1093-1096.

Nelson, E; Rennels, M. Innervation of intracranial arteries. *Brain*, 1970 93, 475-490

Nielsen, KC; Owman, C. Adrenergic innervation of pial arteries related to the circle of Willis in the cat. *Brain Res*, 1967 6, 773-776.

Nichols, FI; Mawad, M; Mohr, J; Stein, B; Hilal, S; Michelsen, J. Focal headache during balloon inflation in the internal carotid and middle cerebral arteries. *Stroke*, 1990 21, 555-559.

Noseda, R; Monconduit, L; Constandil, L; Chalus, M; Villanueva, L. Central nervous system networks involved in the processing of meningeal and cutaneous inputs from the ophthalmic branch of the trigeminal nerve in the rat. *Cephalalgia*, 2008 28, 813-824.

Nozaki, K; Boccalin, P; Moskowitz, M A. Expression of c-fos-like immunoreactivity in brain-stem after meningeal irritation by blood in the subarachnoid space. *Neuroscience*, 1992 49, 669-680.

Nyholt, DR; LaForge, KS; Kallela, M; Alakurtti, K; Anttila, V; Färkkilä, M; Hämaläinen, E; Kaprio, J; Kaunisto, MA; Heath, AC; Montgomery, GW; Göbel, H; Todt, U; Ferrari, MD; Launer, LJ; Frants, RR; Terwindt, GM; de Vries, B; Verschuren, WM; Brand, J; Freilinger, T; Pfaffenrath, V; Straube, A; Ballinger, DG; Zhan, Y; Daly, MJ; Cox, DR; Dichgans, M; van den Maagdenberg, AM; Kubisch, C; Martin, NG; Wessman, M; Peltonen, L; Palotie, A. A high-density association screen of 155 ion transport genes for involvement with common migraine.*Hum Mol Genet*, 2008 17, 3318-3331.

O'Connor, T.P; Van der Kooy, D. Enrichment of a vasoactive neuropeptide (calcitonin gene-related peptide) in the trigeminal sensory projection to the intracranial arteries. *J. Neurosci*, 1988 8, 2468- 2476.

Oku, R; Satoh, M; Fujii, N; Otaka, A; Yajima, H; Takagi, H. Caclitonin gene-related paptide promotes mechanical nociception by potentiating release of substance P from the spinal dorsal horn in rats. *Brain Res*, 1987 403, 350-354.

Olds, ME; Olds, J. Approach avoidance analysis of rat diencephalon. *J. Comp. Neurol*, 1963 120, 259- 295.

Olesen, J; Friberg, L; Olesen, T; Iversen, HK; Lassen, NA; Andersen, AR; Karle, A. Timing and topography of cerebral blood flow, aura, and headache during migraine attacks. *Ann Neurol*, 1990 28, 791-798.

Olesen, J; Thomsen, LL; Lassen, LH; Olesen, IJ. The nitric oxide hypothesis of migraine and other vascular headaches. *Cephalalgia*, 1995 15, 94-100.

Olesen, J; The role of nitric oxide (NO) in migraine, tension-type headache and cluster headache. *Pharmacol Ther*, 2008 120, 157-171.

Olsen, J. Headache Classification Subcommittee of the International Headache Society. The International Classification of Headache Disorders: 2nd edition. *Cephalalgia*, 2004 24 1, 9-160.

Olszewski, J. On the anatomical and functional organization of the trigeminal nucleus. *J. Comp. Neurol,* 1950 92, 401.

Ophoff, RA; Terwindt, GM; Vergouwe, MN; van Eijk, R; Oefner, PJ; Hoffman, SM; Lamerdin, JE; Mohrenweiser, HW; Bulman, DE; Ferrari, M; Haan, J; Lindhout, D; van Ommen, GJ; Hofker, MH; Ferrari, MD; Frants, RR. Familial hemiplegic migraine and episodic ataxia type-2 are caused by mutations in the Ca2+ channel gene CACNL1A4. *Cell*, 1996 87, 543- 552.

Ophoff, RA; Van den Maagdenberg, AM; Roon, KI; Ferrari, MD; Frants, RR. The impact of pharmacogenetics for migraine. *Eur J Pharmacol*, 2001 413, 1-10.

Ositelu, DO; Morris, R; Vaillant, C. Innervation of facial skin but not masticatory muscles or the tongue by trigeminal primary afferents containing somatostatin in the rat. *Neurosci Lett*, 1987 78, 271- 276.

Otsuka, M; Konishi, S. Release of substance P-like immunoreactivity from isolated spinal cord of new born rat. *Nature*, 1976 264, 83-84.

Owman, C; Edvinsson, L; Hardebo, JE. Pharmacological in vitro analysis of amine-mediated vasomotor functions in the intracranial and extracranial vascular beds. *Blood Vessels*, 1978 15, 128-147.

Pan, B; Castro-Lopes, JM; Coimbra, A. Central afferent pathways conveying nociceptive input to the hypothalamic paraventricular nucleus as revealed by a combination of retrograde labeling and c-fos activation. J Comp Neurol, 1999 413, 129-145.

Pardutz, A; Hoyk, Z; Varga, H; Vecsei, L; Schoenen, J. Oestrogen-modulated increase of calmodulin-dependent protein kinase II (CamKII) in rat spinal trigeminal nucleus after systemic nitroglycerin. *Cephalalgia*, 2007 27, 46-53.

Peroutka, SJ. Neurogenic inflammation and migraine: implications for the therapeutics. *Mol Interv*, 2005 5, 304-311.

Pfaller, K; Arvidsson, J. Central distribution of trigeminal and upper cervical primary afferents in the rat studied by anterograde transport of horseradish peroxidase conjugated to wheat germ agglutinin, *J. Comp. Neurol*, 1988 268, 91- 108.

Piercey, M F; Dobry, P J; Schroeder, L A; Einspahr, F J. Behavioural evidence that substance P may be a spinal cord sensory neurotransmitter. *Brain Res*, 1981 210, 407- 412.

Porreca, F; Burgess, SE; Gardell, LR; Vanderah, TW; Malan, TP Jr; Ossipov, MH; Lappi, DA; Lai, J. Inhibition of neuropathic pain by selective ablation of brainstem medullary cells expressing the mu-opioid receptor. *J Neurosci*, 2001 21, 5281-5288.

Portenoy, PK; Kanner RM. Definition and assessment of pain. In: Portenoy, R., Kanner, R. (Editors), *Pain Management: Theory and Practice*. Philadelphia: F.A. Davis; 1996 3-18.

Price, DD. Psychological and neural mechanisms of the affective dimension of pain. *Science*, 2000 288, 1769-1772.

Proietti Cecchini, A; Mea, E; Tullo, V; Peccarisi, C; Bussone, G; Leone, M. Long-term experience of neuromodulation in TACs. *Neurol Sci*, 2008 29 Suppl 1, S62-64.

Ramadan, NM. The link between glutamate and migraine. *CNS Spectr*, 2003 8, 446-449.

Rasmussen, BK; Olesen, J. Migraine with aura and migraine without aura: an epidemiological study. *Cephalalgia*, 1992 12, 221-228.

Randich, A; Gebhart, GF. Vagal afferent modulation of nociception. *Brain Res Brain Res Rev*, 1992 17, 77-99.

Randich, A; Mebane, H; DeBerry, JJ; Ness, TJ. Rostral ventral medulla modulation of the visceromotor reflex evoked by urinary bladder distension in female rats. *J Pain*, 2008 9, 920-926.

Reichling, D. B; Kwait, G. C; Basbaum, A. I. Anatomy and pharmachology of the periaqueductal gray contribution to antinociceptive controls, *Prog. Brain Res*, 1988 77, 31- 46.

Reichling, D; Basbaum, A. Contribution of brainstem GABAergic circuitry to descending antinociceptive controls I. GABA-immunoreactive projection neurons in the periaqueductal gray and nucleus raphe megnus. *J. Comp. Neurol*, 1990 302, 370- 377.

Reynolds, DV. Surgery in the rat during electrical analgesia induced by focal brain stimulation. *Science*, 1969 164, 444- 445.

Ruiz-Gayo, M; Gonzalez, MC; Fernandez-Alfonso, S. Vasodilatory effects of cholecystokinin: new role for an old peptide? *Regul Pept*, 2006 137, 179-184.

Rundek, T; Elkind, MS; Di Tullio, MR; Carrera, E; Jin, Z; Sacco, RL; Homma, S. Patent foramen ovale and migraine: a cross-sectional study from the Northern Manhattan Study (NOMAS). *Circulation*, 2008 118, 1419-1424.

Samsam, M; Knyihár-Csillik, E; Sáry, G; Vécsei, L. Effects of lesions of the Gasserian ganglion on the CGRP immunoreactivity of the caudal trigeminal nucleus. *Neurobiology*, 1996 4 169.

Samsam, M; Coveñas, R; Ahangari, R; Yajeya, J; Narvaéz, JA; Tramu, G. Alterations in neurokinin A, substance P and calcitonin gene-related peptide immunoreactivities in the caudal trigeminal nucleus of the rat following electrical stimulation of the trigeminal ganglion. *Neurosci Let*, 1999 261, 179-182.

Samsam, M; Coveñas, R; Ahangari, R; Yajeya, J; Narvaéz, JA; Tramu, G. Simultaneous depletion of neurokinin A, substance P and calcitonin gene-related peptide from the caudal trigeminal nucleus of the rat during electrical stimulation of the trigeminal ganglion. *Pain*, 2000 84, 389-395.

Samsam, M; Coveñas, R; Csillik, B; Ahangari, R; Yajeya, J; Riquelme, R; Narvaéz, JA; Tramu, G. Depletion of substance P, neurokinin A and calcitonin gene-related peptide from the contralateral and ipsilateral caudal trigeminal nucleus following unilateral electrical stimulation of the trigeminal ganglion: a possible neurophysiological and neuroanatomical link to generalized head pain. *J Chem Neuroanat*, 2001 21, 161-169.

Samsam, M; Coveñas, R; Ahangari, M; Yajeya, J; Narváez, JA; Montes, C; Gonzßález-Barón, S. Implication of the neuropeptides methionine enkephalin, neurotensin and somatostatin of the caudal trigeminal nucleus in the experimental migraine. *Rev Neurol*, 2002 34, 724-729.

Samsam, M; Coveñas, R; Ahangari, R; Yajeya, J; Narváez, JA. Role of neuropeptides in migraine; where do they stand in the latest expert recommendations in migraine treatment? *Drug Development Research*, 2007a, 68: 298- 314.

Samsam, M; Coveñas, R; Ahangari, R; Yajeya, J; Narváez, JA. Role of neuropeptides in migraine headaches, experimental and clinical data. In: Coveñas R, Mangas A, Narváez JA. (Editors), *Focus on Neuropeptide Research*. Trivandrum: Transworld Research Network; 2007b; 273- 298.

Sandor, P; Afra, J; Proietti Cecchini, A; Albert, A; Schoenen, J. From neurophysiology to genetics: cortical information processing in migraine underlies familial influences--a novel approach. *Funct Neurol*, 2005 3, 68-72.

Sano, K; Mayanagi, Y. Posteromedial hypothalamotomy in the treatment of violent, aggressive behaviour. *Acta Neurochir Suppl* (Wien), 1988 44, 145-151.

Sánchez-del-Rio, M; Reuter, U. Migraine aura: new information on underlying mechanisms. *Curr Opin Neurol*, 2004 17, 289-293.

Saria, A; Ma, RC; Dun, NJ. Neurokinin A depolarizes neurons of the guinea pig inferior mesentric ganglia. *Neurosci Lett*, 1985 60, 145-150.

Saria, A; Hauser, K F; Traurig, H H; Turbek, C S; Hersh, L; Gerard, C. Opioid-related changes in nociceptive threshold and in tissue levels of enkephalins after target disruption of the gene for neutral endopeptidase (EC 3.4.24.11) in mice. *Neurosci Lett*, 1997 234, 27-30.

Saxena, PR. Progress in 5-HT receptor classification. *Newsletter of the European Headache Federation (EHF)*, 1994 3, 1-8.

Schoenen, J; Lenaerts, M; Bastings, E. High-dose riboflavin as a prophylactic treatment of migraine: results of an open pilot study. *Cephalalgia*, 1994 14, 328-329.

Schmidt, M; Scheidhauer, K; Luyken, C; Voth, E; Hildebrandt, G; Klug, N; Schicha, H. Somatostatin receptor imaging in intracranial tumors. *Eur J Nucl Med*, 1998 25, 675-686.

Schwerzmann, M; Nedeltchev, K; Lagger, F; Mattle, HP; Windecker, S; Meier, B; Seiler, C. Prevalence and size of directly detected patent foramen ovale in migraine with aura. *Neurology*, 2005 65, 1415-1418.

Seybold, V S; Hylden, J L; Wilcox, G L. Intrathecal substance P and somatostatin in rats: behaviours indicative of sensation. *Peptides*, 198 23, 49-54.

Shiga, H; Yoshino, S; Nakamura, H; Koiwa, M. Role of opioid peptide in rheumatoid arthritis: detection of methionine-enkephalin and leucine-enkephalin in synovial tissue. *Arerugi*, 1993 42, 243-249.

Sicuteri, F; Geppetti, P; Marabini, S; Lembeck, F. Pain relief by somatostatin in attacks of cluster headache. *Pain*, 1984 18, 359-365.

Sicuteri, F; Renzi, D; Geppetti, P. Substance P and enkephalins: a creditable tandem in the pathophysiology of cluster headache and migraine. *Adv Exp Med Biol*, 1986 198, 145-152.

Silberstein, SD. Migraine pathophysiology and its clinical implications. *Cephalalgia*, 2004 2, 2-7.

Skirboll, L; Hökfelt, T; Dockray, G; Rehfeld, J; Brownstein, M; Cuello, AC. Evidence for periaqueductal cholecystokinin-substance P neurons projecting to the spinal cord. *J Neurosci*, 1983 3, 1151-1157.

Smetana, GW. The diagnostic value of historical features in primary headache syndromes: a comprehensive review. *Arch Intern Med*, 2000 160, 2729-2737.

Smith, DJ; Hawranko, AA; Monroe, P J; Gully, D; Urban, M O; Craig, CR; Smith, JP; Smith, D L. Dose dependent pain facilitatory and inhibitory actions of neurotensin are revealed by SR48692, a nonpeptide neurotensin antagonist: Influence on the antinociceptive effect of morphine. *Pharmacol Exp Ther*, 1997 282, 899-908.

Snell, RS. *Clinical Neuroanatomy*. 5th edition. Baltimore: Lippincott Williams & Wilkins; 2001.

Sprenger, T; Valet, M; Hammes, M; Erhard, P; Berthele, A; Conrad, B; Tolle, TR. Hypothalamic activation in trigeminal autonomic cephalgia: functional imaging of an atypical case. *Cephalalgia*, 2004 24, 753-757.

Spierings, ELH. Pathogenesis of the migraine attack. *Clin J Pain*, 2003 19, 255-262.

Spierings, ELH. The aura-headache connection in migraine: a historical analysis. *Arch Neurol*, 2004 61, 794-799.

Sprenger, T; Valet, M; Platzer, S; Pfaffenrath, V; Steude, U; Tolle, TR. SUNCT: bilateral hypothalamic activation during headache attacks and resolving of symptoms after trigeminal decompression. *Pain*, 2005 113, 422-426.

Stovner, LJ; Andrée, C. Eurolight Steering Committee. Impact of headache in Europe: a review for the Eurolight project. *J Headache Pain*, 2008 9, 139-146.

Strecker, T; Dux, M; Messlinger, K. Increase in meningeal blood flow by nitric oxide--interaction with calcitonin gene-related peptide receptor and prostaglandin synthesis inhibition. *Cephalalgia*, 2002 22, 233-241.

Storer, RJ; Akerman, S; Goadsby, PJ. Calcitonin gene-related peptide (CGRP) modulates nociceptive trigeminovascular transmission in the cat. *Br J Pharmacol*, 2004 142, 1171-1181.

Sun-Edelstein, C; Mauskop, A. Complementary and alternative approaches to the treatment of tension-type headache. *Curr Pain Headache Rep*, 2008 12, 447-450.

Szallasi, A; Nilsson, S; Farkas-Szallasi, T; Blumberg, PM; Hökfelt, T; Lundberg, JM. Vanilloid (capsaicin) receptors in the rat: distribution in the brain, regional differences in the spinal cord, axonal transport to the periphery, and depletion by systemic vanilloid treatment. *Brain Res*, 1995 703, 175-183.

Suzuki, N; Hardebo, JE; Owman, C. Origins and pathways of cerebrovascular vasoactive intestinal polypeptide-positive nerves in rat. *J Cereb Blood Flow Metab*, 1988 8, 697-712.

Suzuki, N; Hardebo, JE; Owman, C. Origins and pathways of cerebrovascular nerves storing substance P and calcitonin gene-related peptide in rat. *Neuroscience*, 1989 31, 427-438.

Suzuki, N; Hardebo, JE; Owman, C. Origins and pathways of choline acetyltransferase-positive parasympathetic nerve fibers to cerebral vessels in rat. *J Cereb Blood Flow Metab*, 1990 10, 399-408.

Suzuki, N; Yoshino, S; Nakamura, H. A study of opioid peptides in synovial fluid and synovial tissue in patients with rheumatoid arthritis. *Arerugi*, 1992 41, 615-620.

Tavares, I; Lima, D. Descending projections from the caudal medulla oblongata to the superficial or deep dorsal horn of the rat spinal cord.*Exp Brain Res*, 1994 99, 455-463.

Tavaras, I; Lima, D. From neuroanatomy to gene therapy: searching for new ways to manipulate the supraspinal endogenous pain modulatory system. *J Anat*, 2007 21, 261-268.

Tfelt-Hansen, P; Ashina, M; Olesen, J. Clinical symptoms and pathophysiology of migraine. *Ugeskr Laeger*. 2008 170, 3231-3234.

Thomsen, LL; Olesen, J. Nitric oxide in primary headaches. *Curr Opin Neurol*, 2001 14, 315-321.

Tsimikas, S. Transcatheter closure of patent foramen ovale for migraine prophylaxis: hope or hype? *J Am Coll Cardiol*, 2005 45, 496-498.

Uddman, R; Edvinsson, L. Neuropeptides in the cerebral circulation. *Cerebrovas Brain Metab Rev*, 1989 1, 230-252.

Uddman, R; Edvinsson, L; Ekman, R; Kingman, T; McCulloch, J. Innervation of the feline cerebral vasculature by nerve fibers containing calcitonin gene-related peptide: trigeminal origin and co-existence with substance P. *Neurosci Lett*, 1985 62, 131-136.

Uddman, R; Edvinsson, L; Jansen, I; Stiernholm, P; Jensen, K; Olesen, J; Sundler, F; Peptide-containing nerve fibers in human extracranial tissue: A morphological basis for neuropeptide involvement in extracranial pain? *Pain*, 1986 27, 391-399.

Uddman, R; Goadsby, PJ; Jansen, I; Edvinsson, L. PACAP, a VIP-like peptide: immunohistochemical localization and effect upon cat pial arteries and cerebral blood flow. *J Cereb Blood Flow Metab*, 1993 13, 291-297.

Uddman, R; Tajti, J; Möller, S; Sundler, F; Edvinsson, L. Neuronal messengers and peptide receptors in the human sphenopalatine and otic ganglia. *Brain Res*, 1999 826, 193-199.

Urban, MO; Coutinho, SV; Gebhart, GF. Biphasic modulation of visceral nociception by neurotensin in rat rostral ventromedial medulla. *J Pharmacol Exp Ther*, 1999a 290, 207-213.

Urban, MO; Coutinho, SV; Gebhart, GF. Involvement of excitatory amino acid receptors and nitric oxide in the rostral ventromedial medulla in modulating secondary hyperalgesia produced by mustard oil. *Pain*, 1999b 81, 45-55.

Urban, MO; Zahn, PK; Gebhart, GF. Descending facilitatory influences from the rostral medial medulla mediate secondary, but not primary hyperalgesia in the rat. *Neuroscience*, 1999c 90, 349-352.

Urban, MO; Gebhart, GF. Supraspinal contributions to hyperalgesia. *Proc Natl Acad Sci U S A*, 1999 96, 7687-7692.

van den Maagdenberg, AM; Pietrobon, D; Pizzorusso, T; Kaja, S; Broos, LA; Cesetti, T; van de Ven, RC; Tottene, A; van der Kaa, J; Plomp, JJ; Frants, RR; Ferrari, MD. A Cacna1a knockin migraine mouse model with increased susceptibility to cortical spreading depression. *Neuron*, 2004 41, 701-710.

Vanmolkot, KR; Kors, EE; Hottenga, JJ; Terwindt, GM; Haan, J; Hoefnagels, WA; Black ,DF; Sandkuijl, LA; Frants, RR; Ferrari, MD; van den Maagdenberg, AM. Novel mutations in the Na+, K+-ATPase pump gene ATP1A2 associated with familial hemiplegic migraine and benign familial infantile convulsions. *Ann Neurol*, 2003 54, 360-366.

Varga, H; Párdutz, A; Tajti, J; Vécsei, L Schoenen, J. The modulatory effect of estrogen on the caudal trigeminal nucleus of the rat in an animal model of migraine. *Ideggyogy Sz*, 2006 59, 389-395

Villalón, CM; Centurión, D; Valdivia, LF; de Vries, P; Saxena, PR. An introduction to migraine: from ancient treatment to functional pharmacology and antimigraine therapy. *Proc West Pharmacol Soc*, 2002 45, 199-210.

Wall, PD; Melzack, R. *Textbook of Pain*. 3rd edition. Edinburgh: Churchill Livingstone; 1994.

Wang, D; Wu, JH; Dong, YX; Li, YQ. Synaptic connections between trigemino-parabrachial projection neurons and gamma-aminobutyric acid- and glycine-immunoreactive terminals in the rat. *Brain Res,* 2001 921, 133-137.

Wang, SJ; Lirng, JF; Fuh, JL; Chen, JJ. Reduction in hypothalamic 1H-MRS metabolite ratios in patients with cluster headache. *J Neurol Neurosurg Psychiatry*, 2006 77, 622-625.

Watkins, LR; Wiertelak, EP; McGorry, M; Martinez, J; Schwartz, B; Sisk, D; Maier, SF. Neurocircuitry of conditioned inhibition of analgesia: effects of amygdala, dorsal raphe, ventral medullary, and spinal cord lesions on antianalgesia in the rat. *Behav Neurosci*, 1998 112, 360-378.

Wei, F; Ren, K; Dubner, R. Inflammation-induced Fos protein expression in the rat spinal cord is enhanced following dorsolateral or ventrolateral funiculus lesions. *Brain Res*, 1998 782, 136-141.

Wei, F; Dubner, R; Ren, K. Nucleus reticularis gigantocellularis and nucleus raphe magnus in the brain stem exert opposite effects on behavioral hyperalgesia and spinal Fos protein expression after peripheral inflammation. *Pain*, 1999 80, 127-141.

Weiller, C; May, A; Limmroth, V; Juptner, M; Kaube, H; Schayck, RV; Coenen, HH; Diener, HC. Brain stem activation in spontaneous human migraine attacks. *Nat Med*, 1995 1, 658-660.

Welch, KM; Cao, Y; Aurora, S; Wiggins, G;Vikingstad, EM. MRI of the occipital cortex, red nucleus, and substantia nigra during visual aura of migraine. *Neurology*, 1998 51, 1465-1469.

Welch, KM, Nagesh, V; Aurora, SK; Gelman, N. Periaqueductal gray matter dysfunction in migraine: cause or the burden of illness? *Headache*, 2001 41, 629-637.

Wessman, M; Kaunisto, MA; Kallela, M; Palotie, A. The molecular genetics of migraine. *Ann Med*, 2004 36, 462-473.

Wiertelak, EP; Roemer, B; Maier, SF; Watkins, LR. Comparison of the effects of nucleus tractus solitarius and ventral medial medulla lesions on illness-induced and subcutaneous formalin-induced hyperalgesias. *Brain Res*, 1997 748, 143-150.

Wiesenfeld-Halin, Z; Hökfelt, T; Lundberg, JM; Forssmann, WG; Reinecke, M; Tschopp, FA; Fischer, JA. Immunoreactive calcitonin gene-related peptide and substance P co-exist in sensory neurons to the spinal cord and interact in spinal behavioural responses of the rat. *Neurosci Lett*, 1984 52, 199-204.

Willis, WD; Westlund, KN. Neuroanatomy of the pain system and of the pathways that modulate pain. *J Clin Neurophysiol*, 1997 14, 2-31.

Wilmshurst, PT; Nightingale, S; Walsh, KP; Morrison, WL. Effect on migraine of closure of cardiac right-to-left shunts to prevent recurrence of decompression illness or stroke or for haemodynamic reasons. *Lancet*, 2000 356, 1648-1651.

Wilmshurst, P; Nightingale, S. Relationship between migraine and cardiac and pulmonary right-to-left shunts. *Clin Sci (Lond)*, 2001 100, 215-220.

Wolff, HG. *Headache mechanisms, a summary, Pain*. Research Publication Association of Research and Nervous and Mental Diseases, Vol. 23, Baltimore: William & Wilkins; 1943.

Woolf, C; Wiesenfeld-Hallin, Z. Substance P and calcitonin gene-related peptide synergistically modulate the gain of the nociceptive flexor withdrawal reflex in the rat. *Neurosci Let*, 1986 66, 226-230.

Workman, BJ; Lumb, BM. Inhibitory effects evoked from the anterior hypothalamus are selective for the nociceptive responses of dorsal horn neurons with high- and low-threshold inputs. *J Neurophysiol*, 1997 77, 2831-2835.

Workman, BJ; Lumb, BM. Inhibitory effects evoked from the anterior hypothalamus are selective for the nociceptive responses of dorsal horn neurons with high- and low-threshold inputs. *J Neurophysiol*, 1997 77, 2831-2835.

Yaksh, TL. Spinal systems and pain processing: development of novel analgesic drugs with mechanistically defined models. *Trends Pharmacol Sci* 1999 20, 329-337.

Yaksh, T; Young, C; Rudy, T. systematic examination of the rat brain sites sensitive to direct application of morphin: Observation of differential effects with the periaqueductal gray, *Brain Res*, 1976 114, 83- 103.

Yaksh, T L; Jessell, T M; Gamse, R; Mudge, A W; Leeman, S E. Intrathecal morphin inhibits substance P release from mammalian spinal cord in vivo. *Nature*, 1980 286, 155-157.

Yaksh, TL; Elde, R. Factors governing release of methionine enkephalin-like immune-reactivity from mesencephalin and spinal cord of the cat in vivo. *J. Neurophysiol*, 1981 46, 1056-1075.

Yaksh, T L; Michener, S R; Bailey, J E; Harty, G J; Lucas, D L; Nelson, D K; Roddy, D R; Go, V L. Survey of distribution of substance P, vasoactive intestinal peptide, cholecystokinin, neurotensin, Met-enkephalin, bombesin and PHI in the spinal cord of the cat, dog, sloth and monkey. *Peptides*, 1988 9, 357-372.

Yoshida, A; Chen, K; Moritani, M; Yabuta, NH; Nagase, Y; Takemura, M; Shigenaga, Y. Organization of the descending projections from the parabrachial nucleus to the trigeminal sensory nuclear complex and spinal dorsal horn in the rat. *J Comp Neurol*, 1997 383, 94-111.

Zagami, AS; Goadsby, PJ; Edvinsson, L. Stimulation of the superior sagittal sinus in the cat causes release of vasoactive peptides. *Neuropeptides*, 1990 16, 69-75.

Zhang, RX; Mi, Z P; Qiao, JT. Changes of spinal substance P, calcitonin gene-related peptide, somatostatin, Met-enkephalin and neurotensin in rats in response to formalin-induced pain. *Regul Pept*, 1994 51, 25-32.

Zhang, Z; Winborn, CS; Marquez de Prado, B; Russo, AF. Sensitization of calcitonin gene-related peptide receptors by receptor activity-modifying protein-1 in the trigeminal ganglion. *J Neurosci*, 2007 27, 2693-2703.

Zhao, C; Tao, Z; Xiao, S; Zhao, S; Qiao, J. Histochemical and immunohistochemical studies of distribution of acetylcholinesterase-positive fibers and peptidergic terminals in the nasal mucosa of rats. *Chin Med J (Engl)*, 1998 111, 644-647.

Zhuo, M; Gebhart, GF. Biphasic modulation of spinal nociceptive transmission from the medullary raphe nuclei in the rat. *J Neurophysiol*, 1997 78, 746-758.

In: Neuroanatomy Research Advances
Editors: C. E. Flynn and B. R. Callaghan, pp.59-91

ISBN: 978-60741-610-4
©2010 Nova Science Publishers, Inc.

Chapter II

Architectonic Studies: Past, Present and Future

Peiyan Wong and Jon H. Kaas

Department of Psychology, Vanderbilt University, Nashville, Tennessee, USA

Abstract

The mammalian neocortex has a basic six-layered structure. Modifications to this fundamental design have lead to a diversity of structural and functional areas amongst mammals. Functional borders of certain cortical areas have shown good correspondence to anatomical borders identified by histological methods, the primary visual cortex of squirrels as an example (Kaas et al., 1972). This suggests a link between structure and function, an 'organology' of cortical areas where certain functions are localized in certain areas (Creutzfeldt, 1995). Perhaps through studying the fine anatomy of the neocortex, different functional areas can be identified by their differing fine anatomical structure. Architectonic studies attempt to better understand cortical morphology and parcellate the cortical sheet into distinct areas (Van Essen, 2004). This involves the use of staining methods to visualize various structural features. While architectonic studies came about as early as the 18th century, progress in this field has been hampered by technological limitations. In the past century, architectonic studies have acquired several tools that lead to great progress in the parcellation of the neocortex. This includes the availability of better microscopes, and staining methods that use antibodies with increased specificity and ligands that are able to show the distribution of their respective receptors. In the recent years, architectonic studies have taken on a more quantified, observer-independent approach to reduce variations from individual samples and subjectivity of different researchers. With improved functional imaging methods, there is a need for architectonic studies to come up with reliable spatial cortical maps that can be applied to functional imaging results. This will require the use of multiple approaches, observer-dependent and independent methods, and a battery of staining methods, including the histological, immunohistochemical and receptor-binding methods. In addition, continued efforts to develop better statistical methods for observer-independent methods, software to create spatial maps of the neocortical areas, and more sensitive, area-specific staining methods are necessary.

1. Introduction

Architectonic studies are aimed at parcellating the neocortex through understanding and characterizing the morphology of various cortical areas. Since the discovery of the first anatomical feature that adheres to a discrete location in the neocortex, the white stripe that is now known as the Stria of Gennari (Finger, 1994), there have been many published maps of the human cortex (Zilles et al., 2002). One of the more influential cortical maps is the map by Brodmann (1909), which is still frequently referenced. Brodmann subdivided the human neocortex into areas based on variations in the cytoarchitecture of the cortical sheet. Each defined cortical area had a characteristic histological appearance and was thought to have a specific function to perform (Matelli and Luppino, 2004). Brodmann (1909) viewed these cortical areas as the 'organs' of the neocortex (Creutzfeldt, 1995), working in harmony to ensure the proper functioning of the neocortex. Now, it is widely accepted that the neocortex can be subdivided into distinct functional and anatomical areas (Yamamori, 2006). However, other than the calcarine cortex, which is easily identified in an unstained tissue section due to the presence of the white bands of myelin that form the Stria of Gennari and inner band of Baillarger, most other cortical areas require staining processes before they can be visualized. As a result, progress in our understanding of cortical organization is determined by progress in staining methods, and other technological methods (Cavada, 2004). Currently, our understanding of cortical organization is still rather crude, fraught with ambiguous borders drawn by different investigators (Kaas, 2005). It is essential to come up with improved processing methods that when added to our current repertoire of histological methods, will establish reliable spatial maps upon which functional studies can be based.

A general anatomical and functional design, a *Bauplan*, of the cerebral cortex is common to all neocortical areas (Creutzfeldt, 1995). This principle was derived from classical research done by Brodmann and von Economo on an extensive range of mammalian species, showing that the entire neocortex has an almost identical structure during embryonic life (Brodmann, 1909; Creutzfeldt, 1995). However, embryonic neuroprogenitor cells are not equipotential and they do possess some intrinsic information about their species-specific cortical organization (Rakic, 1988). As such, the basic pattern of cytoarchitectonic areas arises from a combination of intrinsic signals from the cortical neurons and extrinsic signals from inputs by subcortical structures (Rakic, 1988). Modifications to this *Bauplan* in subsequent development have led to the diversity in the structure of the neocortex in mammalian species, which resulted in variations in behavior and cognitive abilities. Identifying and characterizing the various cortical areas in mammalian species would help shed light on the evolutionary processes that have taken place to give rise to the complex neocortex of humans. However, before proceeding to a discussion of various architectonics techniques used in studying the fine structure of neocortex, it is foremost useful to outline the basic features of the neocortex, and consider how variations in the neocortex develop.

1.1 Structural Organization of the Neocortex

If one takes a sample of neocortex from any region of any mammal, be it the small sub-terrainian naked mole rat or human, the same basic 6-layered cortical structure is obtained. Each layer is made up of neurons that have distinct morphologies, connections and functions. The input and output organization between cortex and subcortical structures, and the pyramidal cells orthogonally oriented with respect to cortical layers, are aspects of neocortex that are common across the neocortical sheet and all mammals (Schüz, 2002). The activating input to a cortical area goes mainly into layer 4 of the neocortex, a layer that is populated by granular cells with radial dendrites (Fig. 1). Neurons in layer 4 are highly interconnected to the immediately adjoining layers with short-range connections. In layer 5, pyramidal cells make up the bulk of the neuron population. These pyramidal cells gather information horizontally through their short basilar dendrites and locally across the layers through their long ascending apical dendrite. The neurons then combine the information to provide the major output of the neocortex, mainly to the subcortical areas. Pyramidal cells are also present in layer 3 of the neocortex, the other output layer, but are smaller in size than the ones in layer 5. These cells have shorter apical dendrites and do not make connections with other subcortical structures. Weak, long distance horizontal outputs of pyramidal cells in layer 3 form connections with other columns of neurons and provide a network for cross-talk between regions of the neocortex. Layer 6 is the main feedback layer. Neurons in layer 6 receive information from the upper layers, especially from layer 4, and feedback to neurons where the activating input had originated. Layer 2 is a thin layer that consists of densely packed small neurons that help modify local processing. Layer 1 is mainly a fibrous layer with few neurons. This layer receives input from the brain stem neurons and feedback connections from other cortical areas (Kaas, 2002).

The inputs to the brain undergo segregation or integration by excitatory or inhibitory intracortical connections (Creutzfeldt, 1995). Interactions between the excitatory and inhibitory neurons play a large role in determining the output of the neocortical circuitry (Kaas, 2002). First, these two groups of neurons work to limit the duration of cortical response to an input. An initial excitatory input that activates a neuron in layer 4 is dampened by the inhibition that follows. This allows the neocortex to respond to temporal changes in the surroundings, a property that is important for the survival and adaptation of an animal (Kaas, 2002). Second, excitatory and inhibitory circuits are distributed in a manner that allows them to compare and contrast neighboring inputs. Spatially, inhibitory synapses are distributed locally in a horizontal manner onto neighboring neurons, such that adjacent groups of neurons would inhibit each other if they were activated by the same input. Lateral inhibition would be reduced, however, if the adjacent groups of neurons were responding to different inputs and thus not activated at the same time point. Global features are obtained from repetitive serial computations of temporal and spatial information of local features detected by these neural circuits, leading to the display of more complex behaviors (Kaas, 2002).

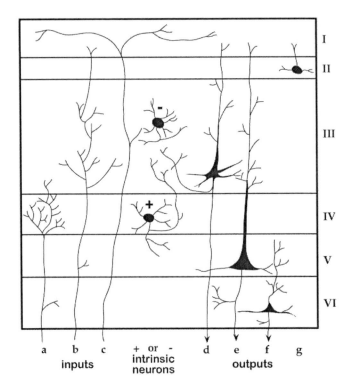

Figure 1. (a) Layer 4 receives most of the input from the thalamus or other cortical areas and the neurons in layer 4 are highly interconnected with adjacent layers. (d) Pyramidal cells in layer 3 form local horizontal connections, forming a network for cross-talk. (e) Layer 5 has large pyramidal cells that project mainly to subcortical structures and is the major output layer. (f) Layer 6 is the main feedback layer and neurons in layer 6 provide feedback to cells where the activating input originates. (g) Layer 2 consists of small neurons involved in local processing. Modified from, Kaas, 2002.

1.2 Variability in the Neocortex

In spite of the common aspects that are present in the neocortices of various species, there is great variability between the cortices of different mammals. An obvious difference between the neocortex of the rat and that of the human is the size of the cortical sheet (Kaas, 2002). However, the size of the neocortical sheet alone does not account for the large diversity in abilities and behaviors of mammals. Brodmann (1909) recognized that primates have a large number of cortical areas, and different mammalian species share some cortical areas, but differ in others.

Close to a century after Brodmann, several common cortical areas have been identified in nearly all mammals examined (Fig. 2) (Krubitzer, 1995; Krubitzer and Kahn, 2003). Such areas include the primary somatosensory area (S1) (Kaas, 1983; Johnson, 1990), the primary visual area (V1) (Inouye, 1909, as cited in Leff, 2003; Sholl, 1955; Rosa and Krubitzer, 1999) and the primary auditory area (A1) (Evans et al., 1965; Ehret, 1997). With evolutionary pressure, environmental factors and functional usage, diversification of cortical phenotypes occurs. However, the three cortical fields mentioned above remain present in mammals, regardless of the morphological or behavioral specializations of the animal (Krubitzer 1995;

Catania, 2000; Henry et al., 2005). Even the lack of apparent usage of a particular sensory system does not eliminate its cortical area. For instance, the presence of a reduced V1 can be architectonically defined even in the blind mole rat (Heil et al., 1991; see Cooper et al., 1993; Bronchti et al., 2002 for more examples). With regards to the diversification of cortical phenotypes, a cortical area may expand, as with the striate and extrastriate cortex of the visually oriented squirrel being respectively four and eight times larger than in rats (Paolini and Sereno, 1998), or reduce in size, as with the barrel field of squirrels being one-third the size of that in rats (Paolini and Sereno, 1998). Formation of new cortical areas can occur as well. These areas may be involved in the integration of sensory information and higher-order processing, including the middle temporal visual (MT) area that appears to be new with primates (Kaas 2005). Neurons in this area seem to be specialized for processing information on visual motion (Maunsell and Van Essen, 1983).

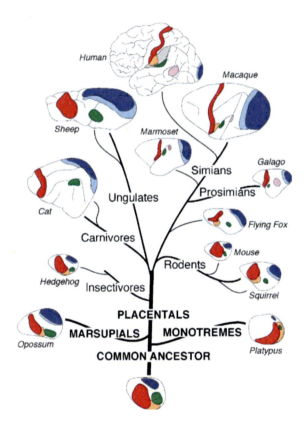

Figure 2. An evolutionary tree showing the phylogenetic relationship of major orders of mammals and the cortical organization of common cortical areas that have been identified. All the species shown here possess common cortical regions such as the primary somatosensory area (S1)(red), second somatosensory area (S2)(orange), primary auditory area (A1)(green), primary visual area (V1)(dark blue) and second visual area (V2)(light blue). Some areas such as the middle temporal area (MT)(pink) have only been observed in primates and may have evolved from an ancestor from the primate branch. Rostral is left, medial is up. Reproduced from Fig. 1, Krubitzer and Kahn, 2003.

The diversity of neocortical areas arises from local transformations in the neocortical sheet. These changes occur within defined boundaries, allowing the delimitation of anatomically distinct cortical areas. These local transformations may involve changes to the laminar structure of the neocortex through two principle processes. The first process is the retraction or disappearance of layers, such as the disappearance of layer 4 that gives rise to the agranular cortex. An example of a decrement of the basic layers would be the agranular motor cortex. The motor cortex is not a primary sensory cortex and lacks the koniocellular appearance of a primary sensory cortex that developed because their primary input is from thalamic projections to layer 4. In contrast, thalamocortical projections to motor cortex are comparatively weaker and are mainly from other sensory areas. This feature allows the delimitation of the motor cortex from adjacent areas, not only in humans but in many other mammals as well (Sherwood et al., 2003). The second process is the sublamination of cortical layers, a way in which the neocortex adds flexibility to its function (Kaas, 2002). In humans, or species that are highly dependent on the visual system, the visual cortex is distinctively laminated and layer 4 is split into sublayers (Brodmann, 1909). Neurons performing the same function are grouped into a sublayer and specialized neurons may develop in a sublayer to carry out particular functions (Kaas 2002). Conversely, for animals with poor vision, such as the rat, the layers in visual cortex are poorly differentiated and the neurons are not morphologically specialized as they need only retain general functions (Kaas, 2002).

Due to the metabolic costs of having more cortical layers, there is a trade-off between the number of cortical layers or sub-layers present and the amount of specialization required. Frequently, the two opposite processes take place in parallel, where some primitive layers may have undergone further differentiation to give rise to sublayers, while other primitive layers may have regressed and fused with each other. The human visual cortex provides a good example of this phenomenon (Fig. 3) (Brodmann, 1909).

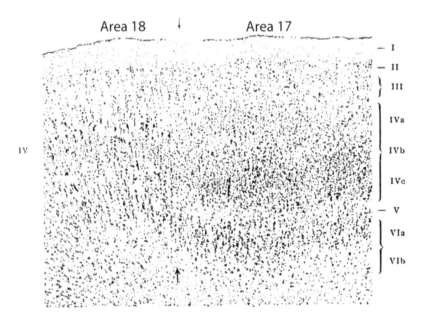

Figure 3. Part of the occipital cortex from an adult human. The border between area 17 and area 18 is shown by the decrease in thickness of layer 4 in area 18. The 6-layered scheme by Brodmann is shown on the left. Scale: 25:1, 10μm. Reproduced from Fig. 12, Brodmann, 1909.

Brodmann had observed that the primitive granular layer 4 splits into three sublayers; two dark cell-dense layers, layer 4A and 4C, and a light cell-poor stripe, layer 4B, also known as the stria of Gennari (1909). While the primitive layer 6 differentiates into two sublayers, 6A and 6B (Brodmann, 1909). A regression of lamination is observed in the supragranular layers, where layer 2 is almost fused with layer 3 (Brodmann, 1909). It should be noted that there is a different nomenclature for sublayers of V1 by Hassler (1966) (Fig. 4).

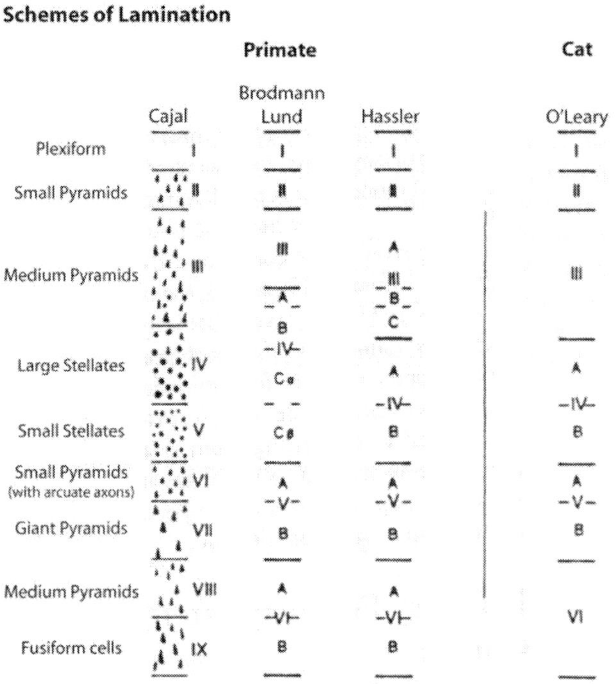

Schemes of Lamination

Figure 4. The relationship between Brodmann's and Hassler's schemes of lamination. Brodmann's scheme shows more similarity with Cajal's 9-layered cortex, while Hassler's scheme allows for comparison across species without having forming composite sub-layers in mammals such as cats. Reproduced from Fig. 9.1, Henry, 1991.

Hassler's scheme regarded Brodmann's layer 4A and 4B to be part of layer 3 and as a result changed layer 4Ca and 4Cb to layer 4A and 4B (Henry, 1991). There are three main pieces of evidence that support Hassler's nomenclature. Firstly, comparing the lamination patterns of V1 across primates, Hassler (1967, as cited in Casagrande and Kaas, 1994) showed that in most New World monkeys, layer 4A and 4B of Brodmann correspond to the less developed sublayers of layer 3, and in prosimians, such as galagos, Brodmann's layer 4A and 4B are nearly indistinguishable as sublayers of layer 3. Secondly, Hassler's scheme provides a simpler explanation for the connections of the layers, where layer 3C neurons of primates and layer 3 neurons in nonprimates both project to extrastriate cortex. However, in Brodmann's scheme, the source of projections to extrastriate cortex in primates would differ from prosimians. In primates, layer 4 cells are the source of projections to the extrastriate cortex in primates, and in prosimians, layer 3 cells are the source of projections (Casagrande and Kaas, 1994). Thirdly, if one were to follow Brodmann's scheme, then layer 4B of monkeys would consist of large pyramidal cells (e.g. Lund et al., 1979), but large pyramidal cells are not a typical feature of layer 4 (Casagrande and Kaas, 1994). In addition, the pyramidal cell layer of V1 is observed to merge with pyramidal cell layer 3C of area 18 (Colonnier and Sas, 1978, as cited in Casagrande and Kaas, 1994). Hassler's scheme allows for more direct comparison between primates and carnivores because it avoids the creation of composite sublayer 4AB for the cat that would be required by Brodmann's scheme (Henry, 1991). With Hassler's scheme, the granular cells of sublayer 4A and 4B are similar across a range of species (Henry, 1991).

Variability within the cortex can come about even when the number of cortical layers remains the same. Changes can take the form of differences in the total thickness of the cortex or differences in the relative thickness of different cortical layers. The variation in total thickness of the cortex allows for parcellation of different cortical areas. For example, the posterior temporal area (Tp) of the grey squirrel is unusually thick compared to the surrounding cortical areas (Fig. 5).

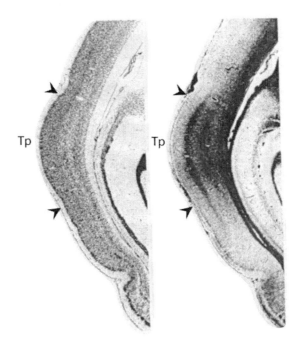

Figure 5. Coronal sections of the grey squirrel processed for Nissl substance (left) and myelin (right). Area temporal posterior (Tp) is shown here. Tp is an example of unusually thick cortex compared to the adjacent area. The myelin section shows well-defined inner and outer bands of Baillarger. Reproduced from Fig. 6. Kaas et al., 1972.

The variability in the thickness of the cortex, or the relative thickness of different cortical layers may be related to experiential and environmental factors. This contributes to individual variability within a species. Rats trained to run mazes of ascending difficulty have been shown to possess thicker cerebral cortices than rats that did not receive training (Diamond, 2001). Arnold Scheibel (1990) has suggested that changes in relative thickness of different cortical layers may occur in the human brain. He noticed that layer 4 of the primary auditory cortical area in the brain of a distinguished violinist was twice as thick as that of normal individuals. Another brain that he examined had an atypically thick layer 4 in the primary visual cortex. This brain belonged to a prominent artist who had a remarkable capacity of intense eidetic imagery (Scheibel, 1990).

Cortical areas also show variation in the density and size of cellular elements. Areas with the primary function of receiving inputs usually possess a thicker layer 4 that is predominantly densely packed with small stellate cells and are thus koniocellular in appearance (Creutzfeldt, 1995). Such areas include the primary sensory areas for visual, auditory and somatosensory inputs (Creutzfeldt, 1995). For areas where the primary function involves output, such as the motor cortex controlling body movements, layer 4 is thinner and less densely packed with neurons, while layer 5 is thicker and packed with large pyramidal cells, such as the Betz cells (Creutzfeldt, 1995).

A final contributor to the variability and specialization of the neocortex is modular organization. The modules are formed from groups of neurons that are carrying out similar functions and located in the same area (Kaas, 2002). These modules form the basis of parallel processing. Information spread through the layers is restricted within the module. This organization allows information sent to the neocortex to be processed simultaneously but separately (Kaas, 2002). Cortical modules help to reduce the length of connections between neurons and allow the different modules to specialize separately according to the needs of the species (Kaas, 1997). This concept of the cortical module was introduced by Vernon Mountcastle, a neurophysiologist who worked on recordings from the somatosensory cortex and noticed that neurons with similar response properties were grouped into regions less than one mm in width across the thickness of cortex (Mountcastle et al., 1955). Similar observations in the primary visual cortex of cats and monkeys showed that inputs from each eye were found to be separated into alternating bands in layer 4. These bands were termed as **"ocular dominance" columns by Hubel and Wiesel in 1977. In 1970, Woolsey and Van der** Loos observed modular organization in layer 4 of rat primary somatosensory cortex. This **modular organization, known as the "barrel field" arose from the segregation** of thalamic inputs from cortical inputs, with the thalamocortical afferents found mainly in the barrels (Agmon et al., 1993; Senft and Woolsey, 1991) and the corticocortical connections terminating around the barrels, forming the septa (Koralek et al., 1990; Miller et al., 2001). Each barrel in layer 4 represents individual mysterical vibrissae on the contralateral face (Simons et al., 1984; Strominger and Woolsey, 1987) and has been described in other rodents such as mice and squirrels (Woolsey et al., 1975; Wong and Kaas, 2008).

In summary, the mammalian neocortex is organized in a vertical and horizontal manner, and the layers and vertical modules of neocortex are essential for neural function. This dual organization increases the computational capacity of the neocortex (Grossberg, 1999), and forms the structural basis for the separation and integration of inputs and outputs, and serial and parallel processing. Due to different evolutionary demands, environments, genetic mutations and experience, diversification and variability of the neocortex arose across species. The size and thickness of neocortex, as well as the thickness of each layer, varies between species and cortical areas. Different cortical areas possess different cellular characteristics, such as density, size and type of neurons. The differences in cytoarchitecture between two given cortical areas may be due to different input-output connections, varying intrinsic connectivity, or both (Matelli and Luppino, 2004). While specializations of cortical areas take place within set boundaries, as Brodmann had pointed out, transitions between areas may be sharp and distinct, an example being the transition from area 17 to 18 (Fig. 6), or may be subtler and take place gradually (1909). These local differences between cortical areas set the criteria for studies involving the parcellation of the neocortex.

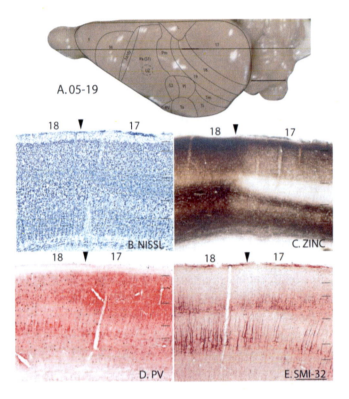

Figure 6. Architectonic subdivisions of the visual cortex in the squirrel brain. A. Subdivision indicated on a dorsal view of the left caudal hemisphere. A horizontal line indicates the approximate location of sagittal brain section shown in B to E. The thick portion of the line corresponds to the portions of the sections that are illustrated. Lines on the sections show the six cell layers in each preparation. Area 17 and 18 are illustrated here. The 17/18 border is sharp and shows correspondence in the four staining methods used here. Scale bar for brain = 5mm, for sections = 0.5mm. Modified from Fig. 4, Wong and Kaas, 2008. Abbreviations used here: 3a/dy, Dysgranular region; F, Frontal area; L, Limbic area; M1, Primary motor cortex; Pa(S1), Parietal anterior area; Pl, Parietal lateral area; Pm, Parietal medial area; Pv, Parietal ventral area; S2, Secondary somatosensory cortex; Ta, Temporal anterior area; Ti, Temporal intermediate area; Tm, Temporal mediodorsal area; Tp, Temporal posterior area; UZ, Unresponsive zone; Areas 17 and 18 are adopted from Brodmann, 1909.

2. Architectonic Studies

Architectonic studies involve the attempt to study the fine anatomy of the cortex by using histological methods to distinguish different cortical areas. Histological stains reveal areal-based variations from the basic cortical architecture, resulting in cortical parcellation. In **1876, Meynert had used the term 'organology' of cortical areas, suggesting a link between** structure and function, that certain functions are localized in certain areas (Creutzfeldt, 1995).

This idea of cortical localization of function probably came about from studies that did not involve actual brain tissue, but instead involved studying bumps and indentations of the skull, or phrenology, an idea put forth by Franz Joseph Gall (Gall and Spurzheim, 1810, as cited in Finger, 1995). Paul Pierre Broca (1824-80) in 1865, Gustav Theodor Fritsch (1838-1927) and Eduard Hitzig (1838-1907) in 1870, and Carl Wernike (1848-1905) in 1874 helped set the stage to show that functions were localized to specific areas in the neocortex (as cited in Finger, 1994). Broca's localization of a centre that controlled the motor expression of speech was probably the first localization of a function in the neocortex that was widely accepted. Fritsch and Hitzig, stimulating small exposed regions of the brain surfaces in awake dogs with small electrical currents, found that stimulation of distinct brain areas elicited different movements from the dogs, providing evidence that different functions may be located in small, localized regions in the neocortex. Wernicke showed that damage to the posterior regions of the left superior temporal lobe led to impairments in speech comprehension (Finger, 1994). Since there is a link between structure and function, using architectonic studies to elucidate the morphology of different cortical areas would provide an anatomical framework for investigating the functional organization of the neocortex.

However, the progress of architectonic studies is highly dependent on methodological developments. As such, it is perhaps essential to first review the problems that architectonic studies faced, the early methods used and their influence on architectonic studies. Followed by the methods that are currently used in architectonic studies, their usefulness and limitations. Speculation about the future of architectonic studies would be attempted, with regards to methodological advancements that may be made, approaches that may be adopted in architectonic studies and how these will contribute to furthering our understanding of the structure and function link of the neocortex.

2.1 Early Architectonic Studies

Near the end of the 18th century, in a laboratory in Parma, Italy, Francesco Gennari, a young medical student, noticed a broad white line running through the calcarine cortex of unfixed, unstained human brain tissue. This broad, white band remained unnamed until a century later in 1888, when Heinrich Obersteiner (1847-1922) named this band the 'Stria of Gennari' in honor of its first observer (as cited in McHenry, 1969, 1983). Gennari's observation established that the cerebral cortex is not uniform in structure and it probably marks the beginning of the field of architectonic studies.

In the early beginnings, progress in architectonic studies was slow, hampered by the lack of proper fixation methods, staining techniques and a microscope with adequate detail resolution (Brazier, 1978). Before Reil used alcohol as a fixative in 1809, the weaker spirits available were largely ineffective. It was not until just before the 20th century that formaldehyde, a fixative still used today, was introduced (Brazier, 1978). Fortunately, the lack of good staining techniques did not prevent findings that formed the foundations of architectonics. In 1840, Jules-Gabriel-François Baillarger (1806-1891, as cited in Brazier, 1978), was studying fine anatomy of the cortex by pressing unfixed, thin slices of brain tissue between two glass plates and holding them up to the light, making observations about the cortex with the naked eye. He noticed a fainter white line running throughout the entire cerebral cortex that was continuous with the more distinct stripe of Gennari (Baillarger, 1840, as cited in Brazier, 1978), and these two white bands are now known as the inner and outer bands of Baillarger. Baillarger also showed that the cortex was made of six layers of cells. This claim was supported in similar findings by Remak (1844, as cited in Brazier, 1978) working, with a magnifying glass, in the posterior lobe of sheep.

Before the 1870s, the available staining methods included carmine dye (Gerlach, 1858, as cited in Brazier, 1978), a bright red dye that revealed cell nuclei. Rudolf Berlin (1858, as cited in Brazier, 1978) used the carmine dye and, like Baillarger, he recognized and numbered the six layers of the neocortex. Additionally, Berlin came up with the terms pyramidal, spindle and granule cell to describe the cellular elements observed (1858, as cited in Brazier, 1978). Amongst the staining methods used in the 1870s, the Golgi stain was probably the most famous. It involved the use of potassium dichromate, followed by silver nitrate and showed the pyramidal cell body and dendrites in beautiful detail (Golgi, 1873, as cited in Brazier, 1978). All the staining methods mentioned so far involved the visualization of the neuron cell bodies, allowing observations concerning the different distribution densities, sizes and types of cell bodies to be made. These criteria allow the cytoarchitectonic distinction between cortical areas to be determined. In 1882, Weigert introduced a stain for myelin sheathes (1882; 1890, as cited in Brazier, 1978), thus introducing a new criteria for parcellation of the neocortex through myeloarchitectonics.

The Nissl method of staining nervous tissue was introduced in 1894 by Franz Nissl and is still widely used as the standard cytoarchitectonic histological stain today. Basic aniline dyes were used on unembedded tissue fixed in 96% alcohol to visualize the Nissl bodies (Nissl, 1894, as cited in Brazier, 1978). Nissl bodies are basophilic granules, mainly made up of ribose nucleic acids and nucleic proteins involved in protein synthesis and metabolism, that are present only in the cell bodies and dendrites. The Nissl stain thus reveals all the cell bodies present in the tissue specimen.

The last problem of access to an adequately functional microscopy was not addressed till the beginning of the 19th century. Until then, neuroanatomists made their observations with the naked eye, with magnifying glasses, or existing microscopes that had poor magnification powers, chromatic effects and spherical aberrations that distorted the images of the cortex (Brazier, 1978). This problem was solved in a breakthrough made by Joseph Jackson Lister in 1827. He designed the first achromatic microscope that had an additional correction for spherical aberration (Brazier, 1978). With Lister's invention, the neuronal cell bodies could be studied in greater detail.

In spite of the technological advances made in the 18th and 19th centuries, there were still many disputes regarding the actual number of layers in the neocortex. Baillarger (1840) and Meynert (1872) had both proposed a six-layered cortex, but this was disagreed upon by Lewis and Clarke (1878, as cited in Brazier, 1978). The latter pair proposed a five-layered cortex, numbering the large pyramidal cells of the motor cortex as the fourth layer instead of the fifth as Meynert had done (Brazier, 1978) (Fig. 8). Much of the controversies surrounding the cortical layers stems from the fact that the neuroanatomists were examining sections from different areas of the brain. Meynert had recognized this and went on to examine brain sections from areas other than those involved in motor functions (Brazier, 1978). Examining more regions of the cortex than his contemporaries, Meynert went on to propose a six-layered precentral cortex and an eight-layered occipital cortex (Brazier, 1978) (Fig. 7A and 7B).

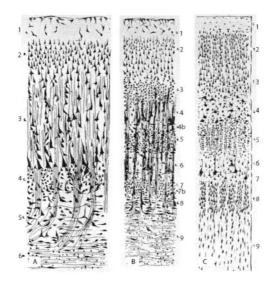

Figure 7. Different schemes of cortical lamination. A and B are Meynert's interpretation of the laminar pattern in the six-layered precentral cortex and eight-layered occipital cortex respectively (From *Psychiatrie*, Braümuller 1884). C is the nine-layered calcarine cortex from Cajal. (From *Histologie du Systeme Nerveux, Vol. 2*, 1911). Reproduced from Brazier, 1978.

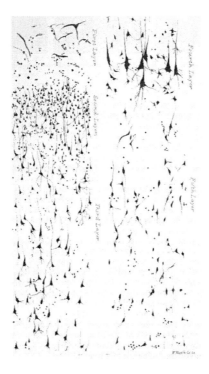

Figure 8. The 5-layered lamination scheme of the frontal cortex by Lewis and Clarke (From *Proc. Roy. Soc.*, 27:38-49, 1878).

2.2 Architectonic Studies of the Early 20th Century

In 1905, Campbell presented the first complete cytoarchitectonic map of the human cerebral cortex, and Brodmann's architectonic map of the human cerebral cortex followed in 1908. Other notable atlases of the human cerebral cortex published in the early 20th century were those done by Elliot Smith in 1907, and Economo and Koskinas in 1925. Vogt and Vogt (1919, as cited in Fleischhauer, 1978) had carried out myeloarchitectonic studies in several mammals. Amongst all the neuroanatomists of the 20th century, it is probably Brodmann who had the greatest and longest lasting impact on the field of architectonic studies. As new techniques of studying the cortex emerged, such as neuroimaging, the maps done by Brodmann and terminology that he had used to describe the cortical areas (1908, 1909) became the basis of description for subsequent cortical studies (Petrides, 2005). This was probably because Brodmann considered all the regions of the cortex and his comparative studies included many mammalian species (Kaas, 2005). In the mid-20th century, Bailey and Bonin (1955), and Sarkissov et al. (1995) published two more atlases of human cerebral cortex. The atlas by Sarkissov was mainly a modified version of the Brodmann map (Petrides, 2005).

While studies of the early 20th century played an important role in the advancement of the field of architectonic studies, the reliability of the borders defined by investigators is rather questionable due to the limited histological stains, lack of stringent parcellation criteria and small sample size used (Lashley and Clark, 1946). As such, the cortical maps have questionable validity, at least for many regions of cortex, and should be treated with caution.

The investigators of the 20th century had to work with limited histological techniques and underdeveloped technology. Additionally, most of the studies done in the early 20th century employed only two main staining methods – the Nissl and myelin stains. In spite of the technological limitations, their work laid the foundations upon which the concepts of subdividing the cortex and relating cortical architecture to function were built. However, subdividing the cortex based on two stains was not rigorous enough to produce consistent, reliable borders. Just as Lorente de Nó (1938) had observed, some cortical regions that were revealed to be functionally dissociated areas by Golgi preparations were not differentiated by other architectonic methods. Additionally, other cortical regions that are defined as homologous areas by architectonic methods are in fact different in origin and structure (Lorente de Nó, 1938). The limited number of histological stains employed in architectonic studies has led to the inconsistent nomenclature used in the architectonic maps of the human cerebral cortex and the monkey cortex by Brodmann (1909). The numerical designations that Brodmann had used for the maps of human cortex were not constant with the maps of monkey cortex, such that the same architectonic designation may refer to two areas that are obviously not homologous in these two species, or two comparable areas in these two species were assigned different numerical designations (Petrides, 2005). This creates a source of confusion when using Brodmann's numerical designations as references and results in a disconnect between animal and human anatomical studies (Petrides, 2005).

Another problem that plagued the architectonic studies during the early 20th century were inconsistent results from different investigators in the same species (Lashley and Clark, 1946; Petrides, 2005). Parcellation of the cortex was carried out by observer-dependent observations of locations of areal borders. The inconsistency in borders drawn by different investigators is more apparent in association areas than in primary sensory areas, as primary sensory areas usually stand out from surrounding cortices. Primary sensory areas can be differentiated by several cytoarchitectonic criteria, such as the presence of a layer 4 that is densely populated by spiny stellate cells, connections from specific sensory thalamic nuclei that can be identified by antibodies including the vesicle glutamate transporter 2 (VGluT2) (Nahmani and Erisir, 2005). Primary sensory areas generally have sharp borders with neighboring areas (Yamamori et al., 2006). On the other hand, association cortices receive less input from specific sensory thalamic nuclei, and are more interconnected with other cortical areas and nuclei (Felleman and Ven Essen, 1991). The lack of thalamic projections to association areas may result in indistinct borders between association areas (Yamamori et al., 2006). As such, delimiting association areas is often difficult. Different investigators had varied criteria for differentiating such areas, and it has been difficult for investigators to replicate the results of another's due to the lack of precise descriptions of the bases for parcellations of cortex (Lashley and Clark, 1946). While Vogt and Vogt had observed "hair-sharp" boundaries between areas (Vogt and Vogt, 1907; 1919, as cited in Lashley and Clark, 1946), von Economo and Koskinas favored transition zones between cortical areas and pointed out that the various criteria for delimiting areal borders do not change concurrently (Economo and Koskinas, 1925, as cited in Lashley and Clark, 1946). Except for area 17, other investigators did not consistently observe such sharp boundaries elsewhere in the cortex (Lashley and Clark, 1946). This large difference in opinions of these two groups of investigators shows how the delimitation of borders in the neocortex are made with a great influence of personal bias (Economo and Koskinas, 1925). Investigators may attempt to maintain a macroscopic view of changes in the cortical sheet, but they may weight the variables of the neocortex differently due to personal knowledge and expectations (Economo and Koskinas, 1925; Lashley and Clark, 1946). Often, investigators consciously, or subconsciously, give the most weight to the variable that is most obvious (Economo and Koskinas, 1925).

There were also concerns on whether architectonic differences between areas indicated functionally different fields. Brodmann had viewed the parcellation of the cortex as a charting of cerebral "organs" (Brodmann, 1909; Lashley and Clark, 1946). Lashley and Clark (1946) held a different view and had suggested that an observable architectonic difference of the cortex need not necessarily indicate functional differences. In addition, they held that there may be functional differences in certain regions of the cortex that do not show structural differences. However, structural changes have associated functional and metabolic consequences, and changes in cortical architecture would not take place if there were no benefits to the organism. A central premise of biology is that structure differences imply functional differences. As such, architectonic differences observed in the cortex provide a strong indication of functional differences. Currently, improved techniques of studying protein distribution and gene expression has given evidence that distinct cell phenotypes and the expression of discrete, unique molecular features is related to functional specialization (Pimenta et al., 2001; for reviews, see Goodman et al., 1984; Levitt, 1985; Jessell, 1988; Hockfield, 1990; Goodman and Shatz, 1993; Bolz and Castellani, 1997). DNA microarray and *in-situ* hybridization studies have found genes that are selectively expressed in areas associated with a specific function. For instance, the *occ1* gene exhibits a species-specific expression in the primary visual cortex of primates (Takahata et al., 2006), while expression of the retinol-binding protein (RBP) gene is complementary to the *occ1* gene, showing high expression in association areas but nearing absence from the primate visual cortex (Komatsu et al., 2005) (Fig. 9).

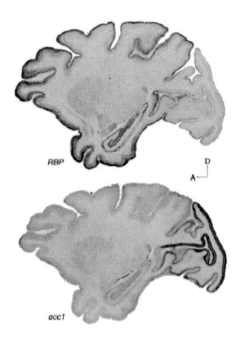

Figure 9. The expression of area-specific genes *occ1* and RBP in primate visual cortex. From Fig. 5A, Komatsu et al., 2005.

On the other hand, the evolution of functional areas of the cortex need not be accompanied by obvious architectonic differences, in terms of cellular types, structure or laminar characteristics. Consequently, histological techniques that are available may be inadequate in making distinctions between those areas. Instead, those areas may be differentiated in other ways, such as by their different afferent and efferent connections. The delimitation of these functional fields, just as Lashley and Clark had pointed out, will require the combination of physiological and anatomical studies (Lashley and Clark, 1946).

2.3 Cytoarchitectonic Methods of the Late 20th Century

Towards the later half of the century, new histological techniques were introduced. In 1979, the cytochrome oxidase (CO) stain (Wong-Riley, 1979) was developed. This stain reveals the presence of cytrochrome oxidase, a transmembrane protein found in mitochondria. The intensity of the CO stain is correlated with the number of mitochondria present and thus the metabolic demands of a cortical area. Areas with higher metabolic demands have a higher population density of mitochondria and as such, would be more intensely stained in the CO stain. Examples of such areas include primary cortical areas (Fig. 10C). Other histochemical methods, made available in the late 20th century, suggest the type of afferent connections that a region in the cortex receives. The Timm stain (Timm, 1958; Danscher, 1981) is one such autometallographic, histochemical technique. The Timm stain involves the precipitation of unbound, free zinc ions in the tissue by the systemic introduction of the amount of sodium sulfide or sodium selenite molecules required to match the amount of zinc ions in the tissues (Danscher and Stoltenberg, 2005). Cortical neurons that contain histochemically detectable zinc ions in their synaptic vesicles are likely to be glutamatergic and have a pyramidal cell appearance (Casanovas-Aguilar, 1995; 1998), and they are predominantly localized to the forebrain structures, such as the hippocampus and neocortex (Perez-Clausell and Danscher, 1985; Valente et al., 2002). This group of cortical neurons is involved in cortico-cortical connections. As such, the Timm stain reveals zones that receive cortico-cortical inputs rather than thalamo-cortical inputs (Fig. 6C; Fig. 13C) (Casanovas-Aguilar et al., 1995; Ichinohe and Rockland, 2004).

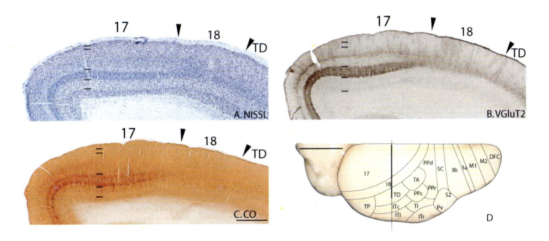

Figure 10. Coronal sections from the tree shrew visual cortex processed for Nissl substance (A), VGluT2 (B), and CO (C). The thick vertical line on the brain (D) indicates the approximate location of the sections that area illustrated. Lines on the sections show the six cell layers in each preparation. The abbreviations used here are: DFC, Dorsal frontal area; M1, Primary motor area; M2, Secondary motor area; 3a/dy, dysgranular zone; 3b, Primary somatosensory area; SC, Somatosensory caudal area; PPd, Posterior parietal dorsal area; PPr, Posterior parietal rostral area; PPc, Posterior parietal caudal area; S2, Secondary somatosensory area; Pv, Parietal ventral area; TA, Anterior temporal area; TD, Dorsal temporal area; Ti, Intermediate temporal area; TP, Posterior temporal areas; ITr, Inferior temporal rostral area; ITi, Inferior temporal intermediate area; ITc, Inferior temporal caudal area; 17 and 18 are adopted from Brodmann (1909). Scale bar for sections = 1mm, for brain = 5mm.

In the 1970s, due to the improvements in molecular biology, particularly in protein isolation and purification techniques, immunocytological methods and hybridoma techniques (Kohler and Milstein, 1975; Goding, 1996) were introduced. Immunohistochemistry makes use of the antibodies produced by molecular biology techniques to visualize the topographic distribution of different classes of molecules (Barnstable, 1980; Zipser and McKay, 1981; Trisler et al., 1981; Hawkes et al., 1982a,b; Hockfield and McKay, 1983). The antibodies bind to specific antigen targets and produce consistent staining patterns. An example would be the parvalbumin antibody (PV) that is immunoreactive for parvalbumin, a calcium-binding protein present in a subpopulation of GABAergic, non-pyramidal cells, including basket interneurons (Condé et al., 1996). PV immunoreactivity also characterizes the cortical terminals of thalamic neurons in sensory nuclei. As such, PV immunoreactivity is densely distributed in primary cortical areas, allowing the delimitation of primary sensory areas from their adjacent cortical areas (Fig. 10, 11). Due to the specificity of the antigen-antibody interaction, immunohistochemical stains are more sensitive. Hence, they often are more useful than conventional histological techniques (Annese and Toga, 2002). The relation between structure and function at the microscopic level is more clearly shown by immunohistochemistry, since it can be assumed that functionally different neuronal populations have different molecular phenotypes.

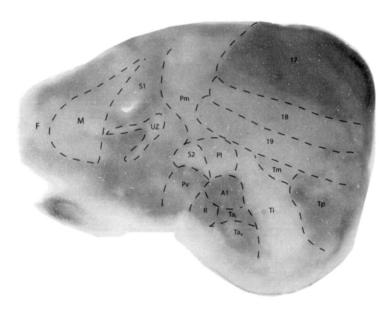

Figure 11. A parvalbumin (PV) stained section cut parallel to the surface of an artificially flattened cerebral hemisphere. Dashed lines show approximate cortical boundaries comparable to the reconstructed dorsal view of the brain in Fig. 13D. The specific antibody-antigen staining shows the topographic distribution of the PV protein in the cortex. There is higher PV staining in primary sensory areas such as area 17, S1 and A1 compared to their surrounding areas. A1, Primary auditory area; R, Rostral auditory area; Ta$_i$, Anterior temporal intermediate area; Ta$_v$, Anterior temporal ventral area; Tp; Temporal posterior area. Please refer to Fig. 6 for the remaining abbreviations used here.

With immunohistochemistry, borders of cortical areas can be defined by the presence of specialized cell morphology. One example is the delineation of the motor cortex by the presence of large Betz cells that are more darkly stained by SMI-32, an antibody that recognizes a neurofilament epitope present in pyramidal cells (Fig. 12) (Lee et al., 1987). Connectivity of a cortical area can be visualized immunohistochemically with antibodies against protein epitopes that are present only in certain neuronal connections. An instance would be the antibody against the VGluT2 protein (Fig. 10B; 13B), which is present in the terminals of a subset of neurons that originate from the thalamus (Nahami & Erisir, 2005). Since primary sensory areas receive dense inputs from the thalamus, these areas show stronger staining for the VGluT2 antibody than adjacent areas (Fig. 10B). Consequently, the different areas visualized by the use of different antibodies may suggest the physiological properties of the various cortical areas (Annese and Toga, 2002).

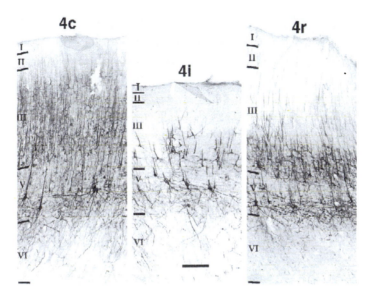

Figure 12. Photomicrographs showing the pyramidal cells stained by SMI-32 antibody in area 4 of the macaque monkey. From left are caudal (4c), intermediate (4i) and rostral (4r) subdivisions. The pyramidal cells visualized by the SMI-32 antibody show different cell morphologies, giving the subdivisions of area 4 different anatomical structures. Scale bar = 250μm. (From Preuss et al., 1997).

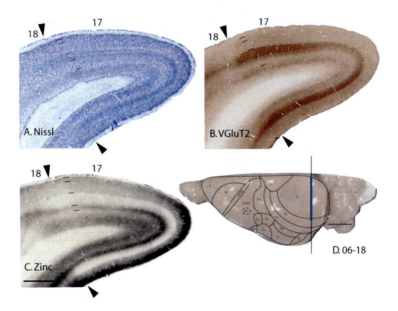

Figure 13. Architectonic subdivisions of the visual cortex in the squirrel brain. D. Subdivision indicated on a dorsal view of the left caudal hemisphere. A vertical line indicates the approximate location of coronal brain section shown in A to C. The thick portion of the line corresponds to the portions of the sections that are illustrated. Lines on the sections show the six cell layers in each preparation. Area 17 and 18 are illustrated here. Area 17 is the primary visual cortex and has high thalamic inputs to layer 4. The dark, thick band in layer 4 of B, the VGluT2 stain, shows this. C. Zinc stain, which stains corticocortical input, shows complementary staining to the VGluT2 stain, with almost no staining in layer 4 of area 17. Scale bar for brain = 5mm, for sections = 2.0mm. Refer to Fig. 7 for the abbreviations used here. Modified from Fig. 1, Wong and Kaas, 2008.

Receptor architecture studies that involve the mapping of the various receptor-binding sites have higher functional relevance than cytoarchitectural studies based on the histological stains, such as Nissl and myelin (Zilles et al., 2004). The distributions of the different receptor types in the brain are visualized by labeling the receptors with their respective radiolabeled neurotransmitters (Zilles et al., 1995, 2002; Geyer et al., 1996, 1997; Zilles and Palomero-Gallagher, 2001). The population density of a receptor type in neocortex is visualized as a color-coded autoradiograph. A range of colors, with red and blue respectively representing regions with the highest and lowest population density, shows the varying density distributions of a receptor type in the cortex and gives a "neurochemical fingerprint" of a cortical area (Matelli and Juppino, 2004). Functionally similar areas, such as motor and premotor areas, have "neurochemical fingerprints" that share a higher degree of similarity than those for functionally dissimilar areas, such as motor and somatosensory areas (Matelli and Juppino, 2004). Grouping cortical areas by their "neurochemical fingerprints" into "neurochemical families" of areas may be useful in defining homologous areas in different species (Matelli and Luppino, 2004). Identification of cortical areas by their "neurochemical fingerprints" may also help to reduce the effect of individual variability, resulting in probablistic maps that are a better representative of a species. The distribution patterns obtained from this technique have shown correspondence to borders established by cyto- and myeloarchitectural methods (Fig. 14).

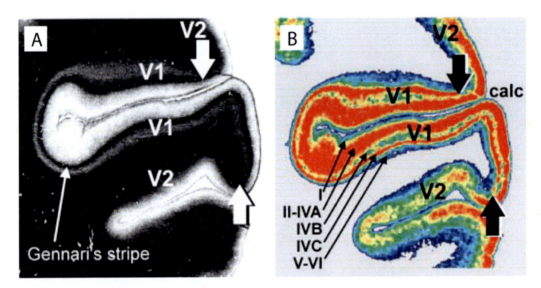

Figure 14. A. Photomicrograph of a myelin-stained section showing the primary visual cortex, V1 and secondary visual cortex, V2 in humans. V1 is characterized by the myelin-dense stripe of Gennari. B. Color-coded autoradiograph of an adjacent section showing the distribution of the $GABA_A$ receptor visualized by using [^{3}H] muscimol. The V1/V2 border is marked by the disppearance of the receptor-dense layer 4C of V1 in B, and the location of this border, which corresponds, with the location where the stripe of Gennari disappears in A. Reproduced from Fig. 1C and 1D, Zilles et al., 2004.

In addition, receptor density studies reveal a further parcellation into areas that were not visible in cyto- or myeloarchitecture (Zilles et al., 2002; Zilles et al., 2004). For example, the distribution pattern of the cholinergic muscarinic M2 receptor reveals modular borders within the cytoarchitectonically defined secondary visual cortex, V2 (Fig. 15)(Zilles et al., 2004).

This suggests that receptor architecture studies allow more detailed study of the microstructure and neurochemical organization of the cerebral cortex (Zilles et al., 2004). However, since a single receptor type does not reveal all the borders of cortex, it is necessary to use a multi-receptor approach when studying areal parcellation of cortex (Zilles et al., 2002; Zilles et al., 2004). Parcellation of cortex based on the receptor-binding method is based on a single criterion of the different patterns of colors shown on the autoradiographs. As autoradiographs do not show other features of neocortex, such as the cell morphology and the relative lamination pattern, receptor-binding studies should include the use of histological methods in order to generate more reliable borders.

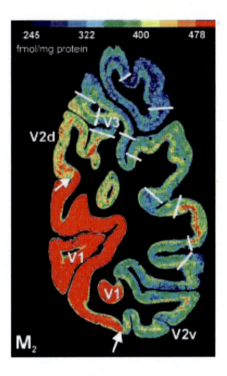

Figure 15. A coronal section through the human occipital cortex showing the distribution of the cholinergic muscarinic M2 receptor. Borders revealed by the M2 receptor expression that were previously unidentified cortical areas are indicated by the white lines. Reproduced from Fig. 4, Zilles et al., 2004.

3. Problems

A recurrent problem in architectonic studies is the presence of histological artifacts. A major cause of histological artifacts is the shrinkage of brain tissue that occurs at the various levels of tissue processing. From fixation (Sadowski et al., 1995; Quester and Schroder, 1997), cryoprotection (Rosene et al., 1986), and histological and immunochemical processings, shrinkage of brain tissue is unavoidable (Annese and Toga, 2002). In addition, tissue sections mounted on a slide have to be dehydrated before coverslipping. In frozen sections, which have not been beforehand dehydrated from fixation processes, the tissue may shrink up to a fifth of its original thickness on the glass slides (Annese and Toga, 2002). This problem is compounded by the irregular shrinkage throughout the thickness of the tissue (Hatton and Von Bartheld, 1999), possibly because different neural structures have different degrees of shrinkage. For instance, during the deacetylation process of myelin staining, lipids from the tissue are removed and this would lead to a greater degree of shrinkage of medullary myelin-rich regions, than that of the cortex, since the cortex is densely packed with cells (Annese and Toga, 2002). Apart from tissue shrinkage, the intensity of tissue staining usually varies between different batches of sections due to a wide range of factors that include: length of fixation, age of the tissue section, length of development during visualization, different batches of reacting solutions and buffers, and the varying immunoreactivity of antibodies from different batches. The irregular tissue shrinkage and variance in staining intensity may affect the judgment of the observer when defining the borders of cortical areas.

Lashley and Clark, in 1946, brought up concerns regarding the lack of proper differentiating criteria when parcellating the cortex, leading to inconsistent results from different investigators. The inconsistent results shed doubt on the reliability of the borders obtained from architectonic studies that lack rigor, and emphasize the importance of employing stringent criteria when defining the borders of cortical areas. The reliability of the borders is dependent on the certainty and precision with which areas can be recognized. Borders that are identified based on a single criterion, especially if they are based on the presence of certain cell types, are likely to be highly unrealiable. An example would be using the changes in density distribution of the giant pyramids in layer 5 as the basis for delimiting the border between area 4 and area 6 in primates. The density distribution of these cells does not change abruptly, but instead reduces progressively across area 4 to the area 4/6 border. Identification of the area 4/6 border based on this single criterion would thus be a subjective one (Matelli and Luppino, 2004). These borders can be made more reliable by employing a battery of staining methods. When there is corroboration across different sections stained for different histological and immunohistochemical stains, there is more evidence for the delimitation of an area. The use of several staining methods should also lead to better descriptions for the basis of areal parcellation, which will in turn allow investigators to understand the criteria for parcellation and replicate the results from other investigators.

A third concern is the significant variability of neocortex across individuals of the same species (Lashley and Clark, 1946; Amunts et al., 1999). Macroscopically, there are variations in the convolutions of the neocortex and the size of each cortical area (Von Economo and Koskinas, 1925, as cited in Lashley and Clark, 1946; Amunts et al., 2001; Van Essen, 2004). Microscopically, the cell density of corresponding cortical areas from different hemispheres can differ by as much as ten percent (Von Economo and Koskinas, 1925, as cited in Lashley and Clark, 1946). In order to reduce the effects of individual variability between animals of the same species, more cases should be included per study, and the neurochemical architecture of various cortical areas should be carefully characterized to form a basis on which a certain area from different individuals can be identified based on their "neurochemical fingerprint".

For nearly a century, architectonic studies of the cerebral cortex involved almost exclusively frontal or sagittal sections (Fleischhauer, 1978). A certain cutting plane may reveal some cortical areas better than others. For example, a coronal cut will show areas along the medial wall better than a sagittal cut. As such, current and future studies should be more rigorous and use all three cutting planes, the coronal, horizontal and sagittal planes. In addition, sections cut parallel to the surface of flattened cortex have proven to be very useful in architectonic studies as they show the topographical relationship between areas in a single section.

4. Observer-Independent Method

While the variance in staining intensities can be kept to a minimum by keeping the variables constant, such as treating all brain tissues with the same length of fixation, developing them consistenly during visualization and obtaining antibodies from the same source, it is impossible to eradicate all histological artifacts. Even if histological artifacts could be prevented, the intersubject differences and the inconsistency of judgments by different observers may still create inconsistent cortical maps. The current concerns surrounding architectonic studies show a need to produce more consistent cortical maps that account for histological artifacts, individual variation in the hemispheres within a species and different parcellation criteria used across different investigators. Accordingly, there is a shift in focus of attention to developing new architectonic methods that are observer-independent and involve some sort of statistically testable procedure for the establishment of cortical borders (Zilles et al., 2004).

Hopf (1966) and Hudspeth et al. (1976) first used densitometry in sections stained for cell bodies (Schleicher et al., 2005). This approach is now used in observer-independent methods. Each cortical region is characterized by the shape of a locally sample intensity profile (Annese et al., 2004). Curvilinear lines are drawn transversely across the neocortical layers of grayscaled images of tissue sections (Zilles and Schleicher, 1993; Schleicher et al., 1999; Hackett et al., 2001; Annese et al., 2004; Schleicher et al., 2005). These lines are not allowed to cross and are drawn such that they are aligned with the vertically organized cell columns and do not traverse across columns of cells (Mountcastle, 1978), reducing the noise of the grey level index (GLI) profiles obtained in 2-dimensional images. However, these lines do not follow the cell columns and as such, layers of the cortex may be misrepresented in areas where the plane of the section is very tangential (Annese et al., 2004). Thus 3-dimensional reconstruction of the brains with these curvilinear lines in place is needed to be fully certain that these lines follow the entire cell column through the cortex (Schleicher et al., 2005). The local intensity profiles obtained from these grayscaled images quantify the laminar pattern of the cortex and through this statistical approach, areal borders of the cortex are drawn (Schleicher et al., 2005). However, the GLI profiles do not account for cell size or cell population density (Schleicher, 2005). Therefore a multiparameter approach that includes parameters such as cell profile count and grey matter density should be used (Sanz-Arigita et al., 2004).

Observer-independent architectonic methods involve the acquisition of digital images of tissue sections and the quantifying of the laminar pattern (Schleicher et al., 2005). Since observer-independent methods remove the subjective nature of observer-dependent methods (Schleicher et al., 2005), it may be possible, for the first time in architectonic studies, to standardize the parcellation scheme used by different investigators for subdividing the cortical sheet into distinct architectonic areas (Van Essen, 2004). Gradually changing borders that were previously arbitrarily identified by investigators due to the lack of definite criteria can now be re-evaluated to result in a common, statistically significant border. This will be an important step in trying to reconcile the cortical maps that were produced by different investigators, such as Brodmann, Vogt and Vogt, and von Economo and Koskinas. Sensitive to sharp areal borders (Schleicher et al., 1999), this method is somewhat able to detect smooth or gradual changes such as those due to cortical folding (Schleicher et al., 1999). By thresholding the digitized images to produce binary images, the observer-independent method also reduces the problem with the effects due to histological artifacts such as inconsistent staining intensities (Wree et al., 1982; Schleicher, 2005). Since observer-independent methods are automated, they are less labor-intensive compared to observer-dependent methods, which require each tissue section to be manually drawn out. One would then expect observer-independent studies to have a larger sample pool size so as to reduce the effect of individual variation.

The borders obtained from the observer-independent method are drawn where there are significant changes in the cortex, but the significance of the change is not identified.

Some anatomical changes need not indicate a different cortical area (Amunts, 2002), which are functionally separate. Instead, the anatomical changes may be subdivisions of an existing cortical area that is responsible for a sub-modality of a certain function, such as the monocular and binocular region of area 17 in squirrels (Kaas et al., 1972). The anatomical variations between the monocular and binocular sub-region of area 17 is obvious enough and would result in the detection of a significant change in the GLI profile, even though both regions are parts of the primary visual cortex. Another instance would be the individual barrels of the barrel field (Woolsey, 1970) that stand out as separate modules in most staining methods, and therefore are likely to show up as significant changes in the GLI profile, but they are not functionally separate areas. On the other hand, some adjoining areas may have transitional zones between them and may not show up as statistically significant changes in the GLI. When employing this method, it remains important to adopt a multimodal approach to ascertain the areal borders (Schleicher et al., 2005), for instance, using combinations of cytoarchitecture, myeloarchitecture and receptor architecture (Zilles et al., 2001). The observer-independent method is highly useful in the study and expansion the areal parcellation of species that have existing cortical maps. However, when establishing a fresh cortical map of a species, results obtained by this method should still be done in conjunction with observer-dependent methods, where location of borders are elucidated by logic and functional areas of the cortex are taken into consideration.

5. The Future

Architectonic brain mapping has changed drastically over the past century, due to better fixation mediums, microscope technology, repertoire of staining methods and quantification methods. The histochemical techniques available for studying the fine anatomy of cortex is set to improve in sensitivity and specificity with advances in the molecular biology and genomic fields. Most recently, the map of gene expression of the mouse brain has been completed and work has started in the human brain (Brill, 2006). Using data from the gene expression map of the brain patterns, protein expression in the brain can be studied to provide further insight into the function of a particular cortical area. Regional distribution of gene expression in the mouse brain was found to be rather selective (Brill, 2006), suggesting that the tightly related protein expression would be regionally selective as well. In primates, the identification of genes with area-specific expression, including the *occ1* gene (Takahata et al., 2006) that is expressed in the primary visual cortex and the RBP gene (Komatsu et al., 2005) that is expressed elsewhere, in association areas, suggests that there are more of such genes to be identified. This may give rise to new antibodies that will allow for the visualization of regional specific areas of the brain, resulting in a more detailed parcellation of the cortex and strengthening the link between fine anatomical structure and function.

A multimodal approach to studying the cortex may be increasingly adopted in the future. More specifically, this multimodal approach will make use of a variety of mapping techniques, such as the cyto-, myelo-, immuno- and receptor architectonic techniques (for examples, see Zilles and Palomero-Gallagher, 2001; Amunts et al., 2002; Sherwood et al., 2003). Architectonic studies will involve the combination of observer-dependent and observer-independent methods (Amunts et al., 2002). The use of this multimodal approach will avoid the problem of over-parcellation of the cerebral cortex that may arise from a single technique approach (Amunts et al., 2002) and increase the reliability of the areal borders obtained. There will also be a shift towards using observer-independent methods for most of the analysis, reducing the amount of manual labor required by observer-dependent methods (Mazziotta and Toga, 2002). However, until there is a validated statistical method to determine the natural number of cortical areas in a distinct cortical region (Schleicher, 2005), observer-dependent analysis will still be required to ensure that areal borders determined by significance measurements are biologically sound.

Anatomical characteristics of regions in the cortex may also be better defined with improved histochemical techniques and the use of multimodal approaches. As such, inconsistencies in nomenclature of classical cortical maps may be resolved (Petrides, 2005). One such discrepancy is between the human and monkey cortical maps by Brodmann (1909). The numerical designations that Brodmann employed were not consistent in his human and monkey cortical maps, even though the areas are comparable (Petrides, 2005). Brodmann (1909) had stated that area 9 in the monkey corresponds to the granular frontal area 9 and frontopolar area 10 in the human brain (Petrides, 2005). However, in his monkey cortical map, Brodmann had named the frontopolar region as area 12 (Petrides, 2005). It is necessary to resolve such discrepancies and reconcile maps between species so that results of research work in monkeys can be meaningfully compared to functional neuroimaging work on human subjects (Petrides, 2005). Detailed characterization of a cortical area will also aid in the identification of homologous areas across species. This will deepen our understanding of the *Bauplan* of the cerebral cortex and the course of brain evolution.

One may expect to see increased integration of architectonic studies with non-invasive microimaging studies. High-field magnetic resonance imaging (MRI) of up to 8 Teslas (T) has already been used on human subjects (Robitaille et al., 1998), and is able to produce sub-millimetric spatial resolution of the human cortex (Annese et al., 2004). In animals, at 11T, a resolution in the range of 10μm can be obtained (Mazziotta and Toga, 2002). MRI scans of histological sections processed for myelin have produced a similar level of detail as the original illustrations of Baillarger (1840) and Elliot Smith (1907) (Annese et al., 2004). In the future, with improved hardware and finer resolution, MRI scans may be used to obtain a myeloarchitectonic map (Annese et al., 2004). The connectivity of cortical areas can be derived from relating architectonic maps to the results of diffusion MRI (dMRI) tractography (Fig. 16) dMRI tractography is a technique that traces fiber bundles *in vivo* (Johansen-Berg and Behrens, 2006; Concha et al., 2005). There are a number of limitations to the dMRI method. For instance, it does not provide information on which fiber tracts are anterograde and which are retrograde, the presence of synapses, or whether a pathway is functional (Johansen-Berg and Behrens, 2006). Within realistic acquisition times and decent signal-to-noise ratio (Watts et al., 2003), the spatial resolution of dMRI is still not fine enough to resolve regions with multiple fiber bundles (Watts et al., 2003), or differentiate crossing fibers (Johansen-Bern and Behrens, 2006; Watts et al., 2003). Nevertheless, dMRI shows the connectivity of cortical areas and relating this to the architectonic maps will enhance the structure and function relationship.

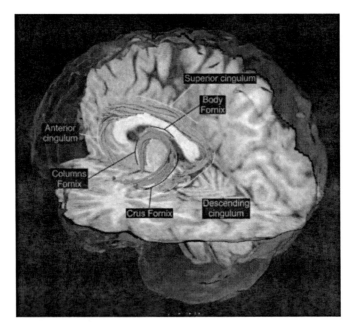

Figure 16. The white matter tracts of fornix and the cingulum of human shown by dMRI tractography. The tracts of the fornix are shown in green and the cingulum shown in orange. Reproduced from Fig. 1, Concha et al., 2005.

Finally, three-dimensional cortical maps may replace current two-dimensional cortical maps obtained from reconstructions of histological sections. The current reconstruction software does not take histological artifacts into consideration, for instance differential tissue shrinkage in the various histochemical techniques (Bouteiller, personal communication), and it would be difficult to do a three-dimensional reconstruction of series of brain sections that have undergone different processing methods. However, the brain is a three-dimensional object and a three-dimensional reconstruction will offer a holistic view of the brain that can be studied from any plane, at any angle (Bouteiller, 2002).

6. Conclusion

Architectonic studies will tend towards a more quantified and objective approach. Integration of observer-independent and observer-dependent methods will increase the objectiveness and decrease the labor-intensiveness of architectonic studies. Multimodal approaches that integrate observer-dependent and observer-independent methods will boost the reliability of cortical borders and lead to the identification of new areas. Identification of cortical areas by their "neurochemical fingerprints" may help to reduce the effect of individual variability, resulting in more accurate probabilistic maps. "Neurochemical families" of cortical areas with similar "neurochemical fingerprints" may aid in the identification of homologous areas in different species and perhaps reconcile differences in classical maps of various species. Advances in molecular biology and the completion of gene expression brain maps of different species will lead to increased availability of antibodies with sensitivity and regional specificity. Improved immunohistochemical methods and receptor architectonics will give functional meaning to architectonically defined areas. The combination of architectonic and imaging techniques, such as dMRI tractography, may enhance our understanding of the connectivity of different cortical areas. There will be increasing pressure to develop methods and software that will produce anatomically accurate three-dimensional brain atlases from histological sections. These three-dimensional atlases will contain information about the structure, function and connections of the cortical areas to allow comparison with results from functional MRI. While architectonic studies have been going on for more than a century, with all the possible improvements that can be made, the future of architectonic studies will be an exciting one.

References

Agmon, A., Yang, L. T., O'Dowd, D. K., & Jones, E. G. (1993). Organized growth of thalamocortical axons from the deep tier of terminations into layer IV of developing mouse barrel cortex. *J Neurosci*, 13(12), 5365-5382.

Amunts, K., Schleicher, A., Burgel, U., Mohlberg, H., Uylings, H. B., & Zilles, K. (1999). Broca's region revisited: cytoarchitecture and intersubject variability. *J Comp Neurol*, 412(2), 319-341.

Amunts, K., & Zilles, K. (2001). Advances in cytoarchitectonic mapping of the human cerebral cortex. *Neuroimaging Clin N Am*, 11(2), 151-169, vii.

Annese, J., Toga, A.W. (2002). Postmortem Anatomy (2 ed.). San Diego: *Academic Press.*

Annese, J., Pitiot, A., Dinov, I. D., & Toga, A. W. (2004). A myelo-architectonic method for the structural classification of cortical areas. *Neuroimage*, 21(1), 15-26.

Bailey, P. a. B., G. (1951). The isocortex of man. *Urbana*: University of Illinois Pr.

Barnstable, C. J. (1980). Monoclonal antibodies which recognize different cell types in the rat retina. *Nature,* 286(5770), 231-235.

Bouteiller, J. M. (2002). 3D Reconstruction from serial non-contiguous sectiosn using variational implicit techniques. *University of Southern California.*

Brazier, M. A. B. (1978). Architectonics of the Cerebral Cortex: *Research in the 19th Century* (Vol. 3). New York: Raven Press.

Brill, D. (2006). Mouse brain map is complete. *Nature,* 443(7110), 380-381.

Brodmann, K. (1909). Brodmann's 'Localisation in the Cerebral Cortex' *(L. J. Garey, Trans.).* London: Eldred Smith-Gordon.

Bronchti, G., Heil, P., Sadka, R., Hess, A., Scheich, H., & Wollberg, Z. (2002). Auditory activation of "visual" cortical areas in the blind mole rat (Spalax ehrenbergi). *Eur J Neurosci,* 16(2), 311-329.

Casagrande, V. A., Kaas, J.H. (1994). The afferent, intrinsic and efferent connections of primary visual cortex in primates *(Vol. 10).* New York: Plenum Press.

Casanovas-Aguilar, C., Christensen, M. K., Reblet, C., Martinez-Garcia, F., Perez-Clausell, J., & Bueno-Lopez, J. L. (1995). Callosal neurones give rise to zinc-rich boutons in the rat visual cortex. *Neuroreport,* 6(3), 497-500.

Casanovas-Aguilar, C., Reblet, C., Perez-Clausell, J., & Bueno-Lopez, J. L. (1998). Zinc-rich afferents to the rat neocortex: projections to the visual cortex traced with intracerebral selenite injections. *J Chem Neuroanat,* 15(2), 97-109.

Castellani, V., & Bolz, J. (1997). Membrane-associated molecules regulate the formation of layer-specific cortical circuits. *Proc Natl Acad Sci U S A,* 94(13), 7030-7035.

Catania, K. C. (2000). Cortical organization in insectivora: the parallel evolution of the sensory periphery and the brain. *Brain Behav Evol,* 55, 311-321.

Cavada, C. (2004). Neuroanatomy in understanding primate brain function: status and challenges. *Cortex,* 40(1), 5-6.

Concha, L., Gross, D. W., & Beaulieu, C. (2005). Diffusion tensor tractography of the limbic system. *Am J Neuroradiol,* 26(9), 2267-2274.

Conde, F., Lund, J. S., & Lewis, D. A. (1996). The hierarchical development of monkey visual cortical regions as revealed by the maturation of parvalbumin-immunoreactive neurons. *Brain Res Dev Brain Res,* 96(1-2), 261-276.

Cooper, H. M., Herbin, M., & Nevo, E. (1993). Visual system of a naturally microphthalmic mammal: the blind mole rat, Spalax ehrenbergi. *J Comp Neurol,* 328(3), 313-350.

Creutzfeldt, O. D. (1995). Cortec Cerebri: Performance, structural and functional organization of the cortex. New York: *Oxford Univ Pr.*

Danscher, G. (1981). Histochemical demonstration of heavy metals. A revised version of the sulphide silver method suitable for both light and electronmicroscopy. *Histochemistry,* 71(1), 1-16.

Danscher, G., & Stoltenberg, M. (2005). Zinc-specific autometallographic in vivo selenium methods: tracing of zinc-enriched (ZEN) terminals, ZEN pathways, and pools of zinc ions in a multitude of other ZEN cells. *J Histochem Cytochem,* 53(2), 141-153.

Diamond, M. C. (2001). Response of the brain to enrichment. *An Acad Bras Cienc.,* 73(2), 211-220.

Ehret, G. (1997). The auditory cortex. *J Comp Physiol,* 181, 547-557.

Evans, E.F., Ross, H.F., Whitfield, I.C. (1964). The spatial distribution of unit charateristic frequency in the primary auditory cortex of the cat. *J. Physiol.* 179, 238-247

Felleman, D. J., & Van Essen, D. C. (1991). Distributed hierarchical processing in the primate cerebral cortex. *Cereb Cortex*, 1(1), 1-47.

Finger, S. (1994). *Origins of Neuroscience*: A History of Explorations into Brain Function. Cary, North Carolina, USA: Oxford Univ Pr.

Fleischhauer, K. (1978). *Cortical Architectonics*: The last 50 years and some problems of today (Vol. 3). New York: Raven Press.

Geyer, S., Ledberg, A., Schleicher, A., Kinomura, S., Schormann, T., Burgel, U., et al. (1996). Two different areas within the primary motor cortex of man. *Nature,* 382(6594), 805-807.

Geyer, S., Schleicher, A., & Zilles, K. (1997). The somatosensory cortex of human: cytoarchitecture and regional distributions of receptor-binding sites. *Neuroimage*, 6(1), 27-45.

Goding, W. J. (1996). Monoclonal antibotides: *Principles and practice*. London: Academic Press.

Goodman, C. S., Bastiani, M. J., Doe, C. Q., du Lac, S., Helfand, S. L., Kuwada, J. Y., et al. (1984). Cell recognition during neuronal development. *Science*, 225(4668), 1271-1279.

Goodman, C. S., & Shatz, C. J. (1993). Developmental mechanisms that generate precise patterns of neuronal connectivity. *Cell,* 72 Suppl, 77-98.

Grossberg, S. (1999). How does the cerebral cortex work? Learning, attention, and grouping by the laminar circuits of visual cortex. *Spat Vis*, 12(2), 163-185.

Hackett, T. A., Preuss, T. M., & Kaas, J. H. (2001). Architectonic identification of the core region in auditory cortex of macaques, chimpanzees, and humans. *J Comp Neurol,* 441(3), 197-222.

Hassler, R. (1966). Comparative anatomy of the central visual systems in day- and night-active primates. *Stuttgart.*

Hatton, W. J., & von Bartheld, C. S. (1999). Analysis of cell death in the trochlear nucleus of the chick embryo: calibration of the optical disector counting method reveals systematic bias. *J Comp Neurol*, 409(2), 169-186.

Hawkes, R., Ng, M., Niday, E., & Matus, A. (1982). Immunocytochemical localization of identified proteins in brain by monoclonal antibodies. *Prog Brain Res*, 56, 77-86.

Hawkes, R., Niday, E., & Matus, A. (1982). Monoclonal antibodies identify novel neural antigens. *Proc Natl Acad Sci U S A,* 79(7), 2410-2414.

Heil, P., Bronchti, G., Wollberg, Z., & Scheich, H. (1991). Invasion of visual cortex by the auditory system in the naturally blind mole rat. *Neuroreport*, 2(12), 735-738.

Henry, E. C., Marasco, P. D., & Catania, K. C. (2005). Plasticity of the cortical dentition representation after tooth extraction in naked mole-rats. *J Comp Neurol*, 485(1), 64-74.

Henry, G. H. (1991). Afferent inputs, receptive field properties and morphological cell types in different laminae of the striate cortex. In A. G. Leventhal (ed.): *The Neural Basis of Visual Function. Boston:* CRC Press, pp. 223-245.

Hockfield, S. (1990). Proteoglycans in neural development. *Semin Dev Biol*, 1, 55-63.

Hockfield, S., McKay, R. D., Hendry, S. H., & Jones, E. G. (1983). A surface antigen that identifies ocular dominance columns in the visual cortex and laminar features of the lateral geniculate nucleus. *Cold Spring Harb Symp Quant Biol*, 48 Pt 2, 877-889.

Hubel, D. H., Wiesel, T. N., & Stryker, M. P. (1977). Orientation columns in macaque monkey visual cortex demonstrated by the 2-deoxyglucose autoradiographic technique. *Nature*, 269(5626), 328-330.

Ichinohe, N., & Rockland, K. S. (2004). Region specific micromodularity in the uppermost layers in primate cerebral cortex. *Cereb Cortex,* 14(11), 1173-1184.

Jessell, T. M. (1988). Adhesion molecules and the hierarchy of neural development. *Neuron,* 1(1), 3-13.

Johansen-Berg, H., & Behrens, T. E. (2006). Just pretty pictures? What diffusion tractography can add in clinical neuroscience. *Curr Opin Neurol*, 19(4), 379-385.

Johnson, J. I. (1990). *Comparative development of somatic sensory cortex.*

Kaas, J. H. (1983). What, if anything, is SI? Organization of first somatosensory area of cortex. *Physiol Rev,* 63(1), 206-231.

Kaas, J. H. (1997). Topographic maps are fundamental to sensory processing. *Brain Res Bull,* 44(2), 107-112.

Kaas, J. H. (2002). *Neocortex.* In Encyclopedia of the Human Brain, San Diego: Academic Press, 291-303.

Kaas, J. H. (2005). The future of mapping sensory cortex in primates: three of many remaining issues. *Philos Trans R Soc Lond B Biol Sci*, 360(1456), 653-664.

Kaas, J. H. (2005). From mice to men: the evolution of the large, complex human brain. *J Biosci*, 30(2), 155-165.

Kaas, J. H., & Catania, K. C. (2002). How do features of sensory representations develop? *Bioessays,* 24(4), 334-343.

Kaas, J. H., Hall, W. C., & Diamond, I. T. (1972). Visual cortex of the grey squirrel (Sciurus carolinensis): architectonic subdivisions and connections from the visual thalamus. *J Comp Neurol,* 145(3), 273-305.

Kohler, G., & Milstein, C. (1975). Continuous cultures of fused cells secreting antibody of predefined specificity. *Nature*, 256(5517), 495-497.

Komatsu, Y., Watakabe, A., Hashikawa, T., Tochitani, S., & Yamamori, T. (2005). Retinol-binding protein gene is highly expressed in higher-order association areas of the primate neocortex. *Cereb Cortex*, 15(1), 96-108.

Koralek, K. A., Olavarria, J., & Killackey, H. P. (1990). Areal and laminar organization of corticocortical projections in the rat somatosensory cortex. *J Comp Neurol*, 299(2), 133-150.

Krubitzer, L. (1995). The organization of neocortex in mammals: are species differences really so different? *Trends Neurosci*, 18(9), 408-417.

Krubitzer, L., & Kahn, D. M. (2003). Nature versus nurture revisited: an old idea with a new twist. *Prog Neurobiol*, 70(1), 33-52.

Lashley, K. S. a. C., G. (1946). The cytoarchitecture of the cerebral cortex of ateles: A critical examination of architectonic studies. *J. Comp Neurol.*, 85, 223-305.

Lee, V. M., Carden, M. J., Schlaepfer, W. W., & Trojanowski, J. Q. (1987). Monoclonal antibodies distinguish several differentially phosphorylated states of the two largest rat neurofilament subunits (NF-H and NF-M) and demonstrate their existence in the normal nervous system of adult rats. *J Neurosci*, 7(11), 3474-3488.

Leff. A., (2004). A historical review of the representation of the visual field in primary visual cortec with special reference to the neural mechanisms underlying macular sparing. *Brain and Language*, 88, 268-278.

Levitt, P. (1985). Relating molecular specificity to normal and abnormal brain development. *Ann N Y Acad Sci*, 450, 239-246.

Lorente de Nó, R. (1938). Architectonics and structure of teh cerebral cortex (1 ed.). *Oxford:* Oxford University Pr.

Lund, J. S., Henry, G. H., MacQueen, C. L., & Harvey, A. R. (1979). Anatomical organization of the primary visual cortex (area 17) of the cat. A comparison with area 17 of the macaque monkey. *J Comp Neurol*, 184(4), 599-618.

Matelli, M., & Luppino, G. (2004). Architectonics of the primates cortex: usefulness and limits. *Cortex*, 40(1), 209-210.

Maunsell, J. H., & van Essen, D. C. (1983). The connections of the middle temporal visual area (MT) and their relationship to a cortical hierarchy in the macaque monkey. *J Neurosci,* 3(12), 2563-2586.

Mazziotta, J. C., Toga, A.W. (2002). Speculations about the Future. *San Diego: Academic Press.*

McHenry, L. C. J. (1969). Garrison's History of Neurology. Springfield, IL: Thomas, *C.C.*

McHenry, L. C. J. (1983). Classics in neurology. *Neurology,* 33, 765.

Miller, B., Blake, N. M., Erinjeri, J. P., Reistad, C. E., Sexton, T., Admire, P., et al. (2001). Postnatal growth of intrinsic connections in mouse barrel cortex. *J Comp Neurol*, 436(1), 17-31.

Mountcastle, V. B., Berman, A.L., Davie, P.W. (1955). Topographic organization and modality representation in first somatic area of cat's cerebral cortex by method of single unit analysis. *Am J Physiol*, 183, 646.

Nahmani, M., & Erisir, A. (2005). VGluT2 immunochemistry identifies thalamocortical terminals in layer 4 of adult and developing visual cortex. *J Comp Neurol*, 484(4), 458-473.

Paolini, M., & Sereno, M. I. (1998). Direction selectivity in the middle lateral and lateral (ML and L) visual areas in the California ground squirrel. *Cereb Cortex*, 8(4), 362-371.

Perez-Clausell, J., & Danscher, G. (1985). Intravesicular localization of zinc in rat telencephalic boutons. A histochemical study. *Brain Res,* 337(1), 91-98.

Petrides, M. (2005). Lateral prefrontal cortex: architectonic and functional organization. *Philos Trans R Soc Lond B Biol Sci,* 360(1456), 781-795.

Pimenta, A. F., Strick, P. L., & Levitt, P. (2001). Novel proteoglycan epitope expressed in functionally discrete patterns in primate cortical and subcortical regions. *J Comp Neurol*, 430(3), 369-388.

Preuss, T. M., Stepniewska I., Jain N., & Kaas J.H. (1997). Multiple divisions of macaque precentral motor cortex identified with neurofilament antibody SMI-32. *Brain Res*, 767, 148-153.

Quester, R., & Schroder, R. (1997). The shrinkage of the human brain stem during formalin fixation and embedding in paraffin. *J Neurosci Methods*, 75(1), 81-89.

Rakic, P. (1988). Specification of cerebral cortical areas. *Science*, 241(4862), 170-176.

Robitaille, P. M., Abduljalil, A. M., Kangarlu, A., Zhang, X., Yu, Y., Burgess, R., et al. (1998). Human magnetic resonance imaging at 8 T. *NMR Biomed*, 11(6), 263-265.

Rosa, M. G., & Krubitzer, L. A. (1999). The evolution of visual cortex: where is V2? Trends *Neurosci*, 22(6), 242-248.

Rosene, D. L., Roy, N. J., & Davis, B. J. (1986). A cryoprotection method that facilitates cutting frozen sections of whole monkey brains for histological and histochemical processing without freezing artifact. *J Histochem Cytochem*, 34(10), 1301-1315.

Sadowski, M., Morys, J., Berdel, B., & Maciejewska, B. (1995). Influence of fixation and histological procedure on the morphometric parameters of neuronal cells. *Folia Morphol* (Warsz), 54(4), 219-226.

Sanz-Arigita, E. J., de Vos K., Pool, C.W., Uylings, H.B.M. (2002). Multivariate quantitative analysis of the microstructure of the cingulate cortex - areas 24 of Brodmann. *Abstracts of the Second Vogt-Brodmann Symposium, the converge of structure and function*, 44.

Sarkissov, S. A., Filimonodd, I.N., Kononowa, E.P., Preobraschenskaja, I.S. and Kukuew, L.A. (1955). Atlas of the cytoarchitectonics of the human cerebral cortex. *Moscoz: Medgiz.*

Scheibel, A. B. (1990). Dendritic correlates of higher cognitive function. New York: *The Guilford Press.*

Schleicher, A., Palomero-Gallagher, N., Morosan, P., Eickhoff, S. B., Kowalski, T., & de Vos, K. (2005). Quantitative architectural analysis: a new approach to cortical mapping. *Anat Embryol (Berl)*, 210(5-6), 373-386.

Schüz, A. (2002). Introduction: Homogeneity and Heterogeneity of Cortical Structure: *A Theme and its Variations (Vol. 5)*. New York: Taylor & Francis.

Senft, S. L., & Woolsey, T. A. (1991). Growth of thalamic afferents into mouse barrel cortex. *Cereb Cortex*, 1(4), 308-335.

Sherwood, C. C., Broadfield, D. C., Holloway, R. L., Gannon, P. J., & Hof, P. R. (2003). Variability of Broca's area homologue in African great apes: implications for language evolution. *Anat Rec A Discov Mol Cell Evol Biol,* 271(2), 276-285.

Sherwood, C. C., Lee, P. W., Rivara, C. B., Holloway, R. L., Gilissen, E. P., & Simmons, R. M. (2003). Evolution of specialized pyramidal neurons in primate visual and motor cortex. *Brain Behav Evol,* 61(1), 28-44.

Sholl, D.A., (1995). The organization of the visual cortex in the cat. *J Anat*. 89(1), 33-46

Shute, C. C. D., & Lewis, P.R. (1961). The use of cholinesterase techniques combined with operative procedures to follow nervous pathways in the brain. *Bibl. Anat.*, 2, 34-49.

Simons, D. J., Durham, D., & Woolsey, T. A. (1984). Functional organization of mouse and rat SmI barrel cortex following vibrissal damage on different postnatal days. *Somatosens Res,* 1(3), 207-245.

Strominger, R. N., & Woolsey, T. A. (1987). Templates for locating the whisker area in fresh flattened mouse and rat cortex. *J Neurosci Methods*, 22(2), 113-118.

Takahata, T., Komatsu, Y., Watakabe, A., Hashikawa, T., Tochitani, S., & Yamamori, T. (2006). Activity-dependent expression of occ1 in excitatory neurons is a characteristic feature of the primate visual cortex. *Cereb Cortex*, 16(7), 929-940.

Timm, F. (1958). [Histochemistry of zinc.*]. Dtsch Z Gesamte Gerichtl Med*, 47(3), 428-431.

Trisler, G. D., Schneider, M. D., & Nirenberg, M. (1981). A topographic gradient of molecules in retina can be used to identify neuron position. *Proc Natl Acad Sci U S A*, 78(4), 2145-2149.

Valente, T., Auladell, C., & Perez-Clausell, J. (2002). Postnatal development of zinc-rich terminal fields in the brain of the rat. *Exp Neurol*, 174(2), 215-229.

Van Essen, D.C. (2004). Towards a quantitative, probabilistic neuroanatomy of cerebral cortex *Cortex,* 40(1), 211-212.

Watts, R., Liston, C., Niogi, S., & Ulug, A. M. (2003). Fiber tracking using magnetic resonance diffusion tensor imaging and its applications to human brain development. *Ment Retard Dev Disabil Res Rev*, 9(3), 168-177.

Wong-Riley, M. (1979). Changes in the visual system of monocularly sutured or enucleated cats demonstrable with cytochrome oxidase histochemistry. *Brain Res*, 171(1), 11-28.

Wong P., & Kaas J. (2008). Architectonic subdivisions of neocortex in the grey squirrel (*Sciurus carolinensis*). *Anat Rec.* 291, 1301-1333.

Woolsey, T. A., & Van der Loos, H. (1970). The structural organization of layer IV in the somatosensory region (SI) of mouse cerebral cortex. The description of a cortical field composed of discrete cytoarchitectonic units. *Brain Res*, 17(2), 205-242.

Yamamori, T., & Rockland, K. S. (2006). Neocortical areas, layers, connections, and gene expression. *Neurosci Res*, 55(1), 11-27.

Zilles, K., Schleicher, A., Palomero-Gallagher N., & Amunts, K. (2002). Quantitative Analysis of cyto- and Receptor Architecture of the human Brain. San Deigo*: Academic Press.*

Zilles, K., & Palomero-Gallagher, N. (2001). Cyto-, myelo-, and receptor architectonics of the human parietal cortex. *Neuroimage,* 14(1 Pt 2), S8-20.

Zilles, K., Palomero-Gallagher, N., Grefkes, C., Scheperjans, F., Boy, C., & Amunts, K. (2002). Architectonics of the human cerebral cortex and transmitter receptor fingerprints: reconciling functional neuroanatomy and neurochemistry. *Eur Neuropsychopharmacol*, 12(6), 587-599.

Zilles, K., Palomero-Gallagher, N., & Schleicher, A. (2004). Transmitter receptors and functional anatomy of the cerebral cortex. *J Anat*, 205(6), 417-432.

Zilles, K., Qu, M., & Schleicher, A. (1993). Regional distribution and heterogeneity of alpha-adrenoceptors in the rat and human central nervous system. *J Hirnforsch*, 34(2), 123-132.

Zilles, K., Schlaug, G., Matelli, M., Luppino, G., Schleicher, A., Qu, M., et al. (1995). Mapping of human and macaque sensorimotor areas by integrating architectonic, transmitter receptor, MRI and PET data. *J Anat*, 187 (Pt 3), 515-537.

Zipser, B., & McKay, R. (1981). Monoclonal antibodies distinguish identifiable neurones in the leech. *Nature,* 289(5798), 549-554.

In: Neuroanatomy Research Advances
Editors: C. E. Flynn and B. R. Callaghan, pp.93-119

ISBN: 978-60741-610-4
©2010 Nova Science Publishers, Inc.

Chapter III

Correlation of Neurotrophin Expression and Survival-Promoting Capacities with Different Programmed Cell Death Periods in the Developing Murine Retina

Elvira Pyziak and Nicole Duenker[*]

Institute for Anatomy, Department of Neuroanatomy, University of Duisburg-Essen, Medical Faculty, 45122 Essen, Germany

Abstract

Programmed cell death (PCD) is a genuine developmental process of the nervous system, affecting not only projecting neurons but also proliferating neural precursors and newly postmitotic neuroblasts. It is widely accepted that during development neurotrophic factors control the survival of different neuronal cell types. In most survival studies published so far, enriched retinal ganglion cell cultures of dissociated cells were used, a system far from being physiological as the neurons lost cell-cell contacts. Besides, in the literature one finds contradictory reports on neurotrophin effects at different time points in retinal development: some studies observed that survival promoting effects of neurotrophins are limited to early neurons, others report effects restricted to differentiated neurons. Last but not least, a multitude of studies analysed survival-promoting effects of neurotrophins under pathological conditions, e.g. the survival of retinal ganglion cells after optic nerve lesion. However, the expression and effect of survival-promoting factors during developmental, naturally occurring PCD has not been investigated so far. In the study presented, we analyzed the cell types expressing neurotrophins and their receptors

---

[*]Corresponding author: Prof. Dr. Nicole Duenker, Institute for Anatomy, Department of Neuroanatomy, University of Duisburg-Essen, Medical Faculty, 45122 Essen, Germany, phone: ++49-(0)201-723-4922, fax: ++49-(0)201-723-5635, e-mail: nicole.duenker@uk-essen.de

by immunocytochemical double labelling with cell type specific markers, correlated the expression profile of neurotrophins and their receptors with naturally occurring PCD periods of the developing retina and compared the survival-promoting capacity of neurotrophin signalling on different cell populations during early and late murine postnatal retinal PCD peaks using an *in vitro* culture system that retains the integrity of the retinal network. We found mRNA levels of the brain derived neurotrophic factor (BDNF) and neurotrophin-4 (NT4) receptor TrkB, insulin and ciliary neurotrophic factor (CNTF) receptors to be up-regulated during murine retinal development and their maximal expression to correlate with the main peaks of postnatal retinal PCD. BDNF, NT4 and insulin exhibited different survival promoting capacities during all postnatal retinal PCD phases affecting early, proliferating neurons as well as different populations of differentiated retinal cells. Although their receptors do not seem to be expressed on photoreceptors, these neurotrophins prevented apoptosis of both retinal ganglion and photoreceptor cells in organotypic murine retinal wholemount cultures. CNTF, by contrast, showed no short-term survival-promoting effect during murine retinal apoptosis, at least not after 24h culture *in vitro*. Thus, this chapter contributes new insights to the controversial discussion about neurotrophin effects on different cell populations and at different time points in retinal PCD.

Introduction

Programmed cell death (PCD) is a genuine developmental process of the nervous system (Buss et al., 2006; Guerin et al., 2006; Danial & Korsmeyer, 2004; Davies, 2003; Lossi & Merighi, 2003; Farkas et al., 2001), affecting not only projecting neurons but also proliferating neural precursors and newly postmitotic neuroblasts (Yeo & Gautier, 2004; Valenciano et al., 2008). In the chick retina, the relative density of PCD *in vivo* is indeed much higher in proliferative and early neurogenic stages of retinal development than during neuronal maturation, innervation and synaptogenesis (Chavarria et al., 2007). In the vertebrate retina, several PCD phases occur, which are controlled by multiple pro-survival signals. In the postnatal mouse retina PCD phases comprise peaks at postnatal day (P) 2, P9 and P15 (Pequignot et al., 2003). At P2, most apoptotic cells are localized in the inner neuroblastic layer, the future ganglion cell layer (GCL). At P9, dying cells comprise neurons of the inner nuclear layer, most likely amacrine cell. Finally, at P15, both the cells of the GCL and outer nuclear layer, comprising photoreceptor nuclei, reveal to contribute to the PCD peak.

As derivatives of the primitive forebrain, the differentiation and maintenance of retinal tissue is conjectured to require neurotrophic support. Among the survival factors active in the nervous system, neurotrophic factors are a class of cell signalling molecules critical for the differentiation and survival of neuronal cells (Vecino et al., 2004; von Bartheld, 1998). One family of neurotrophic factors, the neurotrophins, encompass several proteins that initiate signal transduction through the tyrosine receptor kinase (Trk) family of cell surface receptors. Members of the neurotrophin family and their preferred TrkB receptor include brain-derived neurotrophic factor (BDNF) and neurotrophin-4 (NT 4). Several studies indicate that BDNF as well as NT 4 support the survival of (i) retinal ganglion cells *in vitro* (Johnson et al., 1986; Thanos et al., 1989; Castillo et al., 1994), (ii) target deprived rat retinal ganglion cells after removal of the superior colliculus (Spalding et al., 2004), (iii) retinal interneurons in long-term cultures (Pinzon-Duarte et al., 2004) and rescues photoreceptors from damaging effects of constant light (LaVail et al., 1992). It has been shown that BDNF levels in rat retinal ganglion cells change and that these changes are age-associated. BDNF is up-regulated postnatally in an activity-dependent manner and that visual deprivation diminished the levels of BDNF (Seki et al., 2003). NT4 has been shown to promote survival of developing and adult rat ganglion cells *in vitro* (Cohen et al., 1994; Ary-Pires et al., 1997) and rescues rat ganglion cells from developmental cell death *in vivo* (Cui & Harvey, 1994). Members of the ciliary neurotrophic factor (CNTF) family of cytokines have been shown to influence neuronal differentiation during retinal development and enhance cell survival in various retinal degeneration models (Rhee & Yang, 2003). CNTF is a potent growth factor capable of promoting long-term survival of axotomized retinal ganglion cells (Van Adel et al., 2003) as well as survival after induction of ocular hypertension (Ji et al., 2004). Intravitreal injections of CNTF have been shown to support survival of rat retinal ganglion cells after intraorbital optic nerve transection (Mey & Thanos, 1993). Extrapancreatic (pro)insulin has been shown to stimulate neural development and survival at least in culture (de Pablo & de la Rosa, 1995; Varela-Nieto et al., 2003; for review: Vecino et al., 2004). It has been reported that physiological cell death occurring during the early stages of chick and murine retinal development is regulated by locally produced (pro)insulin (Díaz et al., 1999; 2000; Duenker et al., 2005; Valenciano et al., 2006).

In most survival studies published so far, enriched retinal ganglion cell cultures of dissociated cells were used, a system far from being physiological as the neurons lost cell-cell contacts. When long-term survival was studied, insulin was frequently present in the culture medium used. As we and others showed that insulin has an anti-apoptotic effect by itself (Duenker et al., 2005; Varela-Nieto et al., 2003), it is more than likely that its strong survival-promoting potential obscured the action of neurotrophins tested. Besides, in the literature one can find contradictory reports on neurotrophin effects at different time points in retinal development: some studies observed that survival-promoting effects of neurotrophins are limited to early neurons, other report effects restricted to differentiated neurons. Last but not least, a multitude of studies analysed survival-promoting effects of neurotrophins under pathological conditions, e.g. the survival of retinal ganglion cells after optic nerve lesion or after induction of ocular hypertension. However, to our knowledge, the expression and effect of survival-promoting factors during developmental, naturally occurring PCD has not been investigated so far. Thus, the present study set out to contribute new insights to the controversial discussion about neurotrophin effects at different time points in retinal PCD using an organotypic retinal wholemount culture system close to the *in vivo* situation. For this purpose, we analyzed (a) the cell type, expressing the survival promoting factors BDNF, NT4, insulin and CNTF and their receptors by immunocytochemical double labelling with cell type specific markers, (b) quantified neurotrophin and receptor expression levels during postnatal retinal development and correlated the expression profiles with naturally occurring, developmental cell death periods of the developing murine retina and (c) analyzed and compared the survival-promoting capacity of neurotrophin signalling during murine retinal PCD peaks affecting early, proliferating neurons as well as different populations of differentiated retinal cells.

Material and Methods

Embryos and Tissue Preparation

All experiments were carried out in accordance with the European Communities Council Directive (86/609/EEC) following the Guidelines of the NIH regarding the care and use of animals for experimental procedures. Mouse embryos were collected from timed pregnant C57BL/6 mice (Jackson Laboratory). At postnatal day (P)2, P9, and P15 (= PCD periods) as well as at intermediate stages before and after the cell death peaks (P0, P5, P9, P12, P20) neuroretinas were removed and fixed in 4% paraformaldehyde in 0.1 M phosphate buffer (pH 7.4) for cryo-embedding. Following overnight incubation at 4°C in PBS (pH 7.3) containing 30% sucrose, the tissue was embedded in OCT compound (Tissue-Tek) and sectioned at 10 μm using a cryostat. For Western Blot analysis and RT-PCR (see below) retinas were dissected, removing the connective tissue and the pigment epithelium. From the remaining retinal cup, lens and vitreous body were removed and the neural retina was deep frozen on dry ice. All experiments replicated three times at least in triplicates.

RT-PCR

Series of postnatal murine retinas (P0, P2, P5, P9, P12, P15, P20) were homogenized in 1 ml Trizol (Invitrogen, Karlsruhe, Germany) by manual disruption with an autoclaved plastic pestle and passing the tissue through a 25G needle with a 1 ml insulin syringe several times. The RNA was extracted according to the manufacturer's instructions (Invitrogen). Equal amounts of RNA were subjected to an RT-reaction using oligo(dt)$_{20}$ primers (Invitrogen), employing the SuperScript III reverse transcriptase system (Invitrogen) and following the manufacturer's instructions. An additional DNaseI (Invitrogen) digestion was performed in advance to avoid cross contamination with genomic DNA. 1.5 μl of the RT-reaction product were taken for PCR with BDNF, NT4, TrkB, CNTF, CNTFR, InsR and GAPDH (Glyseraldehyde-3-phosphate dehydrogenase) specific primers, partially already published: BDNF$_{for}$ 5`-ggtatccaaaggccaactga-3`; BDNF$_{rev}$ 5`-cttatgaatcgccagccaat-3`; NT4$_{for}$ 5`-CCCTGCGTCAGTACTTCTTGAGAC-3`; NT4$_{rev}$ 5`-CTGGACGTCAGG CACGGCCTGTTC-3` (Botchkarev et al., 1999; Spears et al., 2003); TrkB$_{for}$ 5`-ATGGCCCAGAGGGTAACCC-3`; TrkB$_{rev}$ 5`-CTCTCTGGAGGCATCCAT-3` (Singh et al., 1997; Spears et al., 2003); CNTF$_{for}$ 5`-gccttgactcagtggatggt-3`; CNTF$_{rev}$ 5`-aggcagaaacttggagcgta-3`; InsR$_{for}$ 5`-tgccagtgatgtgtttccat-3`; InsR$_{rev}$ 5`-tcgatccgttctcgaagact-3`; GAPDH$_{for}$ 5`-CATCACCATCTTGGAGC-3`; GAPDH$_{rev}$ 5`-ATGACCTTGCCC ACAGCCTT-3` (Invitrogen). PCR-products were amplified using an expand high fidelity Taq polymerase (Roche) and employing the following conditions: (i) 10 min at 94°C; (ii) 35 to 37 amplification cycles: 30 sec at 94°C, 45 sec at 60°C (55°C for TrkB), 45 sec at 72°C; (ii) 5 min at 72°C. The PCR products were separated on a 2% agarose gel and stained with ethidium bromide.

Immunoblots

For Western blot analysis, a series of postnatal murine retinas (P0, P2, P5, P9, P12, P15, P20) were homogenized in modified Ripa buffer (0.5% sodium deoxycholate / 0.1% SDS in PBS) and the extracts fractionated in a 7.5-15% SDS-PAGE and transferred to a nitrocellulose membrane by tank blotting with 25 mM Tris/HCl, pH 8.7, 192 mM glycine, 10% methanol as transfer buffer. Membranes were blocked in phosphate buffer saline (PBS; pH 7.4) with 0.1% Tween20 (TBS) and 5% bovine serum albumin and incubated 3hrs at room temperature or overnight at 4°C (for CNTFRα) with the following primary antibodies 1:150 (1:300 for CNTFRα) in TBS with 3% bovine serum albumin: NT4 (Santa Cruz, N-20, sc-545), an affinity purified rabbit polyclonal antibody raised against a peptide mapping within the internal region of NT-4 of human origin; TrkB (Santa Cruz, 794, sc-12), an affinity purified rabbit polyclonal antibody raised against a peptide mapping within a C-terminal cytoplasmic domain of TrkB of mouse origin, CNTF (Santa Cruz, FL-200, sc-13996), a rabbit polyclonal antibody raised against amino acids 1-200 representing full length CNTF of human origin, CNTFRα (BD-Pharmingen; cat# 558891), an affinity purified mouse monoclonal antibody, and InsRβ (Santa Cruz, C-19, sc-711), an affinity purified rabbit polyclonal antibody raised against a peptide mapping at the C-terminus of insulin Rβ of human origin. After three washes with TBS, the membranes were incubated for 1h with the respective secondary antibody (horseradish peroxidase (HRP)-conjugated anti-rabbit IgG (DAKO, Germany) at a dilution of 1:2000 in TBS. Signals were developed by the SuperSignal West Pico Chemiluminescent Substrate (Pierce, Bonn, Germany) and visualized in a chemiluminescence imager (Chemi Genius, Bio Imaging Systems, Syngene). Densitometric measurements were performed by quantifying the density of the bands *vs* the local background using Bio Imaging System software (Syngene). All blots were re-stained with mouse anti-actin (sc-1616, 1:200; Santa Cruz) to verify equal protein loading in all lanes.

ELISA

Retinal BDNF content was analyzed using a BDNF ELISA (enzyme linked immunoassay; Promega) and proinsulin/insulin content was detected by an ultra-sensitive mouse insulin ELISA (enzyme linked immunoassay; Mercodia, Uppsala, Sweden) following the manufacturer's instructions.

Immunocytochemistry

Ten-micrometer cryo-sections were pre-incubated with 10% normal donkey serum (NDS) in phosphate buffer saline (PBS; pH 7.4) for 1h. Immunostaining for NT4, CNTF, TrkB and InsR was performed using the same antibodies used for Western Blotting at dilutions of 1:400. For detection of BDNF, we used a rabbit polyclonal antibody (Santa Cruz; N-20; sc-546; 1:200), raised against a peptide mapping at the amino terminus of the mature BDNF of human origin and for detection of CNTFR on sections, we used an affinity purified goat polyclonal antibody, raised against a peptide mapping at the C-terminus of CNTFRα of rat origin (Santa Cruz, R-20, sc-1914; 1:1:00). For detection of photoreceptor cells in retinal cell suspension, cytospins were incubated with the photoreceptor marker mouse anti-opsin (Sigma) at a dilution of 1:10,000. For detection of ganglion and amacrine cells the respective material was incubated with the ganglion cell-specific, nuclear marker Brn3a (Chemicon; 1:100) or the amacrine cell marker calretinin (Swant; 1:2000) respectively. Following 1h permeabilisation with 3mg/ml BSA/ 100 mM glycine / 0.25% triton, endogenous biotin was blocked using a biotin blocking kit (DAKO). After overnight incubation with the respective maker, the reaction was visualized using the respective biotynylated IgGs (1:200) and streptavidin-conjugated Cy3 or FITC secondary antibodies (MoBiTec; Goettingen, Germany) at a dilution of 1:800. Cytospins and sections were analyzed with a NIKON Eclipse E600 microscope equipped with epifluorescence, a NIKON CCD camera and NIKON Eclipsenet software. As controls, in all cases PBS was substituted for the primary antisera in order to test for nonspecific labeling. No specific cellular staining was observed when the primary antiserum was omitted.

The effect of recombinant BDNF, NT4 and insulin treatment on different cell populations was scored as described previously (Beier et al., 2006). In brief, at least 1000 cells and 10 apoptotic nuclei per DAPI-stained cytospin were counted and the percentage of (i) apoptotic Brn3a-positive RGCs and (ii) apoptotic opsin-positive photoreceptor neurons with condensed nuclei in relation to the total number of pycnotic DAPI-positive cells was calculated.

Retinal Cultures

Eyes were dissected from mice on postnatal days (P) 2, P9, and P15. Lens, vitreous body and pigment epithelium were removed, and the neural retinas pre-incubated with 0.5 mg/ml hyaluronidase for 15 min at 37°C. Retinas were cultured for 24h as organotypic wholemounts in 2 ml chemically defined medium as described previously (Duenker et al., 2005). Cultures were maintained for 24h at 37°C in a 5% CO_2 atmosphere. In dose response experiments cultures were treated with different concentrations (0.1-20 ng/ml; for insulin: 0.1-1000 ng/ml) recombinant human BDNF (tebu-bio), NT4 (tebu-bio), CNTF (tebu-bio), Insulin (Sigma) to determine anti-apoptotic effects. All recombinant factors are produced in *E. coli*, purified by SDS-PAGE gel, high performance S-sepharose column and HPLC analyses to purity greater than 98%. According to the manufacturers, the biological activity of BDNF and NT4 was determined by the dose-dependent (20-50 ng/ml) induction of choline acetyl transferase activity in rat basal forebrain primary septal cell cultures. The biological activity of recombinant CNTF was determined by its ability to stimulate proliferation of human TF-1 cells using concentrations between 50 and 150ng/ml.

Detection of Apoptosis and Proliferation

Apoptotic cell death was determined by counting 4',6-Diamidino-2-phenylindole (DAPI)-stained pyknotic nuclei of retinal single cell suspension after dissociating cultured wholemount retinas. For cell scoring of DAPI stained nuclei, retinas were dissociated into single cell suspension by incubation at 37°C with 5U/ml collagenase (Sigma), 1mg/ml trypsin (Sigma), and 0.125mg/ml hyaluronidase (Sigma), followed by passes through a siliconized Pasteur pipette. Digestion of the tissue was stopped by addition of EDTA and cells were fixed for 1h in 4% paraformaldehyde in 0.1 M phosphate buffer (pH 7.4). An aliquot of the cell suspension was spotted on a slide using a cytospin at 700 rpm for 7 min. Cells were stained and mounted with 4`,6-diamidino-2-phenylindole (DAPI 2 µg/ml; Sigma).

Results

BDNF is Expressed in Retinal Ganglion and Amacrine Cells and Expression is Up-Regulated During Late PCD Periods

Quantifying BDNF expression levels during postnatal retinal development and correlating the expression profiles with naturally occurring, developmental cell death periods of the developing murine retina, we found moderate BDNF mRNA levels from P0 to P5, including the early PCD peak at P2. BDNF mRNA expression was however up-regulated at P9 and P15, the late PCD periods, and these higher levels persist till P20 (Fig. 1A). On protein level, expression of BDNF likewise increased at P9 and persists high with a slight, non-significant decrease at P15 (Fig. 1B). Immunocytochemical double labelling studies with the established ganglion cell marker Brn3a and the amacrine cell marker calretinin revealed that BDNF is expressed on retinal amacrine and dislocated amacrine cells (Fig. 1C) as well as on ganglion cells (Fig. 1D) during retinal PCD periods P2 (data not shown), P9 and P15.

NT4 is Uniformly Expressed Throughout Retinal Development, but Likewise Localized in Retinal Ganglion and Amacrine Cells

In contrast to BDNF, we found NT4, a member of the same family of neurotrophins, to be uniformly expressed throughout postnatal retinal development, on mRNA (Fig. 1E) as well as on protein level (Fig. 1F). No changes in expression correlating with PCD peaks were detectable. Like the expression of BDNF, expression of NT4 is restricted to amacrine and ganglion cell populations during retinal PCD periods (Fig. 1G,H).

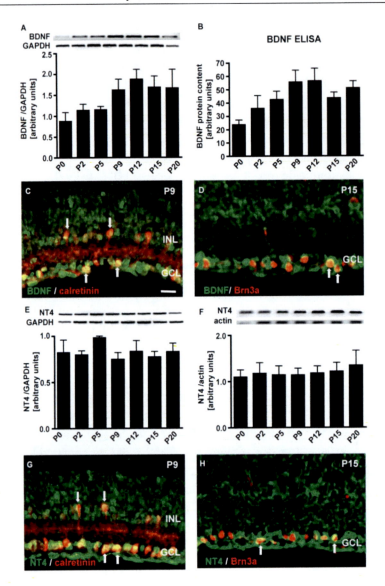

Figure 1. Analysis of BDNF content in the developing postnatal murine retina by RT-PCR (A) and ELISA assay (B). Quantification of RT-PCR on BDNF expression (A) revealed moderate BDNF mRNA levels from murine postnatal (*P*) stage P0 to P5, including the early PCD peak at P2. BDNF mRNA expression was however up-regulated at P9 and P15, the late PCD periods, and these higher levels persist till P20. Protein levels of BDNF likewise increased at P9. (B). All experiments were replicated at least in triplicates. Values are means ± s.e.m. Immunocytochemical double labeling studies with the established amacrine cell marker calretinin and the ganglion cell marker Brn3a (red fluorescence) revealed that BDNF (green fluorescence) is expressed in amacrine, dislocated amacrine and ganglion cells (C,D). Scale bar 20 μm (C) also applies for D,G,H. E,F Analysis of NT4 content in the developing postnatal murine retina by RT-PCR (E) and Western Blot (F). The level of NT4 mRNA (E) and protein (F) remains nearly constant during postnatal murine retinal development. Double labeling study of NT4 (green fluorescence) with Brn3a and calretinin (red fluorescence) revealed that NT4 immunoreactivity is likewise restricted to the ganglion cell layer (*GCL*) and the inner nuclear layer (*INL*) of the developing P9 (G), and P15 (H) retina. White arrows in C,D and G,H point to double labelled neurons in the *GCL* and *INL*, co-localising the respective neurotrophin and the neuron specific marker.

mRNA Levels of TrkB Receptors are Upregulated During Murine Retinal PCD Peaks

Quantification of mRNA levels for the BDNF and NT4 receptor TrkB during murine retinal development revealed a correlation of expression peaks with the maxima of retinal PCD at P2, P9 and P15 (Fig. 2A). On protein level, however, the expression level remains constant (Fig. 2B). Corresponding to the expression profile of its ligands, the TrkB receptor was found to be expressed on the surface of retinal amacrine cells and ganglion cells (Fig. 2C,D).

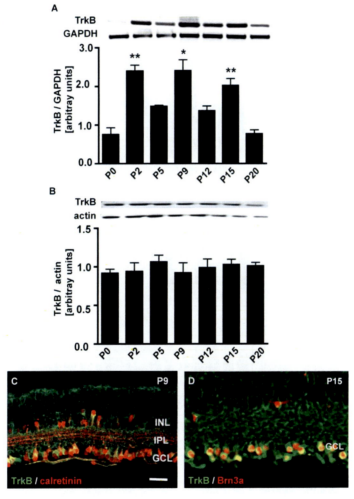

Figure 2. Analysis of TrkB expression by RT-PCR (A), Western blot (B) and immunocytochemical double labelling studies (C,D). During postnatal (*P*) murine retinal development maxima of mRNA levels for the BDNF and NT4 receptor TrkB correlate with the maxima of retinal PCD at P2, P9 and P15 (A). On protein level, however, no correlation between TrkB expression peaks with the maxima of retinal PCD could be observed (B). Values are means ± s.e.m. Immunoreactivity for the TrkB receptor was found in retinal amacrine cells and ganglion cells (C,D), corresponding to the expression profile of its ligands. Scale bar 20 µm (C) also applies for D

BDNF and NT4 have Different Survival Promoting Capacity During Retinal PCD Phases

In dose-response experiments, organotypic murine retinal wholemount cultures were treated for 24h with different concentration of recombinant human BDNF (Fig. 3A,B,C) and NT4 (Fig. 3D,E,F) respectively, to test the effect of the two neurotrophins on the survival of retinal neurons at the main PCD stages P2, P9 and P15. Apoptosis levels were quantified by counting DAPI-stained pyknotic nuclei in cytospins of retinal single cell suspension after dissociating cultured wholemount retinae. No survival promoting effect could be detected for BDNF or NT4 at concentrations lower than 0.1ng/ml (0.01 and 0.05ng/ml; data not shown).

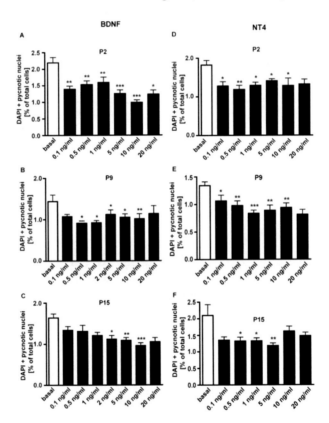

Figure 3. Effect of BDNF and NT4 on the number of apoptotic cells in the developing murine retina. Data gained from DAPI-stained cell counts of cytospins. In dose-response experiments murine P2 (A,D), P9 (B,E) and P15 (C,F) retinal wholemount were treated for 24h with different concentration of recombinant human BDNF (A-C) and NT4 (D-F), respectively. At P2, both, BDNF (A) and NT4 (D) showed a significant survival promoting effect, but the rescue capacity of BDNF appeared to be stronger than the NT4 effect. At P9 (B,E) and P15 (C,F), both BDNF and NT4 showed a similar rescuing effect, but in comparison to the two earlier PCD phases, the survival promoting capacities of both neurotrophins is apparently less effective at this stage. Values are means ± s.e.m. *$P<0.05$; **$P<0.01$; *** $P<0.001$ calculated by one way Annova test and Newman-Keuls Post test comparing all experimental groups.

At P2, both, BDNF and NT4 showed a significant survival promoting effect at a concentration of 0.1ng/ml (Fig. 3A,D). The rescue capacity of BDNF, however, turned out to be stronger than the NT4 effect at this PCD stage, especially at higher concentrations (5, 10 and 20ng/ml). At a concentration of 10ng/ml BDNF treatment has the maximal effect and results in a 1.8-fold decrease in the number of pycnotic neurons (Fig. 3A). Application of NT4, by contrast, only results in a 0.2- (10ng/ml) to 0.5-fold decrease (0.5ng/ml) in the number of apoptotic cells. At P9 BDNF treatment exerted the same survival promoting effect as NT4 application. Although NT4 already rescues neurons at a concentration of 0.1ng/ml (Fig. 3E), application of both, BDNF or NT4 to the cultures maximally results in a 0.5-fold decrease in the number of apoptotic cells (Fig. 3B,E). At P15, BDNF and NT4 likewise showed a similar rescuing effect (Fig. 3C,F). At a concentration of 10ng/ml BDNF treatment has the maximal effect and result in a 0.9-fold decrease in the number of pycnotic neurons (Fig. 3C). Application of NT4 has a maximal 0.6-fold rescuing effect at a concentration of 5ng/ml (Fig. 3F).

Insulin Levels are Uniform During Retinal Development, whereas mRNA Levels of the InsR are Up-Regulated During Murine Retinal PCD Peaks

Quantification of mRNA levels for the InsR during murine retinal development revealed a correlation of expression peaks with the maxima of retinal PCD at P2, P9 and P15 (Fig. 4A), InsR protein levels (Fig. 4B) and insulin content (Fig. 4C) remain, however, constant in all developmental stages investigated. Like the TrkB receptor, during retinal PCD periods, the InsR is likewise expressed on amacrine cells (data not shown) and ganglion cells (Fig. 4D).

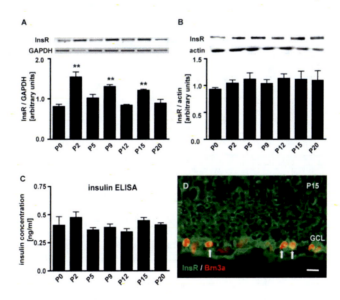

Figure 4. Quantification of mRNA (A) and protein (B) levels for the InsR and insulin (C) during postnatal (P) murine retinal development. Semi-quantitative RT-PCR revealed a correlation of expression peaks of InsR mRNA levels with the maxima of retinal PCD at P2, P9 and P15 (A), whereas Western Blot (B) and ELISA assay (C) showed that InsR protein levels (B) and insulin concentration (C) remain constant in all developmental stages investigated. Values are means ± s.e.m. As revealed by immunocytochemical double labelling studies with the ganglion cell marker Brn3a (red fluorescence), the InsR (green fluorescence) is expressed on cells of the ganglion cell layer (*GCL*; white arrows in D). Scale bar 20 μm (D)

CNTF Expression Gradually Increases During Murine Retinal Development, but Expression Maxima of the CNTFR Correlate with the Main PCD Peaks

Similar to the expression profile of BDNF, we found CNTF mRNA and protein levels to increase, however, more gradually during murine retinal development (Fig. 5A,B). Like TrkB and InsR, the CNTFR mRNA levels exhibit maxima, correlating with the main PCD peaks at P2, P9 and P15 (Fig. 5C), whereas the CNTFR protein level remains constant during postnatal murine retinal development (Fig. 5D). Immunocytochemical double labelling studies of P2 (data not shown), P9 and P15 retinas – corresponding to the PCD phases- revealed that the CNTFR is likewise localized on the surface of calretinin-positive amacrine cells in the INL and displaced amacrine cells of the GCL (Fig. 5E) as well as on the surface of Brn3a-positive ganglion cells of the GCL (Fig. 5F).

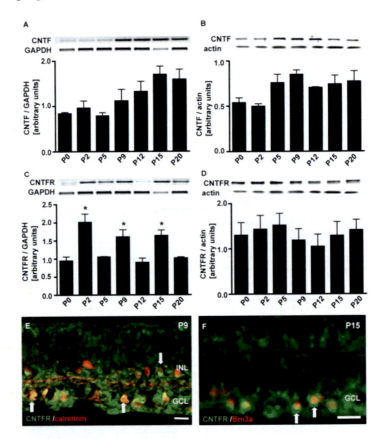

Figure 5. Analysis of CNTF and CNTFR expression by RT-PCR (A,C), Western blot (B,D) and immunocytochemical double labelling studies (E,F). CNTF mRNA (A) and protein levels (B) increase gradually during murine retinal development. CNTFR mRNA levels exhibit maxima, correlating with the main PCD peaks at P2, P9 and P15 (C), whereas the CNTFR protein level remains constant during postnatal murine retinal development (D). Values are means ± s.e.m. Immunocytochemical double labelling studies revealed that the CNTFR (green fluorescence) is likewise localized on the surface of calretinin-positive amacrine cells (red fluorescence) of the inner nuclear layer (*INL*) and ganglion cell layer (*GCL*; white arrows in E) as well as Brn3a-positive cells (red fluorescence) of the *GCL* (white arrows in F). Scale bar 20 µm (E,F)

Insulin Significantly Prevents PCD of Retinal Neurons, whereas CNTF Shows no Survival Promoting Effects During Murine Retinal PCD Periods

In dose-response experiments murine retinal wholemount cultures were treated for 24h with different concentration of recombinant human insulin or CNTF respectively, to determine the survival promoting capacity of the two factors. As revealed by cell counts in DAPI-stained cytospins, application of recombinant insulin to murine organotypic retinal wholemount cultures at the main phases of naturally occurring PCD resulted in a significant

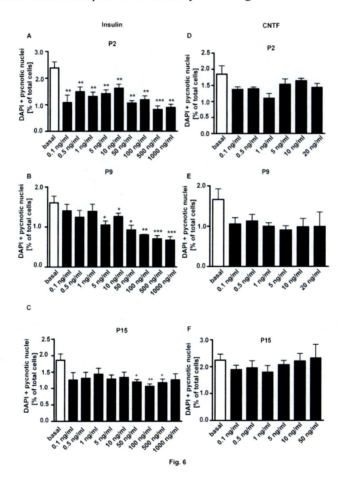

Fig. 6

Figure 6. Effect of insulin and CNTF on the number of apoptotic cells in the developing murine retina. Data gained from DAPI-stained cell counts of cytospins. In dose-response experiments murine P2 (A,D), P9 (B,E) and P15 (C,F) retinal wholemount were treated for 24h with different concentration of recombinant human insulin (A-C) and CNTF (D-F), respectively. Application of recombinant insulin to murine organotypic retinal wholemount cultures at the main phases of naturally occurring significantly prevented PCD of retinal neurons (A-C), whereas no significant survival promoting effect could be observed after CNTF treatment, irrespective of the PCD stage investigated (D-F). At P2, insulin exerted the strongest survival promoting effect with a two-fold decrease in the number of apoptotic bodies already at a concentration of 0.1ng/ml. At P9 and P15, the survival promoting effect was less pronounced and a two-fold significant rescuing effect was visible only after application of 100 ng/ml. Values are means ± s.e.m. *P<0.05; **P<0.01; *** P<0.001 calculated by one way Annova test and Newman-Keuls Post test comparing all experimental groups.

decrease in the number of pycnotic nuclei at P2, P9 and P15 (Fig. 6A-C), whereas no significant survival promoting effect could be observed after CNTF treatment, irrespective of the PCD stage investigated (Fig. 6D-F). At P2, insulin exerted the strongest survival promoting effect with a 1.5-fold decrease in the number of apoptotic bodies already at a concentration of 0.1ng/ml. At P9 and P15, the survival promoting effect was less pronounced and a 1.0-fold significant decrease in the number of pycnotic cells was visible only after application of 100ng/ml. At P9, higher concentrations (500 and 1000ng/ml) could further increase the rescuing effect, whereas at P15, the survival promoting capacity of insulin was strongest at a concentration of 100ng/ml.

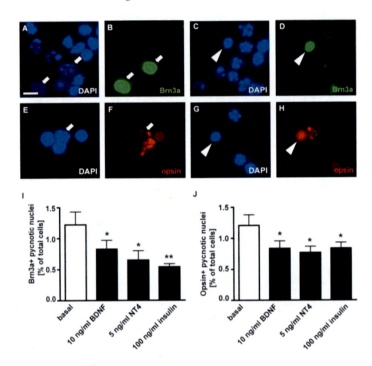

Figure 7. Effect of recombinant BDNF, NT4 and insulin treatment on the number of ganglion and photoreceptor cells in P15 murine retinal wholemount cultures. The Brn3a antibody specifically labelled retinal ganglion cells (RGC; white arrows in A,B). Opsin immunocytochemistry was used to specifically label photoreceptor cells (white arrows in E,F) in DAPI counterstained cytospins. Brn3a and opsin immunoreactivity was frequently found in apoptotic nuclei (white arrowhead in C,D and G,H). Scale bar in (A) = 20μm also applies for B-H. Quantification of cell counting from cytospins after treatment of murine retinal cultures with recombinant BDNF, NT4 and insulin resulted in a significant decrease in the total number of Brn3a-positive RGCs (I) and opsin-positive photoreceptor cells (J). Values are means ± s.e.m. ** P<0.01 statistical differences compared to basal group, calculated by one way Anova test and Newman-Keuls Post test comparing all experimental groups.

BDNF, NT4 and Insulin Prevent Apoptosis of Ganglion Cells and Photoreceptors During Late PCD of the P15 Murine Retina

To test the survival promoting effect of BDNF, NT4 and insulin treatment on different cell populations in the P15 murine retina, where ganglion and photoreceptor cells are susceptible to die during the late postnatal PCD period, a Brn3a antibody was used to specifically label retinal ganglion cells (Fig. 7A-D), and an opsin antibody to detect photoreceptor cells (Fig. 7E-H) in DAPI-counterstained cytospins from murine retinal cultures. Quantification of cell counting from cytospins after treatment of murine retinal cultures with recombinant BDNF, NT4 and insulin showed a significant decrease in the total number of apoptotic Brn3a-positive RGCs (Fig. 7I) and pycnotic opsin-positive photoreceptor cells (Fig. 7J). Thus, all three neurotrophic factors exert a survival promoting effect on both retinal neuron populations, ganglion cells and photoreceptor cells.

Conclusion

Many of the reported effects of neurotrophins in the central nervous system have been established on dissociated cell cultures. However, conclusions gathered from these experiments cannot always be transferred to the *in vivo* situation. Differences are at least to some extent due to the disintegration of the neuronal network and a loss of normal cell-cell interactions. Knock-out animals would provide an ideal animal model to test the effects of neurotrophins on retinal development; their use is limited, however, by low survival and the many peripheral problems related to pleiotropic effects of the neurotrophin gene mutation. In the present study, we used organotypic retinal wholemount cultures to investigate the survival promoting capacity of different neurotrophins. This *in vitro* system retains the integrity of the retinal network (Pinzon-Duarte et al., 2004) and constitutes an optimal model to study the effect of exogenous applied substances of cell types in the retina.

In the study presented, we investigated and compared the expression and survival-promoting capacities of BDNF, NT4, insulin and CNTF and their receptors during the three main programmed cell death (PCD) phases of the developing postnatal murine retina. Former studies mainly focussed on one or two developmental stages, mostly without referring to naturally occurring PCD peaks. In this context, it has been reported that the influence of neurotrophic factors on retinal cell survival depends on the stage of development of the retina (Vecino et al., 2004). In the literature, controversial statements on neurotrophin effects at different time points in retinal development can be found. Some authors describe survival promoting effects limited to early stages of neuronal development, others state neurotrophic actions restricted to differentiated neurons.

Expression and Survival Promoting Effect of BDNF

In previous studies, BDNF expression has been observed in the ganglion cell layer (GCL) and inner nuclear layer (INL) of the developing and adult rodent (Perez & Caminos, 1995; Bennett et al., 1999; Pollock et al., 2001; Rohrer et al., 2001; Vecino et al., 1998; 2002) and chick retina (Vecino et al., 1998; Das et al., 1997). In situ hybridisation combined with retrograde labelling of RGCs revealed that displaced ACs rather than RGCs are the main source of BDNF mRNA in the GCL of the chick retina (Herzog & von Bartheld, 1998). Seki et al. (2003) examined the distribution of BDNF in the developing rat retina. Double-labelling studies with neuron specific MAP2 antibody, however, only allow distinguishing between

RGCs and displaced AC by size. We used cell type specific markers for RGCs (Brn3a) and ACs (calretinin) and found BDNF to be localized in both populations of retinal neurons, RGCs and ACs at all retinal stages analysed. Di Polo et al. (2000) found BNDF and immunoreactivity for its TrkB receptor co-localized in cone outer segments. We, however, could not detect any immunosignal for BDNF or TrkB (see below) in the outer retina at any developmental stage investigated.

Frost et al. (2001) reported on changes in BDNF protein levels in the developing hamster retina. Immunoassays revealed that BDNF protein concentration remains low through postnatal day (P) 12 and then increases 4.5-fold to attain its adult level on P18. This expression profile nearly reflects our results from BDNF ELISA assays and RT-PCR experiments. The developmental changes in the hamster retina correlated with structural and functional maturation events of the developing retinal projection system. The authors state that most of the normal developmental elimination of RGCs occurs during the epoch when BDNF protein levels are at their peak in the superior colliculus and low in the retina of the hamster visual system (Frost et al., 2001). In line with these results, murine RGC death takes place at P2, when we found BDNF levels to be low. In the rat retina both protein and mRNA levels of BDNF increase after P14 (Seki et al., 2003). As the level of BDNF protein in the retinas of visually deprived eyes was lower than in control eyes the authors concluded that BDNF expression in RGCs is up-regulated in an activity-dependent manner (Seki et al., 2003). Pollock et al. (2001) likewise found BDNF protein levels in the rat retina to be higher during the light phase of the circadian cycle than during the dark phase. They suggested early sensory experience alters the trafficking and synthesis of the BDNF protein. Along this line, it has been demonstrated that in the chick retina BDNF expression peaks around E12-E15 and mRNA levels are up-regulated by light exposure (Hallböök et al., 1996; Karlsson & Hallböök, 1998). In the present study, we did not detect a correlation between BDNF expression and light exposure: mice open their eyes around P15 and an increase in BDNF mRNA and protein content was observed already around P9.

Previous studies showed that BDNF, through TrkB activation, acts as a trophic factor controlling the survival of retinal neurons (Vecino et al., 2004). On the one hand, it has been reported that BDNF controls PCD that affects early postmitotic neuroblasts (Frade et al., 1999). In the chick retina, the application of BDNF to embryos *in ovo* prevented retinal cell death during the early period of developmental cell death (E5-E7). The addition of exogenous applied BDNF to embryos resulted in an approximately 70% increase in the number of RGCs in both E6 and E9 chick retinas (Frade et al., 1997). Drum et al. (1996), however, found that exogenous administration of BDNF to chick embryos *in ovo* did not prevent normal chick RGC death (Drum et al., 1996). One possible explanation for this phenomenon is that the protective effect of BDNF is merely transient. In line with this explanation, in BDNF null mutants, no effect on the final number of axons in the optic nerve could be detected (Cellerino et al., 1997; Rohrer et al., 2001) and BDNF [-/-] mice have normal numbers of RGCs (Jones et al., 1994; Cellerino et al., 1997). Besides, Johnson et al. (1986) reported that within dissociated cultures from E17 rat retinas, the number of surviving neurons, positive for the RGC marker Thy-1 could be kept constant for at least 4 days, whereas the survival of postnatal rat retinal neurons was only transiently increased by the application of BDNF. Rodriguez-Tebar et al. (1989), by contrast, found BDNF to promote the survival of differentiated RGCs. They found that at E5, when naturally occurring PCD peaks but RGC axons have not yet reached their target, chick RGCs survived *in vitro* irrespective of the presence or absence of BDNF, contradicting the results of Frade et al. (1999). With increasing age the BDNF dependency for survival of chick RGC increased, and the authors concluded that RGCs *in vitro* depend on BDNF for survival only when their axons have reached their targets *in vivo* (Rodriguez-Tebar et al., 1989). These contradictory results might also be explained in terms of different experimental set ups: *in ovo* application (Frade et al., 1999) vs. *in vitro* cell culture (Rodriguez-Tebar et al., 1989). Thus, the role of neurotrophic factors at the later stages of PCD is far from being transparent (Guerin et al., 2006) and up to now it was unclear whether neurotrophic factors are crucial to RGC survival at all during later stages of RGC death (Bähr, 2000).

Using a murine retinal wholemount culture system, an experimental setting close to the *in vivo* situation, we re-addressed this question, comparing the survival-promoting capacity of BDNF application at different PCD stages. We found BDNF to exert the strongest survival-promoting effects at P2, the early RGC death period, resembling the results of Frade et al. (1999) for the chick retina. At later stages of PCD, when apoptosis mostly affects cells of the INL (P9), and differentiated RGCs and photoreceptors (PR; P15), the rescuing effect of BDNF application was less pronounced, but still evident.

Cusato et al. (2002) showed that providing 50 ng/ml BDNF in P5 and P7 rat whole-retina culture assays modulates the frequency of dying cells in the amacrine cell layer, but had no effect upon cells of the GCL at this developmental retinal stage (Cusato et al., 2002). Pinzon-Duarte et al. (2004) reported that the application of 100ng/ml BNDF to organotypic rat retinal cultures promotes the survival of cells in the GCL and in the INL, but was not enough to prevent cell loss of photoreceptors. It has, however, been demonstrated that BDNF can prevent photoreceptor cell degeneration caused by mutation and damaging effects of constant light (La Vail et al., 1992; 1998). The neuroprotective effect of BDNF on photoreceptors and the confinement of its receptors to the inner retina (see below) make it likely that BDNF can act via direct and indirect pathways (Pinzon-Duarte et al., 2004). Wahlin et al. (2000) investigated if the survival-promoting effects of BDNF occur by direct action of the factor on PRs or indirectly through the activation of other cells. The results of the study support the hypothesis that BDNF acts indirectly through the activation of Müller cells and perhaps other non-photoreceptor cells (Wahlin et al., 2000).

Comparison of BDNF and NT4 Effects

It has been shown that NT4 like BDNF increases the survival of developing and adult rat RGCs *in vitro* (Cohen et al., 1994; Ary-Pires et al., 1997). Besides, several studies showed that *in vivo* intraocular injection of recombinant BDNF and NT4 into rat eyes reduce naturally occurring RGC death (Cui & Harvey, 1994; Spalding et al., 2004). Knockout analysis by Harada et al. (2005), however, showed that NT4 alone plays no significant role in retinal development. Analysis of null mutations of BDNF in combination with NT4 increased the peak rate of developmental RGC death, but null mutation of NT4 alone was ineffective (Pollock et al., 2003; Harada et al., 2005). Studies using combinatorial neurotrophin deletions reveal that while BDNF and NT4 subserve distinct neuron populations in most cases, other neuron sub-populations can be supported by either BDNF or NT4, providing evidence for compensatory actions between these neurotrophins (Conover & Yancopoulos, 1997). Knocking the NT4 gene into the BDNF locus rescued BDNF deficient mice and likewise revealed distinct NT4 and BDNF activities (Fan et al., 2000). Kashiwagi et al. (2000) investigated the effects of BNDF and NT4 on isolated cultured P2 rat RGCs by FACS analysis. Testing different concentrations of BDNF, the authors found BDNF to improve the survival rate of RGCs at the highest concentration tested (100ng/ml), whereas NT4 did not significantly improved the survival rate irrespective of the concentration used (0.1, 1, 10 and 100ng/ml). Along this line, a previous study showed that BDNF has an increasing effect upon survival of RGCs from newborn rat retinas at doses ranging from 1 to 100ng/ml, while NT4 had a maximum trophic effect at 10–20ng/ml, and no trophic effect at 100ng/ml (Ary-Pires et al., 1997). We likewise observed different survival-promoting capacities for NT4 and BDNF: at P2, the rescue capacity of BDNF was stronger than the NT4 effect. It has been suggested that the distinct activities of NT4 and BDNF may result from differential activation of the TrKB receptor and its downstream signals (Fan et al., 2000). We, however, could not detect any immunosignal for TrkB in the outer retina at any developmental stage investigated.

In the present study, the use of cultures of different stages of development indirectly implicate effects on different neuronal populations as at P2 PCD affects RGCs, at P9 cells of the INL and at P15 RGCs and PRs (Pequignot et al., 2003). Additionally, we investigated the survival-promoting effect of BDNF and NT4 on certain cell populations by immuncytochemical staining of cytospins with specific markers after culture, allowing distinguishing between dying PR and RGCs at P15. We found BDNF and NT4 to prevent apoptosis of both RGCs and PR during the late PCD period of the P15 retina.

Thus, the present study contributes new insights to the controversial discussion about BNDF and NT4 survival-promoting capacities at different time points in retinal PCD and their effect on different neuronal populations.

TrkB Expression

Expression of the BDNF and NT4 receptor TrkB has been localized immunocytochemically or by in situ hybridisation in RGC and a subpopulation of ACs of the INL in the embryonic, postnatal and adult rodent retina (Ernfors et al., 1992; Jelsma et al., 1993; Rickman & Brecha, 1995; Koide et al., 1995; Perez & Caminos, 1995; Ugolini et al., 1995; Garner et al., 1996; Cellerino & Kohler, 1997; Karlsson & Hallböök, 1998; Cellerino et al., 1997; Vecino et al., 2002) and in chicken retinas (Cellerino et al., 1995; Garner et al., 1996; Hallböök et al., 1996), but not on bipolar cells and rod and cone photoreceptors (Ugolini et al., 1995; Cellerino & Kohler, 1997; Rohrer et al., 2001; Di Polo et al., 2000). In the newborn and postnatal rat retina, the TrkB receptor is localized in the INL as well as in cells of the GCL (Rickman & Brecha, 1995). We confirmed this expression pattern for the developing mouse retina, using immunocytochemical double-labelling techniques to identify the specific cell types expressing TrkB receptors as ACs and RGCs. We likewise did not detect any staining in the PR layer.

Ugolini et al. (1995) found TrkB mRNA expression to parallel the time of differentiation and the beginning of PCD in various retinal layers. In line with these results, we found TrkB mRNA maxima to correlate with the main PCD peaks, indicating an involvement of BDNF and NT4 signalling—via the TrkB receptor—in developmental death dynamics, also suggested by TrkB knockout studies (Klein et al., 1993; Pollock et al., 2003).

InsR Expression and Insulin Rescuing Effect

Extrapancreatic (pro) insulin and the insulin receptor seem to play an important role in the regulation of proliferative stages of retinal neurogenesis. It has been reported that neural development is regulated, at least in culture, by (pro)insulin (de Pablo & de la Rosa, 1995; Varela-Nieto et al., 2003; for review: Vecino et al., 2004). Thus, it has been suggested that these factors are important autocrine and paracrine signals during development of the CNS.

(Pro)insulin mRNA is broadly expressed in the early embryonic chick retina, and decreases later between days 6 and 8 of embryonic development (Díaz et al., 2000). It has therefore been speculated that the control of early processes in chick neurogenesis rely on insulin. Insulin-like immunoreactivity in the human and murine retina has been observed in the INL, GCL, outer and inner plexiform layers (Das et al., 1984). Hyndman (1993) detected insulin receptor immunoreactivity in the developing chick retina at all stages studied. Beginning at E12, amacrine cells in the INL were strongly immunoreactive. By E19, there was a decrease in immunoreactivity throughout the retina, with the exception of the GCL and a few amacrine cells. This distribution was also present in 3-day-old posthatched chick retinas (Hyndman, 1993). The results of the immunohistochemical double-labelling experiments of the present study resemble these staining patterns, detecting strong signals in the GCL and INL.

In the present study, we not only found insulin to be expressed constantly throughout murine retinal development but, even more interesting, observed a correlation between insulin receptor (InsR) expression peaks and PCD maxima. Insulin receptor expression has been detected early in the developing chick retina (de la Rosa et al., 1994) and in line with our results it has been shown that the levels of the InsR are regulated during chick retinal development (Kyriakis et al., 1987). Investigating retinal neurons from 7-day old chick embryos *in vitro* the authors report on an increase in receptor numbers between day 1 and 4 in culture, with a peak expression at day 4 corresponding to the late PCD stage in the chick retina at P11. Rajala & Anderson (2003) reported that light regulates the insulin receptor in the retina. It has been concluded that it is likely that changing receptor level with a constant level of insulin – reflecting the situation found in the present study - is the actual regulator of developmental death dynamics in the retina (Kyriakis et al., 1987).

In human ocular tissue the InsR was clearly demonstrated immunohistochemically in inner and outer segments of rods and cones (Naeser, 1997; Rajala et al., 2006). Besides, it has been shown that insulin receptor substrates, integrating signals from InsRs with other processes to control cellular growth, function and survival, are mainly localized to photoreceptors and are essential for the maturation and survival of PRs (Yi et al., 2005).

It has been reported that physiological cell death occurring during the early stages of chick retinal development is regulated by locally produced (pro) insulin (Díaz et al., 1999; 2000). In organotypic cultures of E5 and E9 chick retinas exogenous applied insulin attenuates apoptosis (Díaz et al., 1999; Chavarria et al., 2007). Along this line, *in ovo* treatment with specific antibodies against (pro) insulin or the insulin receptor induced apoptosis in chick neuroretinas (Díaz et al., 2000). Insulin has likewise been demonstrated to reduce apoptosis in R28 cells, a neural cell line derived from neonatal rat retina (Barber et al., 2001). It has however, been reported that high concentrations (over 1 μM) of insulin were required to promote survival of amacrine cells in rat retinal cultures (Politi et al., 2001). At murine developmental stage P9, the PCD stage where mostly cell of the INL, including amacrine cells die, we likewise observed that higher concentrations of insulin where required to exert a survival promoting effect.

Valenciano et al. (2006) showed that addition of 100 nM insulin to E15 organotypic murine retinal cultures significantly prevented early neural cell death. A previous study by our group already showed that application of exogenous insulin is likewise capable to prevent PCD in the P2 murine retina (Duenker et al., 2005). In the present study, we extended the characterization of insulin effects on cell death at later stages of naturally occurring PCD and confirmed a significant, yet less pronounced survival promoting effect for P9 and P15. Although we did not detect any immunosignal for the InsR in the PR layer or the ONL at all murine retinal stages investigated, application of recombinant insulin to P15 retinal cultures not only prevented apoptosis of RGCs, but also significantly reduced programmed cell death of PR.

CNTFR Expression and Missing CNTF Effects

Members of the CNTF family of cytokines have been shown to influence neuronal differentiation during retinal development and enhance cell survival in various retinal degeneration models (Rhee & Yang, 2003). Rhee & Yang (2003) characterized the expression profile of the CNTFR in the developing mouse retina. They found the CNTFR signal present in the GCL, the two plexiform layers, and the INL. In contrast to the present study, the authors did not use double labelling with cell type specific markers to identify the nature of the neurons but relied on positional information and /or DAPI counter staining. Kirsch et al. (1997) investigated the expression of CNTF and CNTF receptor (CNTFR) in the developing postnatal rat retina by RT-PCR, immunocytochemistry and in situ hybridisation. In sections of P0 retinas in situ hybridisation with a probe for the CNTFR yielded strong labelling of neurons in the GCL, most likely representing differentiated RGCs. At P6, an additional signal was visible in ACs and horizontal cells. In line with the results of the present study, an up-regulation in CNTF mRNA and protein expression from P8 to adult was observed. In contrast to the present study, where we found the CNTFR mRNA levels to exhibit maxima, correlating with the main PCD peaks, Kirsch et al. (1997) found a constant up-regulation in expression level for CNTFR mRNA levels. However, no apoptosis stages have been investigated and thus, no correlation with retinal apoptosis peaks were found.

Similar to our findings, other studies likewise reported an unexpected discrepancy between the developmental time course of CNTFR protein and mRNA (Kirsch et al., 1997). We found a discrepancy between protein and mRNA expression profiles not only for the CNTFR but for all neurotrophin receptors investigated. There are several possible explanations for the divergence of retinal mRNA and protein levels. First, there could be a translational or posttranslational control of receptor protein levels. Second, receptor protein produced by mature ganglion cells, which show high mRNA expression, may be preferentially transported to the optic nerve and its target regions.

It has been shown that CNTF promotes the long-term survival of RGCs (Meyer-Franke et al., 1995) and prevents photoreceptor cell degeneration caused by mutation and light-induced damages in various rodent models (LaVail et al., 1998; Cayouette et al., 1998; Rhee & Yang, 2003). Kirsch et al. (1997) found that in cultures grown for 7 days in the presence of recombinant CNTF the number of immunocytochemically labelled horizontal cells and amacrine cells did not significantly changed, whereas a dramatic effect on the number of surviving opsin-positive photoreceptors were observed. Ikeda et al. (2004) likewise confirmed that CNTF enhances cell viability in rat retinal cultures after 3 days. Injection of an inhibitor for the PI3K pathway together with CNTF into the vitreous of rat eyes 2 days before constant light exposure revealed that CNTF also promotes cell survival *in vivo* (Ikeda et al., 2004).

We did not detect any survival promoting effect, when we treated organoytpic retinal wholemounts for 24h with various concentrations of recombinant CNTF. An explanation for this discrepancy might be found in terms of culture duration. This hypothesis is supported by the fact, that although it has been shown that CNTF stimulates retinal cultures from newborn rat and embryonic chick, in both systems CNTF became effective only after several days (Kirsch et al., 1997; Hofmann, 1988), indicating that the neurotrophic protein did not act as a survival factor but promote later stages of differentiation.

Summarizing, one can state that the present study for the first time sheds light on the expression and gradual survival-promoting capacities of different neurotrophic factors during developmental, naturally occurring PCD not been investigated so far and contributes new insights to the controversial discussion about neurotrophin effects at different time points and on different cell populations in retinal development.

Acknowledgments

The authors would like to thank A. Paunel-Görgülü for help with Western blots, U. Laub and U. Jonetat for excellent technical assistance, and S. Braun for careful proofreading of the manuscript.

References

Ary-Pires, R., Nakatani, M., Rehen, S.-K. & Linden, R. (1997). Developmentally regulated release of intraretinal neurotrophic factors in vitro. *Int J Dev Neurosci, 15*, 239-255.

Bähr, M. (2000). Live or let die - retinal ganglion cell death and survival during development and in the lesioned adult CNS. *Trends Neurosci, 23*, 483-490.

Barber, A. J., Nakamura, M., Wolpert, E. B., Reiter, C. E. N., Seigel, G. M., Antonetti, D. A. & Gardner, T. W. (2001). Insulin rescues retinal neurons from apoptosis by a phosphatidylinositol 3 kinase/Akt-mediated mechanism that reduces the activation of capsase-3. *J Biolog Chem, 276*, 32814-32821.

Beier, M., Franke, A., Paunel-Görgülü, A. N., Scheerer, N. & Dünker, N. (2006). Transforming growth factor beta mediates apoptosis during all postnatal programmed cell death periods of the developing murine retina. *Neuroscience Research, 56*, 193-203.

Bennett, J. L., Zeiler, S. R. & Jones, K. R. (1999). Patterned expression of BDNF and NT-3 in the retina and anterior segment of the developing mammalian eye. *Invest Ophthalmol Vis Sci, 40*, 2996-3005.

Botchkarev, V. A., Botchkareva, N. V., Welker, P., Metz, M., Lewin, G. R., Subramaniam, A., Bulfone-Paus, S., Hagen, E., Braun, A., Lommatzsch, M., Renz, H. & Paus, R. (1999). A new role for neurotrophins: involvement of brain–derived neurotrophic factor and neurotrophin-4 in hair cycle control. *FASEB, 13*, 395-410.

Buss, R. R., Sun, W. & Oppenheim, R. W. (2006). Adaptive roles of programmed cell death during nervous system development. *Annu Rev Neurosci, 29*, 1-35.

Castillo, B. Jr., del Cerro, M., Breakfield, X. O., Frim, D. M., Barnstable, C. J., Dean, D. O. & Bohn, M. C. (1994). Retinal ganglion cell survival is promoted by genetically modified astrocytes designed to secrete brain-derived neurotrophic factor (BDNF). *Brain Res, 647*, 30-36.

Cayouette, M., Behn, D., Sendtner, M., Lachapelle, P. & Gravel, C. (1998). Intraocular gene transfer of ciliary neurotrophic factor prevents death and increases responsiveness of rod photoreceptors in the retinal degeneration slow mouse. *J Neurosci, 18*, 9282-9293.

Cellerino, A., Strohmaier, C., & Barde, Y. A. (1995). Brain-derived neruotrophic factor and the developing chick retina. In C. F. Ibanez (ed.), *Life and death in the nervous system* (pp. 131-139). Oxford, U.K.: Elsevier Science LTD.

Cellerino, A., Carroll, P., Thoenen, H. & Barde, Y. A. (1997). Reduced size of retinal ganglion cell axons and hypomyelination in mice lacking brain-derived neurotrophic factor. *Mol Cell Neurosci, 9*, 397-408.

Cellerino, A. & Kohler, K. (1997). Brain-derived neurotrophic factor /Neurotrophin-4 receptor TrKB is localized on ganglion cells and dopaminergic amacrine cells in the vertebrate retina. *J Comp Neuro, 386*, 149-160.

Chaum, E. (2003). Retinal neuroprotection by growth factors: a mechanistic perspective. *J Cell Biochem, 88*, 57-75.

Chavarria, T., Valenciano, A. I., Mayordomo, R., Egea, J., Comella, J. X., Hallböök, F., de Pablo, F. & de la Rosa, E. (2007). Differential, age-dependent MEK-ERK and PI3K-Akt activation by insulin acting as a survival factor during embryonic retinal development. *Dev Neurobiol, 67*, 1777-1788.

Cohen, A., Bray, G. M. & Aguayo, A. J. (1994). Neurotrophin 4 (NT-4/5) increases adult rat ganglion cell survival and neurite outgrowth in vitro. *J Neurobiol, 25*, 953-959.

Conover, J. C. & Yancopoulos, G. D. (1997). Neurotrophin regulation of the developing nervous system: analyses of knockout mice. *Rev Neurosci, 8*, 13-27.

Cui, Q. & Harvey, A. R. (1994). NT-4/5 reduces naturally occurring retinal ganglion cell death in neonatal rats. *NeuroReport, 5*, 1882-1884.

Cusato, K., Bosco, A., Linden, R. & Reese, B. E. (2002). Cell death in the inner nuclear layer of the retina is modulated by BDNF. *Dev Brain Res, 139*, 325-330.

Danial, N. N. & Korsmeyer, S. J. (2004). Cell death: Critical control points. *Cell, 116*, 205-219.

Das, A., Pansky, B., Budd, G. C. & Kollarits, C. R. (1984). Immunocytochemistry of mouse and human retina with antisera to insulin and S-100 protein. *Curr Eye Res, 3*, 1397-1403.

Das, I., Hempstead, B. L., MacLeish, P. R. & Sparrow, J. R. (1997). Immunohistochemical analysis of the neurotrophins BDNF and NT-3 and their receptors trk B, trk C, and p75 in the developing chick retina. *Vis Neurosci, 14*, 835-842.

Davies, A. M. (2003). Regulation of neuronal survival and death by extracellular signals during development. *EMBO J, 22*, 2537-2545.

De Pablo, F. & de la Rosa, E. J. (1995). The developing CNS: a scenario for the action of proinsulin, insulin and insulin-like growth factors. *Trends Neurosci, 18*, 143-150.

De la Rosa, E. J., Bondy, C. A., Hernandez-Sanchez, C., Wu, X., Zhou, J., Lopez-Carranza, A., Scavo, L. M. & de Pablo, F. (1994). Insulin and insulin-like growth factor system components gene expression in the chicken retina from early neurogenesis until late development and their effect on neuroepithelial cells. *Eur J Neurosci, 6*, 1801-1810.

Díaz, B., Pimentel, B., de Pablo, F. & de la Rosa, E. J. (1999). Apoptotic cell death of proliferating neurepithelial cells in the embryonic retina is prevented by insulin. *Eur J Neurosci, 11*, 1624-1632.

Díaz, B., Serna, J., de Pablo, F. & de la Rosa, E. J. (2000). In vivo regulation of cell death by embryonic (pro)insulin and the insulin receptor during early retinal neurogenesis. *Development, 127*, 1641-1649.

Di Polo, A., Cheng, L., Bray, G. M. & Aguayo, A. J. (2000). Colocalization of TrkB and brain-derived neurotrophic factor proteins in green-red-sensitive cone outer segments. *Invest Ophthalmol Vis Sci, 41*, 4014-4021.

Drum, K., Forbes, M., Wang, S. W. & Johnson, J. E. (1996). Treatment with bdnf does not prevent normal chick rgc death in ovo. *Soci Neuroscience, Abstr, 22*, 397.25.

Duenker, N., Valenciano, A. I., Franke, A., Hernandez-Sanchez, C., Dressel, R., Behrendt, M., de Pablo, F., Krieglstein, K., & de la Rosa, E. J. (2005). Balance of pro-apoptotic transforming growth factor-beta and anti-apoptotic insulin effects in the control of cell death in the postnatal mouse retina. *Eur J Neurosci, 22*, 28-38.

Ernfors, P., Merlio, J. P. & Persson, H. (1992). Cells expressing mRNA for neurotrophins and their receptors during embryonic rat development. *Eur J Neurosci, 4*, 1140-1158.

Fan, G., Egles, C., Sun, Y., Minichiello, L., Renger, J. J., Klein, R., Liu, G. & Jaenisch, R. (2000). Knocking the NT4 gene into the BDNF locus rescues BDNF deficient mice and reveals distinct NT4 and BDNF activities. *Nat Neurosci, 3*, 350-357.

Farkas, R. H. & Grosskreutz, C. L. (2001). Apoptosis, neuroprotection, and retinal ganglion cell death: an overview. *Int Ophthalmol Clin, 41*, 111-130.

Frade, J. M., Bovolenta, P., Martinez-Morales, J. R., Arribas, A., Barbas, J. A. & Tebra, A. R. (1997). Control of early cell death by BDNF in the chick retina. *Development, 124*, 3313-3320.

Frade, J. M., Bovolenta, P. & Rodriguez-Tebar, A. (1999). Neurotrophins and other growth factors in the generation of retinal neurons. *Microsc Res Techn, 45*, 243-251.

Frost, D. O., Ma, Y. T., Hsieh, T., Forbes, M. E. & Jonson, J. E. (2001). Developmental changes in BDNF protein levels in the hamster retina and superior colliculus. *J Neurobiol, 49*, 173-187.

Garner, A. S., Menegay, H. J., Boeshore, K. L., Xie, X. Y., Voci, J. M., Johnson, J. E. & Large, T. H. (1996). Expression of TrkB receptor isoforms in the developing avian visual system. *J Neurosc, 16*, 1740-1752.

Guerin, M. B., McKernan, D. P., O`Brien, C. & Cotter, T. G. (2006). Retinal ganglion cells: dying to survive. *Int J Dev Biol, 50*, 665-674.

Hallböök, F. A., Bäackström, K., Kullander, T., Ebendal, T. & Carri, N. G. (1996). Expression of neurotrophins and trk receptors in the avian retina. *J Comp Neurol, 364*, 664-676.

Harada, C., Harada, T., Quah, H. M. A., Namekata, K., Yoshida, K., Ohno, S., Tanaka, K. & Parada, L. F. (2005). Role of neurotrophin-4/5 in neural cell death during retinal development and ischemic retinal injury in vivo. *Invst Opthalmol Vis Sci, 46*, 669-673.

Herzog, K. H. & von Bartheld, C. S. (1998). Contributions of the optic tectum and the retina as sources of brain-derived neurotrophic factor for retinal ganglion cells in the chick embryo. *J Neurosci, 18*, 2891-2906.

Hofmann, H. D. (1988). Ciliary neurotrophic factor stimulates choline acetyltransferase activity in cultured chicken neurons. *J Neurochm, 51*, 109-113.

Hyndman, A. G. (1993). Identification of a population of amacrine cells rich in insulin receptors. *Brain Res Dev Brain Res, 75*, 289-292.

Ikeda, K., Tatsuno, T., Noguchi, H. & Nakayama, C. (2004). Ciliary neurotrophic factor protects rat retina cells in vitro and in vivo via PI3 kinase. *Curr Eye Res, 29*, 349-355.

Jelsma, T. N., Freidman, H. H., Berkelaar, M., Bray, G. M. & Aguayo, A. J. (1993). Different forms of the neurotrophin receptor trkB mRNA predominate in the rat retina and optic nerve. *J Neurobiol, 24*, 1207-1214.

Ji, J. Z., Elyaman, W., Yip, H. K., Lee, V. W. H., Yick, L. W., Hugon, J. & So, K. F. (2004). CNTF promotes survival of retinal ganglion cells after induction of ocular hypertension in rats: the possible involvement of STAT3 pathway. *Eur J Neurosci, 19*, 265-272.

Johnson, J. E., Barde, Y. A., Schwab, M. & Thoenen, H. (1986). Brain-derived neurotrophic factor supports the survival of cultured rat retinal ganglion cells. *J Neurosci, 6*, 3031-3038.

Jones, K. R., Farinas, I., Backus, C. & Reichardt, L. F. (1994). Target disruption of BDFN gene perturbs brain and sensory neuron development but not motor neuron development. *Cell, 76*, 989-999.

Karlsson, M. & Hallböök, F. (1998). Kainic acid, tetrodotoxin and light modulate expression of brain-derived neurotrophic factor in developing avian retinal ganglion cells and their tectal target. *Neurosci, 83*, 137-150.

Kashiwagi, F., Kashiwagi, K., Iizuka, Y. & Tsukahara, S. (2000). Effects of brain-derived neurotrophic factor and neurotrophin-4 on isolated cultured retinal ganglion cells: Evaluation by flow cytometry. *Invest Ophthalmol Vis Sci, 41*, 2373-2377.

Kirsch, M., Lee, M. Y., Meyer, V., Wiese, A. & Hofmann, H. D. (1997). Evidence for multiple, local fucntions of ciliary neurotrophic factor (CNTF) in retinal development: expression of CNTF and its receptor and in vitro effects on target cells. *J Neurochem, 68*, 979-990.

Klein, R., Smeyne, R. J., Wurst, W., Long, L. K., Auerbach, B. A., Joyner, A. L. & Barbacid, M. (1993). Target disruption of the trkB neurotrophin receptor gene results in nervous system lesions and neonatal death. *Cell, 75*, 113-122.

Koide, T., Takahashi, J. B., Hoshimaru, M., Kojima, M., Otsuka, T., Asahi, M. & Kikuchi, H. (1995). Localization of trkB and low-affinity nerve growth factor receptor mRNA in the developing rat retina. *Neurosci Letters, 185*, 183-186.

Kyriakis, J. M., Hausman, R. E. & Peterson, S. W. (1987). Insulin stimulates choline acetyltransferase activity in cultured embryonic chicken retina neurons. *Proc Natl Acad Sci USA, 84*, 7463-7467.

LaVail, M. M., Unoki, K., Yasumura, D., Matthes, M. T., Yancopoulos, G. D. & Steinberg, R. H. (1992). Multiple growth factors, cytokines, and neurotrophins rescue photoreceptors from the damaging effects of constant light. *Proc Nat Acad Sci USA, 89*, 11249-11253.

LaVail, M. M., Yasumura, D., Matthes, M. T., Lau-Viliacorta, C., Unoki, K., Sung, C. H. & Steinberg, R. H. (1998). Protection of mouse photoreceptors by survival factors in retinal degeneration. *Invest Ophthalmol Vis Sci, 39*, 592-602.

Lossi, L. & Merighi, A. (2003). In vivo cellular and molecular mechanisms of neuronal apoptosis in the mammalian CNS. *Prog Neurobiol, 69*, 287-312.

Meyer-Franke, A., Kaplan, M. R., Pfrieger, F. W. & Barres, B. A. (1995). Characterization of the signalling interactions that promote the survival and growth of developing retinal ganglion cells in culture. *Neuron, 14*, 805-819.

Mey, J. & Thanos, S. (1993). Intravitreal injections of neurotrophic factors support the survival of axotomized retinal ganglion cells in adult rats in vivo. *Brain Res, 602*, 304-317.

Naeser, P. (1997). Insulin receptors in human ocular tissues. Immunohistochemical demonstration in normal and diabetic eyes. *Ups J Med Sci, 102*, 35-40.

Pequignot, M. O., Provost, A. C., Salle, S., Taupin, P., Sainton, K. M., Marchant, D., Martinou, J. C., Ameisen, J. C., Jais, J. P. & Abitbol, M. (2003). Major role of BAX in apoptosis during retinal development and in establishment of a functional postnatal retina. *Dev Dyn, 228*, 231-238.

Perez, M. T. & Caminos, E. (1995). Expression of brain-derived neurotrophic factor and of its functional receptor in neonatal and adult retina. *Neurosci Lett, 183*, 96-99.

Pinzon-Duarte, G., Arango-Gonzalez, B., Guenther, E. & Kohler, K. (2004). Effects of brain-derived neurotrophic factor on cell survival, differentiation and patterning of neuronal connections and Müller glia cells in the developing retina. *Eur J Neurosci, 19*, 1475-1484.

Politi, E. L., Rotstein, N. P., Salvador, G., Giusto, N. M. & Insua, M. F. (2001). Insulin-like growth factor-I is a potential trophic factor for amacrine cells. *J Neurochem, 76*, 1199-1211.

Pollock, G. S., Vernon, E., Forbes, M. E., Yan, Q., Ma, Y. T., Hsieh, T., Robichon, R., Frost, D. O. & Johnson, J. E. (2001). Effects of early visual experience and diurnal rhythm on BDNF mRNA and protein levels in the visual system, hippocampus, and cerebellum. *J Neurosci*, *21*, 3923-3931.

Pollock, G. S., Robichon, R., Boyd, K. A., Kerkel, K. A., Kramer, M., Lyles, J., Ambalavanar, R., Khan, A., Kaplan, D. R., Wiliams, R. W. & Forst, D. O. (2003). TrkB receptor signalling regulates developmental death dynamics, but not final number, of retinal ganglion cells. *J Neurosci*, *23*, 10137-10145.

Rajala, R. V. & Anderson, R. E. (2003) Light regulation of the insulin receptor in the retina. *Mol Neurobiol* 28, 123-138.

Rajala, R. V., Elliott, M. H., McClellan, M. E. & Anderson, R. E. (2006). Localization of the insulin receptor and phosphoinositide 3-kinase in detergent-resistant membrane rafts of rod photoreceptor outer segments. *Adv Exp Med Biol*, *572*, 491-497.

Rhee, K. D. & Yang, X. J. (2003). Expression of cytokine signal transduction components in the postnatal mouse retina. *Mol Vis*, *9*, 715-722.

Rickman, D. W. & Brecha, N. C. (1995). Expression of the proto-oncogene, trk, receptors in the developing rat retina. *Vis Neurosci*, *12*, 215-222.

Rodriguez-Tebar, A., Jeffrey, P. L., Thoenen, H. & Barde, Y. A. (1989). The survival of chick retinal ganglion cells in response to branin-derived neurotrophic factor depends on their embryonic age. *Dev Biol*, *136*, 296-303.

Rohrer, B., LaVail, M. M., Jones, K. R. & Reichardt, L. F. (2001). Neurotrophin receptor TrkB activation is not required for the postnatal survival of retinal ganglion cells in vivo. *Exp Neurology*, *172*, 81-91.

Seki, M., Nawa, H., Fukuchi, T., Abe, H. & Takei, N. (2003). BDNF is upregulated by postnatal development and visual experience: quantitative and immunohistochemical analyses of BDNF in the rat retina. *Inv Ophthalmol Vis Sci*, *44*, 3211-3218.

Singh, T. D., Mizuno, K., Kohno, T. & Nakamura, S. (1997). BDNF and trkB mRNA expression in neurons of the neonatal mouse barrel field cortex: normal development and plasticity after cauterizing facial vibrissae. *Neurochem Res*, *22*, 791-797.

Spalding, K. L., Rush, R. A. & Harvey, A. R. (2004). Target-derived and locally derived neurotrophins support retinal ganglion cell survival in the neonatal rat retina. *Inc J Neurobiol*, *60*, 319-327.

Spears, N., Molinek, M. D., Robinson, L. L. L., Fulton, N., Cameron, H., Shimoda, K., Telfer, E. E., Anderson, R. A. & Price, D. J. (2003). The role of neurotrophin receptors in female germ-cell survival in mouse and human. *Development*, *130*, 5481-5491.

Thanos, S., Bähr, M., Barde, Y. A. & Vanselow, J. (1989). Survival and axonal elongation of adult rat retinal ganglion cells. *Eur J Neurosci*, *1*, 19-26.

Ugolini, G., Cremisi, F. & Maffei, L. (1995). TrkA, TrkB and p75 mRNA expression is developmentally regulated in the rat retina. *Brain Res*, *704*, 121-124.

Valenciano, A. I., Corrochano, S., de Pablo, F., de la Villa, P. & de la Rosa, E. (2006). Proinsulin /insulin is synthesized locally and prevents caspase- and cathepsin-mediated cell death in the embryonic mouse retina. *J Neurochem*, *99*, 524-536.

Valenciano, A. I., Boya, P. & de la Rosa, E. J. (2008). Early neural cell death: numbers and cues from the developing neuroretina. *Int J Dev Biol*, *52*, [in Press].

Van Adel, B. A., Kostic, C., Deglon, N., Ball, A. K. & Arsenijevic, Y. (2003). Delivery of ciliary neurotrophic factor via lentiviral-mediated transfer protects axotomized retinal ganglon cells for an extended period of time. *Hum Gene Rher*, *14*, 103-115.

Varela-Nieto, I., de al Rosa, E. J., Valenciano, A. I. & Leon, Y. (2003). Cell death in the nervous system: Lessons from insulin and insulin-like growth factors. *Mol Neurobiol*, *28*, 23-49.

Vecino, E., Caminos, E., Ugarte, M., Martin-Zanca, D. & Osborne, N. N. (1998). Immunohistochemical distribution of neurotrophins and their receptors in the rat retina and the effects of ischemia and reperfusion. *Gen Pharmacol*, *30*, 305-314.

Vecino, E., Garcia-Greso, D., Garcia, M., Martinez-Millan, L., Sharma, S. C. & Carrascal, E. (2002). Rat retinal ganglion cells co-express brain derived neurotrophic factor (BDNF) and its receptor TrKB. *Vision Res*, *42*, 151-157.

Vecino, E., Hernandez, M. & Garcia, M. (2004). Cell death in the developing vertebrate retina. *Int J Dev Biol*, *48*, 965-974.

von Bartheld, C. S. (1998). Neurotrophins in the developing regenerating visual system. *Histol Histopathol*, *13*, 437-459.

Wahlin, K. J., Campochiaro, P. A., Zack, D. J. & Adler, R. (2000). Neurotrophic factors cause activation of intracellular signaling pathways in Muller cells and other cells of the inner retina, but not photoreceptors. *Invest Ophthalmol Vis Sci*, *41*, 927-936.

Yeo, W. & Gautier, J. (2004). Early neural cell death: dying to become neurons. *Dev Biol*, *274*, 233-244.

Yi, X., Schubert, M., Peachey, N. S., Suzuma, K., Burks, D. J., Kushner, J. A., Suzuma, I., Cahill, C., Flint, C. L., Dow, M. A., Leshan, R. L., King, G. L. & White, M. F. (2005). Insulin receotr substrate 2 is essential for maturation and survival of photoreceptor cells. *J Neurosci*, *25*, 1240-1248.

In: Neuroanatomy Research Advances ISBN: 978-60741-610-4
Editors: C. E. Flynn and B. R. Callaghan, pp.121-143 ©2010 Nova Science Publishers, Inc.

Chapter IV

Comparative Distribution of Orexin-like Immunoreactivity in the Brain of Vertebrates

Kristan G. Singletary, Christopher R. Hayworth and Yvon Delville

Psychology Department and Institute for Neuroscience, University of Texas,
Austin, Texas, USA

Abstract

Orexin neuropeptides are highly conserved among vertebrates. This conservation extends to neuroanatomy and perhaps function. Orexin is thought to be involved in feeding, the sleep/wake cycle, stress and reproduction in mammals. However, its role in most vertebrates is unclear. In an effort to gain a better understanding of the function of orexin we compared orexin immunoreactive like (-lir) cell bodies and fiber distributions across tetrapods. Our studies support previous findings that orexin-lir neurons are concentrated in the vertebrate hypothalamus. In addition, there is a high degree of conservation of orexin-lir innervation across vertebrates.

While orexin cell bodies are located in the hypothalamus across vertebrates, there are slight differences in hypothalamic area. Discrepancies between species may be due to phylogenetic differences, and this could reflect diverging roles for the orexin system. It is interesting to note that in these vertebrates, aside from mammals, these orexin cell bodies are associated with neurosecretory areas and likely involved in homeostasis.

Examining orexin-lir fiber distribution can also help elucidate the function of orexins. Generally, there is moderate to dense orexin-lir innervation of the hypothalamus, midline thalamic areas, and ventral telencephalon. Overall similarities suggest that the orexin system is involved in general physiological or homeostatic roles, although slight differences could reflect a lineage relationship in vertebrate evolution and help to track phylogenies. As such, this short commentary will provide a comparative overview of the distribution of orexin cells and fibers across the brains of vertebrates in relation to function.

1. Introduction

The orexins (hypocretins) are neuropeptides in the incretin peptide superfamily [Alvarez and Sutcliffe 2002] that regulate many processes in mammals. Studies have shown orexin to regulate feeding, stress responsivity, reproduction, and nociception [de Lecea et al. 1998; Pu et al. 1998; Sakurai et al. 1998; van den Pol 1999; Dube et al. 1999; Ida et al. 2000; Kuru et al. 2000; Bingham et al. 2001; Archer et al. 2002; Karteris et al. 2005; Muschamp et al. 2007]. In recent years, primary interest in the orexins has grown given their involvement in mammalian sleep/wake behavior. The sleep/wake cycle is stabilized by a key neuropeptide, orexin [Saper et al. 2001]. Reduced orexin expression in mammalian brains is associated with severe disturbances to their sleep/wake cycle including symptoms of narcolepsy, such as extended drowsiness and occasional periods of sleep during the day, as well as enhanced arousal and short onset of REM sleep at night [Chemelli et al. 1999; Lin et al. 1999; Peyron et al. 2000; Thannickal et al. 2000; Downs et al. 2007].

There are two forms of orexin, orexin A and orexin B as well as two orexin receptors identified in mammals. Orexin A and orexin B are cleaved separately [de Lecea et al. 1998; Sakurai et al. 1998] from a single precursor prepro-orexin. Of the two receptors, orexin receptor 1 has a higher affinity for orexin A and orexin receptor 2 binds both A and B equally [Sakurai et al. 1998]. The role of orexin on the sleep/wake cycle appears to be mediated through orexin-2 receptors, as indicated by studies with electrophysiological thalamic recordings, receptor-saporin lesions, deletion mutations and rescue studies [Lin et al. 1999; Gerashchenko et al. 2001; Bayer et al. 2002; Fujiki et al. 2003; Willie et al. 2003; Akanmu and Honda 2005].

Orexin A and B amino acid sequences have been characterized in fish, amphibians, birds and mammals and are highly conserved among these vertebrates [Sakurai et al. 1998, Shibahara et al. 1999; Alvarez and Sutcliffe 2002; Ohkubo et al. 2002; Kaslin et al. 2004]. Orexin A is identical in human, rat, mouse, and pig. Orexin B in mice and rats differs from human orexin B by only two amino acids [Sakurai et al. 1998]. It has been shown that chicken orexin A and B are 85% and 65% homologous to human orexin A and B, respectively [Ohkubo et al. 2002]. In *Xenopus laevis* prepro-orexins are 56% homologous to the human sequence [Shibahara et al. 1999]. In zebrafish orexin A and B are 32% and 50% homologous to human orexins A and B [Kaslin et al. 2004].

If this conservation also extends to neuroanatomy, perhaps the function of the orexin system is also similar. The orexin system has been extensively studied and is involved in many processes in mammals. However, its role in other vertebrates is unclear. In an effort to confirm the conservation of the distribution of orexin we examined and compared orexin-like immunoreactive (-lir) cell bodies and fiber distributions among various vertebrates. This includes a description of a reptile (*Anolis carolinensis*). Also, orexin distribution in various closely related passerines is described. Using this information we can gain a better understanding of the possible functions of the orexin system across evolution. As such, this short commentary will provide a comparative overview of the distribution of orexin cells and fibers across the brains of vertebrates with reference to function.

2. Methods and Materials

2.1 Animal Care

Syrian Hamsters (*Microcetus auratus*): Adult male (*n*=8) hamsters were purchased from Harlan Sprague–Dawley (Indianapolis, IN, USA). All animals were housed in a reversed daylight cycle (14L, 10D, lights on at 9:00 a.m.) and received food and water *ad libitum*.

House Finch (*Carpodacus mexicanus*): Adult males (n=5) were caught in Tempe, Arizona in September (latitude: 33.414N; longitude: 111.908W). They were housed in an outdoor aviary exposed to ambient temperature and natural photoperiod (10L:14D at time of sacrifice), and received food and water *ad libitum*. Finches were all sacrificed on the same day in December. The Arizona State University Institutional Animal Care and Use Committee preapproved all experimental procedures.

House Sparrow (*Passer domesticus*): Adults n=5, males=2, females=3 were caught in Tempe, Arizona in March (latitude: 33.414 N; longitude: 111.908 W) and received the same treatment as the House Finch but was exposed to an 8L:16D light cycle.

White-crowned Sparrow (*Zonotrichia leucophrys leucophrys*): Adults n=7, males=4, females=3 and Harris Sparrow (*Zonotrichia querula*): Adults n= 13 were caught in Austin, Texas in February. Sparrows were brought to the laboratory and housed in single cages (16"w x 11" d x 21"h) under short day photoperiod (8L:16D). The animals remained in visual and auditory contact with each other and received food and water *ad libitum*. Temperature in the animal room was approximately 65°F.

Green Tree Frog (*Hyla cinerea*): Adult male frogs (n=5), supplied through Charles Sullivan Inc. (Nashville, TN) were housed in a controlled environment (12L:12D, 21°C) for at least two weeks before sacrifice. The frogs were kept in ten-gallon glass tanks with free access to water. Food (crickets) was provided twice a week. All studies were approved by the IACUC of the University of Texas at Austin and the animals were kept in an AALAC-accredited facility.

2.2 Immunocytochemistry

All orexin A and B antibodies were obtained from Santa Cruz Biotechnology, Santa Cruz, CA. The goat polyclonal orexin A and B antibodies are raised against an epitope within the last 100 amino acids of the C-terminus of prepro-orexin and affinity purified. The prepro-orexin epitope is of human origin and identical to the corresponding sequence of mouse origin. The secondary donkey anti-goat was bought from Jackson Immunoresearch, West Grove, PA.

Syrian hamsters under anesthesia (Nembutal) were perfused with saline followed by 4% paraformaldehyde in 0.1M phosphate-buffered saline. Brains were extracted, postfixed at 4 °C overnight and immersed in 20% sucrose in phosphate-buffered saline (wt/vol). Brains were then sliced into 40μm thick sections for free floating immunostaining. Sections were stained with Orexin A (1:4000) or B (1:4000) using a protocol adapted from previous studies [Wommack and Delville 2002].

Birds received an intramuscular injection of 0.1 ml sodium pentobarbital (200 mg/kg; Nembutal, Abbott Laboratories, North Chicago, IL). All birds were perfused transcardially with 0.9% saline containing 0.1% sodium nitrite, followed by 4% paraformaldehyde in 0.1 M phosphate buffer. The brains were taken out of the skull and postfixed in 4% paraformaldehyde overnight at 4° C. Afterwards, the brains were embedded in gelatin following a procedure modified from previous descriptions [Saldanha et al. 1994; Deviche et al. 2000]. First, the brains were placed in 0.1 M phosphate buffer overnight at 4°C, followed by immersion in a 4% gelatin (175 bloom, Sigma Chemical Co., St Louis, MO) solution for 30 minutes. Afterwards, they were embedded in an 8% gelatin mold and allowed to solidify overnight. Later, brains were immersed in 10% and 20% sucrose solutions for 24 hours each, ending with 48 hours in 30% sucrose solution. They were then frozen on dry ice and cut on a cryostat into 40 μm-thick coronal sections. Three parallel sets of sections were collected for each brain and saved at -20°C in a cryoprotectant [Watson et al. 1986].

Free-floating sections were processed by immunocytochemistry for orexin A and B following a protocol adapted from previous studies [Singletary et al. 2005; 2006]. After washing in 0.1M phosphate buffer saline, sections were treated with 0.5% hydrogen peroxide to eliminate endogenous peroxidase activity. Sections were washed in 0.1M PBS and blocked in a 10% normal donkey serum solution in 0.1M PBS. Sections were successively incubated in orexin A or B antiserum (1:4000) in a 0.1M PBS/ 0.3% Triton X-100 solution to ensure permeabilization. Sections were washed again and incubated in donkey anti-goat immunoglobulin (1:400). Sections were labeled with 0.5 μg/ml diaminobenzidine (Sigma, St. Louis, MO) after incubation in an avidin-biotinylated peroxidase conjugate (1:100, VectaStain ABC kit, Vector Labs, Burlingame, CA). Sections were then mounted on gelatin coated slides, dried overnight, dehydrated in gradient alcohols, defatted with xylene (Sigma, St. Louis, MO), and coverslipped with Permount (Fisher Scientific, Hampton, NH). Some stained sections were counterstained with thionin to confirm neuroanatomical identification. Brain regions were identified using avian brain atlases and other descriptive studies [Stokes et al. 1974; Aste et al. 1998; Medina and Reiner 2000; Brandstatter and Abraham 2003; Krutzfeldt and Wild 2004; Kuenzel 2004; Reiner et al. 2004; 2005].

Green tree frogs were rapidly decapitated and brains fixed by immersion in 4% paraformaldehyde in 0.1M phosphate buffer (PB) for 24 hours. The brains were then transferred to a 30% sucrose solution in 0.1M PB for 24 hours. Brains were frozen in an embedding medium (M1 embedding matrix, Thermal Shandon, Pittsburgh, PA) on dry ice and then sectioned in the transverse plane on a cryostat (20μm: thaw-mounted or 40 μm: free-floating sections) at -17°C and mounted onto subbed slides. Each brain was divided into 3 sets of serial slices.

Tissue on slides and free-floating sections were washed in 0.1M phosphate buffered saline (PBS), and immersed in 0.1% $NaBH_4$ for 15 minutes in order to clear the tissue of any residual fixative. Slices were next rinsed again in PBS and preincubated in a 10% normal donkey serum, 0.3% Triton-X 100, 3% H_2O_2 and PBS solution for one hour. Sections were then incubated 24 hours in orexin A or B antiserum (1:4000), two serial sets from each brain receiving either antiserum. Afterward, sections were rinsed in PBS and then incubated in a donkey anti-goat secondary antibody (1:400) for one hour. Again, sections were rinsed in PBS and then incubated in an avidin-biotinylated conjugate (1:100, VectaStain ABC kit, Vector Labs, Burlingame, CA) for one hour. Sections were rinsed in a 0.1M phosphate buffered (PB) solution and immersed in a DAB solution. Subsequently mounted slices were rinsed in PB and then dehydrated in order to coverslip, and free floating gelatin embedded slices were organized in series, mounted on subbed slides, dehydrated, and coverslipped. Some series of orexin A and B slides were counterstained with cresyl violet or thionin. The distribution of immunoreactive neurons and fibers was mapped through a camera lucida attached to the microscope. The quality of the labeling was similar for both orexin A and B. Neural areas were identified using previous descriptions of frog brains [Wilczynski et al. 1983; Allison et al. 1994; Neary et al. 1995].

The specificity of all tetrapod immunostaining was tested through omission of the primary antibody and pre-absorption of the antibody to orexin A or B. For this, the orexin B antibody was incubated overnight in the presence of orexin A or B (sc-8070P or sc-8071P, 40 µg/ml, Santa Cruz Biotechnology, Santa Cruz, CA) before application to tissue sections. Omission of the primary antibodies and peptide pre-absorption eliminated all immunostaining.

3. Results

3.1 Distribution of Orexin-lir Somata

In the Syrian hamsters orexin A and B immunoreactive (-ir) cell bodies were found in a discrete population in the lateral hypothalamus and perifornical area extending caudally towards the dorsomedial hypothalamus (Fig. 1D). In the House finch (Fig. 1B), House sparrow, White-crowned sparrow and Harris' sparrow, orexin A and B-lir neurons were located in a single population centered on the paraventricular nucleus of the hypothalamus (PVN) extending out to the stratum cellulare externum or posterior lateral hypothalamus. In the green treefrog orexin A and B-lir perikarya formed a discrete population centered on the suprachiasmatic nucleus (SCN) (Fig. 1A). Orexin-lir cells extended from the caudal SCN rostrally into the caudal edge of the preoptic area (POA), and a few extended dorsally to the magnocellular preoptic nucleus. On the rostral end of their distribution, orexin-lir cells were located along the walls of the third ventricle. Caudally, the cells were gradually located toward the lateral edge of the SCN. Orexin-lir perikarya had few dendrites and appeared either ovoid or piriform. Orexin-lir cell bodies were found in a narrow population in the periventricular hypothalamus (PVH) of the Green anole lizard (Fig. 1C, 3B).

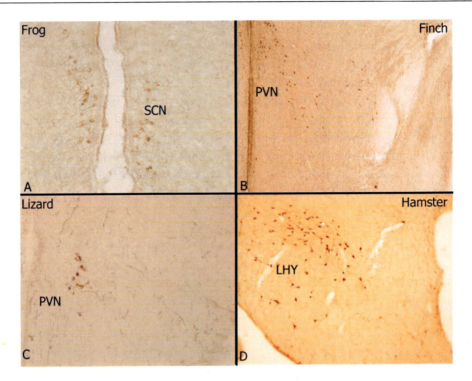

Figure 1. Photomicrographs showing orexin immunoreactive neurons in the hypothalamus of various vertebrates.

3.2 Distribution of Orexin-lir Processes

Orexin A and B-ir fibers were found throughout the brain in concordance with previous findings in the Syrian hamster [Mintz et al. 2001]. Highest densities were found in the hypothalamic area surrounding the cells and the midline thalamic area including the paraventricular nucleus of the thalamus (PVT) and habenular region. Moderate densities of fibers were found in the PVN, the tuberomammillary nucleus (TMN) and the preoptic area. The locus coeruleus (LoC) was also heavily innervated as well as the dorsal raphe. Rostrally, fibers were found extending to the septum and ventral cortex.

In all the birds mentioned here, the distribution of orexin A and B-lir fibers were similarly visible across the brain with the highest density seen within the preoptic area (POA), hypothalamus, thalamus and LoC. Previous research in the house finch details the innervation [Singletary et al. 2006]. Orexin-lir projections extended rostrally from the paraventricular nucleus of the hypothalamus (PVN) to the POA, laterally towards the medial striatum, nidopallium, and dorsally along the lateral ventricle towards the mesopallium. Ventrolaterally the fibers project to the optic tectum. Caudally, the highest densities of orexin-lir fibers were found along the third ventricle. The periaqueductal grey, substantia nigra pars compacta and the LoC also showed a high density of orexin-lir fibers. The red nucleus (Ru) is highly innervated on the medial edge, decreasing to a low density towards the lateral edge. Heaviest densities were found in the PVN and along the midline dorsally and ventrally.

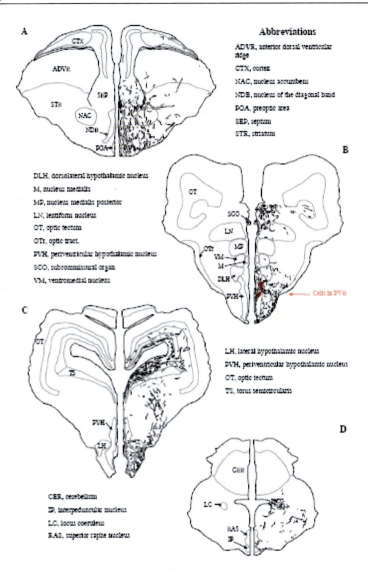

Figure 2. Schematic tracings representing the distribution of orexin-lir cells (red filled) and fibers in the brain of the green anole lizard (*Anolis carolinensis*) on the right. Nomenclature on the left.

In the anolis, orexin-lir fibers were most prevalent in the ventral medial forebrain and periventricular midbrain (Fig. 2). Orexin-lir projections extended from the PVH to the telencephalon. Here the densest projections were found within and ventral to the septum (Fig. 3A), including the area between the nucleus accumbens and the nucleus of the diagonal band. A medium density of orexin-lir fibers was seen extending laterally to the striatum and dorsolaterally to the hyperstriatum and cortex. From the PVH orexin-lir fibers projected dorsally along the ventricle toward the dorsomedial nucleus of the thalamus and habenula (Fig. 3C) and dorsolaterally to the lateral hypothalamus (LH). A high density of fibers was also seen dorsolateral to the subcommissural organ with a few fibers extending toward the optic tectum. Caudally, a high density of orexin-lir projections were found in the posterior PVH and LH, extending to the stratum album periventricular and medial torus semicircularis with a low density of orexin-lir projections in the stratum griseum periventricular and stratum album centrale (Fig 3D). In the hindbrain a high density of orexin-lir fibers were found in the LoC, with a few found ventrolateral to the LoC and at the very edge of the superior raphe nucleus (RAS).

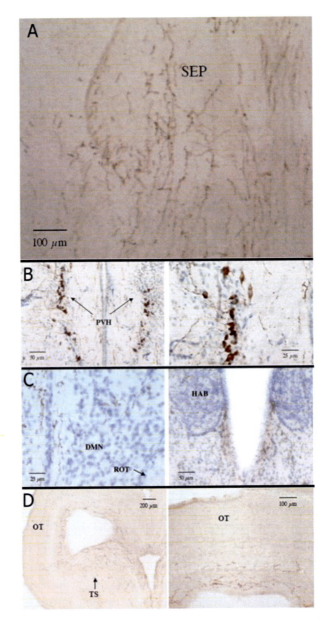

Figure 3. *Anolis carolinensis* (A) Orexin-lir fibers within and adjacent to the septum (SEP). (B) Photomicrographs depicting orexin-lir cells and fibers at the level of the periventricular hypothalamic nucleus (PVH). (C) Orexin-lir fibers within the dorsomedial nucleus of the thalamus (left) and adjacent to the habenula (right). DMN, dorsomedial nucleus of the thalamus; HAB, habenula; ROT, nucleus rotundus. (D) Orexin-lir fibers within the torus semicircularis (TS) and optic tectum (OT).

In the green treefrog, orexin-lir fibers were visible from the telencephalon to the medulla, with the highest concentrations within the preoptic area and hypothalamus. Previous research in the treefrog details the innervation [Singletary et al. 2005]. Rostrally, fibers were observed in the septal areas, the medial and lateral pallium and nucleus accumbens. In the diencephalon, dense orexin-lir fibers were seen in the periventricular and dorsal medial portions of the thalamus. Caudally, moderate orexin-lir innervation was noted in the laminar nucleus of the torus, the deep layers of the optic tectum, the pretectal gray and extending into the medulla. Fewer orexin-lir fibers were seen in the telencephalon and the metencephalon.

4. Conclusion

4.1 Functional Implications of Orexin-lir Neuronal Distribution

Our studies on the distribution of orexin-lir neurons in the Syrian hamster, passerines, and the green tree frog support previous findings for the conservation of the orexin system across vertebrates. However orexin-lir distribution varies slightly across vertebrates, suggesting the orexin system may support different functions based on diverging physiological needs. For example, in rodent brains orexin neurons are centered on the lateral hypothalamus (LHy) including the perifornical area, which is involved in feeding behavior and the sleep/wake cycle [Peyron et al. 1998; Cutler et al. 1999; Nambu et al. 1999; McGranaghan et al. 2001; Mintz et al. 2001]. However, in sheep, only a few are seen in the lateral hypothalamus [Iqbal et al. 2001] and the orexin neurons in this LHy subpopulation project to the preoptic area apparently to regulate gonadotropin releasing hormone (GnRH). The majority of orexin cells are concentrated on the dorsomedial hypothalamus (DMH), which regulates feeding, the sleep/wake cycle and the baroreceptor reflex [McDowall et al. 2006]. It is possible that the orexin system may have different primary functions in different animals. It is also likely that due to differences in brain morphology several brain areas in one animal may accomplish the same functions as one area in another animal. Studies show that administration of orexin B does induce feeding in sheep [Sartin et al. 2001] and in the pig [Dyer et al. 1999] as in rodents. In the pig, orexin neurons are seen in the perifornical areas, DMH and posterior hypothalamus with a few seen in the anterior hypothalamus (AH) and POA suggesting a division of roles in feeding, arousal, reproduction or fluid homeostasis [Su et al. 2008]. Is orexin an overarching gatekeeper to homeostatic maintenance? Does the orexin system divide into several differing functional subpopulations as the evolution of more complex behavior emerges? If so, the mammalian species would likely have the most diverse and complex functions regulated by the orexin system. Indeed, the mammalian orexin sequence is thought to have evolved more rapidly than other vertebrates [Alvarez and Sutcliffe et al. 2002].

We also have to consider that neighboring areas and connectivity may dictate how orexin neurons function. Depending on the area of the brain, different neurotransmitters or neuropeptides are present and co-localize with orexin neurons, influencing separate or supplemental function. In rats, 94% of orexin neurons are co-localized with dynorphin in the LHy, which suppresses GABAergic input to the tuberomammillary neurons. These histaminergic neurons are known to increase arousal via orexin input [Bayer et al. 2001; Huang et al. 2001]; therefore, dynorphin facilitates the effect of the orexin excitatory stimulus [Chou et al. 2001; Eriksson et al. 2004]. Separate glutamate and orexin immunoreactive vesicles are present in the orexin projections to the tuberomammillary nucleus, which may increase the excitatory input depending on concurrent release [Torrealba et al. 2003]. Orexin cells are also co-localized with Narp, a neuronal pentraxin known to regulate AMPA glutamate receptor clustering and excitatory synaptogenesis [Reti et al. 2002]. At least 50% of orexin cells are considered to be glutamatergic based on VGLUT2 immunostaining in the rat. The authors of that study also consider that the function of subsets of orexin neurons may be dependent on the neurochemical phenotypes [Rosin et al. 2003]. Other examples indicate that the orexin system may be important in reproduction in some mammalian species. Six percent of orexin cells are co-localized with GnRH neurons in the pig hypothalamus [Su et al. 2008]. Many studies have also shown orexin to modulate reproduction in rodents [Pu et al. 1998; Kohsaka et al. 2001; Campbell et al. 2003] as in other mammals. Considering the co-localization and connectivity of orexin neurons though, it is likely orexin plays a larger role in the sleep/wake cycle or energy metabolism. Therefore, although orexin is highly conserved across these mammals it is not homogeneous and may suggest separate or additional functions.

Also, environmental pressures unique to a species may facilitate evolution of systems in order to adapt. The threat of predation or the timing of food availability can alter the sleep durations and cycles of animals. Sleep stages and durations are different in a predator vs. prey, where the predator can afford to enter deeper stages of sleep but the prey needs to remain vigilant [Lima et al. 2005]. Though the proteins regulating these behaviors may be somewhat conserved the sensitivity to receptors or protein expression may vary depending on circadian or circannual states or sensory information [Richardson et al. 1995; Taheri et al. 2000; Archer et al. 2002; Chen and Randeva 2004]. Receptor selectivity may also change over the course of evolution, which may alter the potency and therefore function of the orexins [Shibahara et al. 1999].

Terrestrial vs. aquatic vertebrates have different environments so would likely have differing behavioral homeostatic fluid balance mechanisms [Feder and Burggren 1992] or neuromotor patterns during feeding [van der Leeuw et al. 2001]. Understanding the specialization of function of the orexin system or the addition of functions can also be used to tease out phylogenetic lineages.

In most species, orexin-lir cells are periventricular and found in neurosecretory areas. The PVN is a neurosecretory area in reptiles and mammals with connections to the median eminence and pituitary [Kawata and Sano 1982; Smeets et al. 1990; Propper et al. 1992; Luo et al. 1995]. The rostral PVN in birds also contains neurosecretory cells [Panzica et al. 1982; Kiss et al. 1987; Panzica et al. 1999; Absil et al. 2002]. In fish and amphibians, neurosecretory areas are found in the POA and SCN [Goossens et al. 1977; Conway and Gainer 1987; Smeets and Gonzalez 2001; Duarte et al. 2001]. The fact that areas containing orexin-lir cells in non-mammalian vertebrates have a neurosecretory function suggest that the neuropeptide, although found in different brain regions, play a similar role. Orexin-ir cells in many mammals are found outside of the neurosecretory PVN in the LHy. It is interesting to note that both areas contain neurons that regulate feeding behaviors. There are second-order target neurons in the PVN that inhibit feeding [Olson et al. 1991; Kow et al. 1991], but in the LHy the second-order neurons, which include orexin, induce feeding [Sakurai et al. 1998; Dube et al. 1999]. It is likely that in other vertebrates both inhibition and activation of feeding are primarily regulated by areas that differ in specialization in comparison to mammals. Indeed, though the avian brain is organized somewhat differently than mammals, studies have shown the neuronal populations to be comparable to mammals [Karten 1997; Medina and Reiner 2000; Jarvis et al. 2005].

In birds, orexin-lir neurons are located in one paraventricular population that expands to the stratum cellulare externum or posterior lateral hypothalamus [Rattenborg et al. 2002; Ohkubo et al. 2002; Singletary et al. 2006]. Orexin-lir neurons were located in similar areas regardless of phylogeny or domestication in birds. Given the location of cells, studies were done to determine if orexin was involved in the regulation of feeding as in mammals. However, while food deprivation up-regulates prepro-orexin in rats [Cai et al. 1999; Karteris et al. 2005], fasting does not enhance orexin expression in Japanese quail [Phillips-Singh et al. 2003]. Furthermore, while injections of orexin A increase feeding in rats [Dube et al. 1999], and infusions of orexin A increase feeding in goldfish [Volkoff et al. 1999], no orexigenic effect has been seen in chicken or pigeons [Furuse et al. 1999; Simao de Silva et al. 2008]. It is also interesting to note that unlike mammals, a receptor that preferentially binds orexin A in chickens has not yet been identified [Ohkubo et al. 2003]. Though only one receptor has been found in birds, it is the most similar to orexin receptor 2 which binds A or B with the same affinity. Several studies in mammals suggest a role for orexin A as orexigenic and orexin B as a modulator of the sleep/wake cycle [Sakurai et al. 1998; Fujiki et al. 2003], but these roles could be dependent on the receptors that have evolved in different vertebrates [Chen and Randeva, 2004]. In addition, orexin A injections in pigeons increase arousal [Simao de Silva et al. 2008] and orexin receptor antagonist injections increase sleep behavior in sparrows [Singletary et al. 2009] similar to mammals. It is possible that as the orexin system evolved in birds, the regulation of the sleep/wake cycle was conserved but feeding modulation was lost.

In green anole lizards, orexin-lir cells have been found more caudally as a single population located along the third ventricle within the periventricular nucleus [Farrell et al. 2003]. In turtles, orexin-lir neurons are predominantly found in the median eminence (ME) extending to the periventricular hypothalamic nucleus [Eiland et al. 2001]. This closely resembles the population seen in birds, but in birds this neuronal population extends laterally. Studies determining structure or function have not been completed in reptiles but from cell and fiber location it is likely that orexin regulates homeostasis.

In goldfish, while there is a consensus that a group of orexin-lir cell bodies is located along the third ventricle, some studies reported an additional group in a more lateral brain region [Huesa et al. 2005; Nakamachi et al. 2006]. In medaka, orexin-lir cell bodies have a similar distribution to the goldfish [Amiya et al. 2007]. There is inconsistency among the findings in zebrafish as well. In one zebrafish study, orexin cells are distributed into two separate populations, one along the third ventricle within the preoptic area and SCN, and the other within the anterior hypothalamus [Kaslin et al. 2004]. Recently however, researchers have shown only one population in the rostral medial hypothalamus using a species-specific antibody [Faraco et al. 2006]. Discrepancies between species may be due to phylogenetic differences, although within species this could reflect different techniques or species-specific antibodies available.

Studies have shown that injections of orexins increase feeding in goldfish [Volkoff et al. 1999; Nakamachi et al. 2006] and locomotor activity [Nakamachi et al. 2006]. In fasted goldfish the expression of orexin mRNA is increased as well as the number of orexin-lir cells [Nakamachi et al. 2006]. The orexin system has been more thoroughly studied in zebrafish. Similar to birds, there is only one orexin receptor found in zebrafish that is most homologous to the mammalian orexin receptor 2 [Prober et al. 2006]. The orexin system has also been implicated in the regulation of the sleep/wake cycle in zebrafish. In orexin receptor mutant zebrafish, a decrease in sleep is found with sleep fragmentation. Additionally when orexin A was injected decreased locomotion and increased sleep was observed [Yokogawa et al. 2007]. In contrast, overexpression of orexin in zebrafish larva decreases sleep [Prober et al. 2006]. This is conflicting but may be explained by the age of the zebrafish, the development of the orexin system and the balance of sleep/wake neuronal systems.

4.2 Functional Implications of Orexin-lir Fiber Distribution

4.2.1 Mammals

In addition to orexin cell body location, orexin-ir fiber distribution can help further elucidate the physiological roles of orexin. Generally, in mammals, there is dense orexin-ir innervation of the hypothalamus, midline thalamic areas, and locus coeruleus, whereas, the hippocampus, cortex and cerebellum are sparsely innervated. However in some cases, orexin-ir fiber distribution differs slightly depending on species. For example, dissimilar to rats, orexin projections are absent in the hamster SCN though they are seen in the surrounding areas [Mintz et al. 2001; this study]. This result is interesting given the overwhelming evidence for the role of orexin in the sleep/wake cycle and the circadian function of the SCN.

4.2.2 Birds

The apparently conserved neural distribution of orexins suggests that these peptides play similar roles among birds including galliformes, columbiformes and passeriformes. The distribution of immunoreactive neurons and fibers in this study was consistent with previous descriptions in birds using various methods of mRNA analysis and immunohistochemistry with different orexin antibodies [Rattenborg et al. 2002; Ohkubo et al. 2002, 2003; Phillips-Singh et al. 2003; Singletary et al. 2006].

High densities of orexin-lir fibers were observed across the hypothalamus, thalamus, and preoptic area similar to mammals. In addition, the auditory system is highly innervated, with the highest densities seen in the nucleus intercollicularis (ICo) and torus semicircularis (located just rostral to the ICo). In lizards and frogs, the torus semicircularis is moderately innervated [Farrell et al. 2003; Galas et al. 2001; Singletary et al. 2005]. The SCN and LHN are also highly innervated, areas thought to have circadian and visual functions in birds similar to the mammalian SCN [Brandstatter and Abraham 2003]. This is also consistent in lizards and frogs [Farrell et al. 2003; Galas et al. 2001; Singletary et al. 2005]. In addition, areas known to be involved in vigilance and movement in mammals, such as the LoC, the periaqueductal grey (PAG), Ru and substantia nigra pars compacta (SNc) are highly innervated in the passerine brain by orexin-lir fibers. Taken collectively, the results suggest that orexin is important for sensory and motor processing and circadian function in birds and other vertebrates.

There are a few discrepancies in orexin-lir fiber distribution between birds and mammals. For example, in passerines the Ru is innervated where fibers are scarce in mammals [Peyron et al. 1998]. Also, virtually no fibers were seen in the pedunculopontine tegmentum (PPT) in passerines, but this area in mammals is highly innervated [Peyron et al. 1998; Cutler et al. 1999; Nambu et al. 1999; McGranaghan et al. 2001; Mintz et al. 2001]. However, as a moderate density of orexin-lir fibers surrounds the periphery of the PPT in house finches, one cannot rule out the possibility of synaptic contact just outside the area. The PPT regulates atonia during REM sleep in mammals [Takakusaki et al. 2004; Takakusaki et al. 2005]. Interestingly, the nuchal (neck) muscles in birds, but not mammals, elicit electromyographic activity during REM sleep [Rattenborg et al. 2004]. An association between the absence of orexin-lir fibers in the PPT and the absence of atonia may not be limited to nuchal muscles, but also exist in other muscle groups.

4.2.3 Reptiles

In reptiles, the orexin-lir fibers are most prevalent in the medial and periventricular areas of the hypothalamus [Eiland et al. 2001; Farrell et al. 2003]. To date there are no physiological studies of the effects of orexin on reptiles and amphibians. Therefore, we can only speculate the function of orexin based solely on orexin-lir cell location and fiber distribution. In turtles orexin-lir neurons located in the ME send processes that protrude and likely secrete orexin directly into the CSF where it may be involved in endocrine function [Eiland et al. 2001]. In addition, in the anolis, orexin-lir fiber distribution also extended into thalamic areas, mainly the midline thalamus and habenula, which are thought to relay sensory information to the cortex. These areas are also important in the maintenance of biological rhythms in mammals and have similar connections. The optic tectum and torus semicircularis in the lizard were also innervated similar to amphibians [Galas et al. 2001; Singletary et al. 2005; Suzuki et al. 2008]. Orexin-lir fibers were not found in the cerebellum similar to other vertebrates. Despite the fact that there is a greater quantity and lateral extent of orexin-lir fibers in birds compared to lizards there was overall a similar distribution near the midline. This may mean a conservation of function between birds and lizards but that in birds, the larger innervation pattern would indicate additional functions of orexin.

4.2.4 Amphibians

In anurans, most of the orexin-lir innervation was located in the diencephalon and mesencephalon whereas the hippocampus, cerebellum and cortex are sparsely innervated. The distribution of orexin-lir innervation in the brain of *Hyla* is consistent with other vertebrates. In *Hyla*, as in mammals, orexin-lir fibers innervate the hypothalamus, preoptic area, thalamus, septum, and parts of the striatum, midbrain and hindbrain [Nambu et al. 1999; Mintz et al. 2001]. This innervation was also similar to the *Rana* and *Xenopus* but was more expansive [Shibahara et al. 1999; Galas et al. 2001]. However, few orexin-lir fibers were found in the *Rana* septum in contrast to the green tree frog and *Xenopus*. Also, orexin-lir projections were absent in the anterior and central thalamic nuclei of the *Xenopus*, which were moderate to dense in the *Rana* and *Hyla*. These latter frogs are considered terrestrial frogs and belong to the same superfamily of Neobatrachia, but the *Xenopus* is considered aquatic and belongs to the Mesobatrachia superfamily.

In the urodele axolotl, the orexin-lir is found predominantly in the hypothalamus and mesencephalon but not the thalamus [Suzuki et al. 2008]. Also, innervation of the SCN was scarce in contrast to what has been reported in the anurans. However, there was a higher density of orexin-lir innervation found in the urodele mesencephalon than in anurans. Further investigation of the variations in the amphibian orexin system could yield evidence of additional functions, although the overall similarity of orexin-lir innervation across vertebrates suggests that the orexin system is involved in general physiological regulation.

4.2.5 Fish

This degree of conservation of the orexin system is interesting considering the differing specializations of these various vertebrates. For example mammals and birds thermoregulate internally; mammals, birds and reptiles are amniotic; mammals, birds, reptiles and amphibians are tetrapods. Considering that the earliest evidence of the emergence of the orexin system is seen in fish [Alvarez and Sutcliffe 2002], these studies are fundamental to understanding the role of the orexin system.

In goldfish orexin-lir fibers are predominantly found in the ventral telencephalon, diencephalon and dorsal white zone of the optic tectum. Few fibers are found in the vicinity of the locus coeruleus and dorsal raphe [Huesa et al. 2005; Nakamachi et al. 2006], which indicates that orexin may be involved in feeding but not the control of vigilance, arousal or serotonergic modulation. However, orexin may be involved in only hunger-related arousal in goldfish, as these areas are not activated during mammalian food anticipatory behavior [Torrealba et al. 2003].

This is in contrast to the innervation seen in one zebrafish study [Kaslin et al. 2004] and in mammalian studies [Date et al. 1999; Brown et al. 2001]. In the zebrafish, orexin-lir innervation was found in the aminergic systems including the locus coeruleus, dorsal raphe, histaminergic neurons and cholinergic systems [Kaslin et al. 2004] but more recent studies show that that may be the result of non species-specific antibodies [Yokogawa et al. 2007]. Furthermore, the sole orexin receptor found in the zebrafish is not expressed in the locus coeruleus, serotonergic or histaminergic neurons. This lack of orexin-lir innervation and absence of orexin receptor in these wake promoting areas are crucial in explaining the surprising role of orexin on the sleep/wake cycle in zebrafish.

4.3 Further Considerations

The orexin peptides have highly conserved sequences across vertebrates. However, the receptors for these peptides are not as conserved or have not been found yet. Interestingly, *Xenopus* orexin B has a higher affinity *in vitro* for human receptor 1 and 2 than human orexin B but *Xenopus* orexin receptors have not been characterized yet. Only one receptor has been found in birds and in zebrafish, both of which are most homologous to the mammalian orexin

2 receptor. The functions of the orexin system are also dependent on the receptor type and distribution, the co-localization of orexin cells, and the areas the cells project to.

Additionally, behavioral state may modulate the system according to the species' unique adaptations or gender. Peripherally there are sex differences in the orexin system as well [Ohkubo et al. 2003; Silveyra et al. 2007]. In white crowned sparrows, levels of orexin fiber innervation change when birds are in the migratory condition [unpublished observations]. Cerebral spinal fluid levels of orexin change diurnally, and the activity of orexin neurons change throughout the day [Estabrooke et al. 2001; Martinez et al. 2002]. Orexin and orexin receptor expression changes in response to food deprivation [Nakamachi et al. 2006; Chen and Randeva, 2004] or photoperiod in sheep [Archer et al. 2002].

Overall, it is important to consider that differences in the orexin system within and between species could arise due to these factors. Many of the studies done thus far do not include information on the time of sacrifice or time of injection of drugs made to alter the orexin system. Many of the studies include animals in different photoperiods and different reproductive stages. Antibodies and techniques vary and can become problematic if comparisons are not all done with species specific antibodies and sensitive imaging techniques, though the obvious limitation is availability. Despite the fact that many caveats exist, any information that can be garnered proves beneficial for furthering the basic understanding for the role of orexin in human and all vertebrate physiology.

4.4 Summary

Because there are general similarities in cell location it is logical to assume some similar function of orexin across vertebrates. In the increasing complexity of the homeostatic mechanisms within and across each taxon, or introduction to unique environmental pressures, it is likely that the orexin system became more complex. The orexin system can be better explained by understanding the function of the areas that the orexin cells, fibers and receptors are found. In this study, we have contributed a detailed description of the orexin cell and fiber distribution in the reptilian brain. Though much work needs to be completed to determine the receptors in non-mammalian vertebrates, we can begin to narrow down function by comparing distributions of cells and fibers, orexin sequences, and the few physiological studies available. Given the information today the orexin system seems to regulate general homeostatic function across vertebrates, with specialization of function depending on the species.

Acknowledgments

The authors would like to thank Dr. William Farrell and Dr. Walt Wilczynski for expert advice and use of their figures. We would also like to thank Mimi Huang, Geri Vine, Jeannie Banh, Sherry Lim and Cari Sagum for excellent technical assistance. Dr. Christy Strand was also kind to critically read the manuscript. This work was supported by NSF IOB 0518272 to YD.

References

Absil, P., Papello, M., Viglietti-Panzica, C., Balthazart, J., Panzica, G.C. (2002). The medial preoptic nucleus receives vasotocinergic inputs in male quail: a tract-tracing and immunocytochemical study. *J. Chem. Neuroanat.* 24, 27-39.

Akanmu, M.A., Honda, K.(2005). Selective stimulation of orexin receptor type 2 promotes wakefulness in freely behaving rats. *Brain Res.* 1048 (1-2), 138-145.

Allison, J.D., Wilczynski, W. (1994). Efferents from the suprachiasmatic nucleus to basal forebrain nuclei in the Green Treefrog (*Hyla cinerea*), *Brain Behav. Evol.* 43,129-139.

Alvarez, C.E., Sutcliffe, J.G. (2002). Hypocretin is an early member of the incretin gene family. *Neurosci. Lett.* 324, 169-172.

Amiya, N., Amano, M., Oka, Y., Iigo, M., Takahashi, A., Yamamori, K. (2007). Immunohistochemical localization of orexin/hypocretin-like immunoreactive peptides and melanin-concentrating hormone in the brain and pituitary of medaka. *Neuroscience Letters* 427: 16-21.

Archer, Z.A., Findlay, P.A., Rhind, S.M., Mercer, J.G., Adam, C.L. (2002). Orexin gene expression and regulation by photoperiod in the sheep hypothalamus. *Regul. Pept.* 104(1-3): 41-45.

Aste, N., Balthazart, J., Absil, P., Grossman, R., Mülhbauer, E., Viglietti-Panzica, C. Panzica, G.C. (1998). Anatomical and neurochemical definition of the nucleus of the stria terminalis in Japanese Quail (*Coturnix japonica*). *J. Comp. Neurol.* 396, 141-157.

Bayer, L., Eggermann, E., Serafin, M, Saint-Mleux, B., Machard, D., Jones, B., Mühlethaler, M. (2001). Orexins (hypocretins) directly excite tuberomammillary neurons. *Eur. J. Neurosci.* Nov; 14(9): 1571-5.

Bayer, L., Eggermann, E., Saint-Mleux, B., Machard, D., Jones, B.E., Mühlethaler, M., Serafin, M. (2002). Selective action of orexin (hypocretin) on nonspecific thalamocortical projection neurons. *J. Neurosci.* 22(18):7835-7839.

Bingham, S., Davey, P.T., Babbs, A.J., Irving, E.A., Sammons, M.J., Wyles, M., Jeffrey, P., Cutler, L., Riba, I., Johns, A., Porter, R.A., Upton, N., Hunter, A.J., Parsons, A.A.(2001). Orexin-A, an hypothalamic peptide with analgesic properties. *Pain.* 92(1-2):81-90.

Brandstatter, R., Abraham, U. (2003). Hypothalamic circadian organization in birds. I. Anatomy, functional morphology, and terminology of the suprachiasmatic region. *Chronobiol. Int.* 20, 637-655.

Brown, R.E., Sergeeva, O., Eriksson, K.S., Haas, H.L. (2001). Orexin A excites serotonergic neurons in the dorsal raphe nucleus of the rat. *Neuropharmacology.* Mar;40(3):457-9.

Cai, X.J., Widdowson, P.S., Harrold, J., Wilson, S., Buckingham, R.E., Arch, J.R.S., Tadayyon, M., Clapham, J.C., Wilding, J., Williams, G. (1999). Hypothalamic orexin expression modulation by blood glucose and feeding. *Diabetes* 48, 2132-7.

Campbell, R.E., Grove, K.L., Smith, M.S. (2003). Gonadotropin-releasing hormone neurons coexpress orexin 1 receptor immunoreactivity and receive direct contacts by orexin fibers. *Endocrinology* 144(4): 1542-1548.

Chemelli, R.M., Willie, J.T., Sinton, C.M., Elmquist, J.K., Scammell, T., Lee, C., Richardson, J.A.,Williams, S.C., Xiong, Y., Kisanuki, Y., Fitch, T.E., Nakazato, M., Hammer, R.E., Saper, C.B., Yanagisawa, M.(1999). Narcolepsy in orexin knockout mice: molecular genetics of sleep regulation. *Cell* 98(4):437-451.

Chen, J., Randeva, H.S. (2004). Genomic organization of mouse orexin receptors:

characterization of two novel tissue-specific splice variants. *Mol. Endocrinol.* 18, 2790-2804.

Chou, T.C., Lee, C.E., Lu, J., Elmquist, J.K., Hara, J., Willie, J.T., Beuckmann, C.T., Chemelli, R.M., Sakurai, T., Yanagisawa, M., Saper, C.B., Scammell, T.E. (2001). Orexin (hypocretin) neurons contain dynorphin. *J. Neurosci.* 21(19):RC168.

Conway, K.M., Gainer, H. (1987). Immunocytochemical studies of vasotocin, mesotocin, and neurophysins in the Xenopus hypothalamo-neurohypophysial system. *J. Comp. Neurol.* 264, 494-508.

Cutler, D.J., Morris, R., Sheridhar, V., Wattam, T.A.K., Holmes, S., Patel, S., Arch, J.R.S., Wilson, S., Buckingham, R.E., Evans, M.L., Leslie, R.A., Williams, G. (1999). Differential distribution of orexin-A and orexin-B immunoreactivity in the rat brain and spinal cord. *Peptides* 20, 1455-1470.

Date, Y., Ueta, Y., Yamashita, H., Yamaguchi, H., Matsukura, S., Kangawa, K., Sakurai, T., Yanagisawa, M., Nakazato, M. (1999). Orexins, orexigenic hypothalamic peptides, interact with autonomic, neuroendocrine and neuroregulatory systems. *Proc. Natl. Acad. Sci.* 96(2):748-753.

de Lecea, L., Kilduff, T.S., Peyron, C., Gao, X.B., Foye, P.E., Danielson, P.E., Fukuhara, C., Battenberg, E.L.F., Gautvik, V.T., Bartlett, F.S., Frankel, W.N., van den Pol, A.N., Bloom, F.E., Gautvik, K.M., Sutcliffe, J.G. (1998). The hypocretins: hypothalamus-specific peptides with neuroexcitatory activity. *Proc. Natl. Acad. Sci. USA* 95, 322-327.

Deviche, P., Saldanha, C.J., Silver, R. (2000). Changes in brain gonadotropin-releasing hormone- and vasoactive intestinal polypeptide-like immunoreactivity accompanying reestablishment of photosensitivity in male dark-eyed juncos. (*Junco hyemalis*). *Gen. Comp. Endocrinol.* 117(1):8-19.

Downs, J.L., Dunn, M.R., Borok, E., Shanabrough, M., Horvath, T.L., Kohama, S.G., Urbanski, H.F. (2007) Orexin neuronal changes in the locus coeruleus of the aging Rhesus macaque. *Neurobiol. Aging* 28(8):1286-1295.

Duarte, G., Segura-Noguera, M.M., Martin del Rio, M.P., Mancera, J.M. (2001). The hypothalamo-hypophyseal system of the white seabream *Diplodus sargus*: immunocytochemical identification of arginine-vasotocin, isotocin, melanin-concentrating hormone and corticotropin-releasing factor. *Histochem. J.* 33, 569-578.

Dube, M.G., Kalra, S.P., Kalra, P.S. (1999). Food intake elicited by central administration of orexins/hypocretins: identification of hypothalamic sites of action. *Brain Res.* 842, 473-477.

Dyer, C.J., Touchette, K.J., Carroll, J.A., Allee, G.L., Matteri, R.L. (1999). Cloning of porcine prepro-orexin cDNA and effects of an intramuscular injection of synthetic porcine orexin-B on feed intake in young pigs. *Dom. Anim. Endocrinol.* 16, 145-148.

Eiland, M.M., Thannickal, T.C., Siegel, J. (2001). Distribution of hypocretin (orexin) and MCH containing cells in the turtle. *Actas de Fisiol.* 7, 263.

Eriksson, K.S., Sergeeva, O.A., Selbach, O., Haas, H.L. (2004). Orexin (hypocretin)/ dynorphin neurons control GABAergic inputs to tuberomammillary neurons. European *Journal of Neuroscience* 19,1278-1284.

Espana, R.A., Plahn, S., Berridge, C.W. (2002). Circadian-dependent and circadian-independent behavioral actions of hypocretin/orexin. *Brain Res.* 943(2), 224-236.

Estabrooke, I.V., McCarthy, M.T., Ko, E., Chou, T.C., Chemelli, R.M., Yanagisawa, M., Saper, C.B., Scammell, T.E. (2001) Fos expression in orexin neurons varies with behavioral state. *J. Neurosci.* Mar 1;21(5), 1656-62.

Faraco, J.H., Appelbaum, L., Marin, W., Gaus, S.E., Mourrain, P., Mignot, E. (2006). Regulation of hypocretin (orexin) expression in embryonic zebrafish. *J. Biol. Chem.* 281, 29753-29761.

Farrell, W.J., Delville, Y., Wilczynski, W. (2003). Immunocytochemical localization of orexin in the brain of the green anole lizard (*Anolis carolinensis*). *Soc. Neur. Abstr.* 33, 828.4.

Feder, M.E., Burggren, W.W., (eds.). (1992). *Environmental Physiology of the Amphibians.* University of Chicago Press., 646 pages.

Fujiki, N., Yoshida, Y., Ripley, B., Mignot, E., Nishino, S. (2003). Effects of IV and ICV hypocretin-1 (orexin A) in hypocretin receptor-2 gene mutated narcoleptic dogs and IV hypocretin-1 replacement therapy in a hypocretin-ligand-deficient narcoleptic dog. *Sleep* 26, 953-959.

Furuse, M., Ando, R., Bungo, T., Ao, R., Shimojo, M., Masuda, Y. (1999). Intracerebroventricular injection of orexins does not stimulate food intake in neonatal chicks. *Br. Poult. Sci.* 40, 698-700.

Galas, L., Vaudry, H., Braun, B., van den Pol, A.N., de Lecea, L., Sutcliffe, J.G., Chartrel, N. (2001). Immunohistochemical localization and biochemical characterization of hypocretin/orexin-related peptides in the central nervous system of the frog *Rana ridibunda*. *J. Comp. Neurol.* 429, 242-252.

Gerashchenko, D., Kohls, M.D., Greco, M., Waleh, N.S,. Salin-Pascual, R., Kilduff, T.S., Lappi, D.A., Shiromani, P.J. (2001). Hypocretin-2-saporin lesions of the lateral hypothalamus produce narcoleptic-like sleep behavior in the rat. *J. Neurosci.* 21(18), 7273-7283.

Goossens, N., Dierickx, K., Vandesande, F. (1977). Immunocytochemical demonstration of the hypothalamo-hypophyseal vasotocinergic system of *Lampetra fluviatilis*. *Cell Tiss. Res.* 177, 317-323.

Huang, Z.L., Qu, W.M., Li, W.D., Mochizuki, T., Eguchi, N., Watanabe, T., Urade, Y., Hayaishi, O. (2001). Arousal effect of orexin A depends on activation of the histaminergic system. *Proc. Natl. Acad. Sci. USA*; 98: 9965–70.

Huesa, G., van den Pol, A.N., Finger, T.E. (2005). Differential distribution of hypocretin (orexin) and melanin-concentrating hormone in the goldfish brain. *J. Comp. Neurol.* 488, 476-491.

Ida, T., Nakahara, K., Murakami, T., Hanada, R., Nakazato, M., Murakami, N. (2000). Possible involvement of orexin in the stress reaction in rats. *Biochem. Biophys. Res. Commun.* 270(1), 318-23.

Iqbal, J., Pompolo, S., Sakurai, T., Clarke, I.J. (2001). Evidence that orexin-containing neurons provide direct input to gonadotropin-releasing hormone neurons in the ovine hypothalamus. *J. Endocrinol.* 13, 1033-1041.

Jarvis, E.D., Güntürkün, O., Bruce, L., Csillag, A., Karten, H., Kuenzel, W., Medina, L., Paxinos, G., Perkel, D.J., Shimizu, T., Striedter, G., Wild, M., Ball, G.F., Dugas-Ford, J., Durand, S., Hough, G., Husband, S., Kubikova, L., Lee, D., Mello, C.V., Powers, A., Siang, C., Smulders, T.V., Wada, K., White, S.A., Yamamoto, K., Yu, J., Reiner, A.,

Butler, A.B. (2005). Avian brains and a new understanding of vertebrate brain evolution. *Nat. Rev. Neurosci.* 6, 151-159.

Karten, H.J. (1997). Evolutionary developmental biology meets the brain: The origins of mammalian cortex. *Proc. Natl. Acad. Sci. USA* 94, 2800-2804.

Karteris, E., Machado, R.J., Chen, J., Zervou, S., Hillhouse, E.W., Randeva, H.S. (2005). Food deprivation differentially modulates orexin receptor expression and signaling in rat hypothalamus and adrenal cortex. *AJP-Endo.* 288, 1089-1100.

Kawata, M., Sano, Y. (1982). Immunohistochemical identification of the oxytocin and vasopressin neurons in the hypothalamus of the monkey (*Macaca fuscata*). *Anat. Embryol.* (Berl). 165, 151-167.

Kaslin, J., Nystedt, J.M., Östergård, M., Peitsaro, N., Panula, P. (2004). The orexin/hypocretin system in zebrafish is connected to the aminergic and cholinergic systems. *J. Neurosci.* 24, 2678-2689.

Kiss, J.Z., Voorhuis, T.A., van Eekelen, J.A., de Kloet, E.R., de Wied, D. (1987). Organization of vasotocin-immunoreactive cells and fibers in the canary brain. *J. Comp. Neurol.* 263, 347-364.

Kohsaka, A., Watanobe, H., Kakizaki, Y., Suda, T., Schioth, H.B., (2001). A significant participation of orexin-A, a potent orexigenic peptide, in the preovulatory luteinizing hormone and prolactin surges in the rat. *Brain Res.* 898: 166-170.

Kow, L.M., Pfaff, D.W. (1991). The effects of the TRH metabolite cyclo(His-Pro) and its analogs on feeding. *Pharmacol. Biochem. Behav.* 38, 359-364.

Krutzfeldt, N.O.E., Wild, J.M. (2004). Definition and Connections of the Entopallium in the Zebra Finch (*Taeniopygia guttata*). *J. Comp. Neurol.* 468, 452-465.

Kuenzel,W.,(2004). Chicken atlas for nomenclature forum. *http://www.avianbrain.org/atlases.html*

Kuru, M., Ueta, Y., Serino, R., Nakazato, M., Yamamoto, Y., Shibuya, I., Yamashita, H. (2001). Centrally administered orexin/hypocretin activates HPA axis in rats. *Neuroreport.* 11(9), 1977-80.

Lima, S. L., Rattenborg, N.C., Lesku, J.A., Amlaner, C.J. (2005). Sleeping under the risk of predation. *Anim. Behav.* 70, 723-736.

Lin, L., Faraco, J., Li, R., Kadotani, H., Rogers,W., Lin, X., Qiu, X., de Jong, P.J., Nishino, S., Mignot, E. (1999). The sleep disorder canine narcolepsy is caused by a mutation in the hypocretin (orexin) receptor 2 gene. *Cell* 98(3):365-376.

Luo, Y., Peng, N., Yang, W., Zhang, W. (1995). Studies on the distribution of vasopressin-immunoreactive neuronal perikarya and their fibers in the hypothalamus of *Tupaia belangeri. Brain Res.* 687, 191-193.

Martinez, G.S., Smale, L., Nunez, A.A. (2002). Diurnal and nocturnal rodents show rhythms in orexinergic neurons. *Brain Res.* 955, 1-7.

McDowall, L.M., Horiuchi, J., Killinger, S., Dampney, R.A.L. (2006). Modulation of the baroreceptor reflex by the dorsomedial hypothalamic nucleus and perifornical area. *AJP-Regul. Integr. Physiol.* 290, 1020-1026.

McGranaghan, P.A., Piggins, H.D. (2001). Orexin A-like immunoreactivity in the hypothalamus and thalamus of the Syrian hamster (*Mesocricetus auratus*) and Siberian hamster (*Phodopus sungorus*), with special reference to circadian structures. *Brain Res.* 904, 234-244.

Medina, L., Reiner, A. (2000). Do birds possess homologues of mammalian primary visual, somatosensory and motor cortices? *Trends Neurosci.* 23, 1-12.

Mintz, E.M., van den Pol, A.N., Casano, A.A., Albers, H.E. (2001). Distribution of hypocretin-(orexin) immunoreactivity in the central nervous system of Syrian hamster (*Mesocricetus auratus*). *J. Chem. Neuroanat.* 21, 225-238.

Muschamp, J.W., Dominguez, J.M., Sato, S.M., Shen, R.Y., Hull, E.M. (2007). A role for hypocretin (orexin) in male sexual behavior. *J. Neurosci.* 27(11), 2837-45.

Nakamachi, T., Matsuda, K., Maruyama, K., Miura, T., Uchiyama, M., Funahashi, H., Sakuri, T., Shioda, S. (2006). Regulation by Orexin of Feeding Behaviour and Locomotor Activity in the Goldfish. *J. Neuroendo.* vol. 18, 290-297.

Nambu, T., Sakurai, T., Mizukami, K., Hosoya, Y., Yanagisawa, M., Goto, K. (1999). Distribution of orexin neurons in the adult rat brain. *Brain Res.* 827, 243-260.

Neary, T.J. (1995). Afferent projections to the hypothalamus in Ranid frogs, *Brain Behav. Evol.* 46 1-13.

Ohkubo, T., Boswell, T., Lumineau, S. (2002). Molecular cloning of chicken prepro-orexin cDNA and preferential expression in the chicken hypothalamus. *Biochim. Biophys. Acta* 1577, 476-480.

Ohkubo, T., Tsukada, A., Shamoto, K. (2003). cDNA cloning of chicken orexin receptor and tissue distribution: sexually dimorphic expression in chicken gonads. *J. Mol. Endocrinol.* 31, 499-508.

Olson, B.R., Drutarosky, M.D., Chow, M.S., Hruby, V.J., Stricker, E.M., Verbalis, J.G. (1991). Oxytocin and an oxytocin antagonist administered centrally decrease food intake in rats. *Peptides* 12, 113-118.

Panzica, G.C., Viglietti-Panzica, C., Contenti, E. (1982). Synaptology of neurosecretory cells in the nucleus paraventricularis of the domestic fowl. *Cell Tiss. Res.* 227, 79-92.

Panzica, G.C., Plumari, L., Garcia-Ojeda, E., Deviche, P. (1999). Central vasotocin-immunoreactive system in a male passerine bird (*Junco hyemalis*). *J. Comp. Neurol.* 409, 105-117.

Peyron, C., Tighe, D.K., van den Pol, A.N., de Lecea, L., Heller, H.C., Sutcliffe, J.G., Kilduff, T.S. (1998). Neurons containing hypocretin (orexin) project to multiple neuronal systems. *J. Neurosci.* 18, 9996-10015.

Peyron, C., Faraco, J., Rogers, W., Ripley, B., Overeem, S., Charnay, Y., Nevsimalova, S., Aldrich, M., Reynolds, D., Albin, R., Li, R., Hungs, M., Pedrazzoli, M., Padigaru, M., Kucherlapati, M., Fan, J., Maki, R., Lammers, G.J., Bouras, C., Kucherlapati, R., Nishino,S., Mignot, E. (2000). A mutation in a case of early onset narcolepsy and a generalized absence of hypocretin peptides in human narcoleptic brains. *Nat. Med.* 1286(9):991-997.

Phillips-Singh, D., Li, Q., Takeuchi, S., Ohkubo, T., Sharp, P.J., Boswell, T. (2003). Fasting differentially regulates expression of agouti-related peptide, pro-opiomelanocortin, prepro-orexin, and vasoactive intestinal polypeptide mRNAs in the hypothalamus of Japanese quail. *Cell Tiss. Res.* 313, 217-225.

Prober, D.A., Rihel, J., Onah, A.A., Sung, R-J., Schier, A.F. (2006). Hypocretin/orexin overexpression induces an insomnia-like phenotype in zebrafish. *J. Neurosci.* 26(51): 13400-13410.

Propper, C.R., Jones, R.E., Lopez, K.H. (1992). Distribution of arginine vasotocin in the brain of the lizard Anolis carolinensis. *Cell Tiss. Res.* (1992) 267, 391-398.

Pu, S., Jain, M.R., Kalra, P.S., Kalra, S.P. (1998). Orexins, a novel family of hypothalamic neuropeptides, modulate pituitary luteinizing hormone secretion in an ovarian steroid-dependent manner. *Regul. Pept.* Nov 30;78(1-3):133-6.

Rattenborg, N.C., Gerstner, J.R., Landry, C.F., Obermeyer, W.H., Benca, R,M. (2002). Hypocretin immunoreactive neurons in normal and roller pigeons (*Columbia livia*) Sleep: 25 *abstract Supplement* 211.F.

Rattenborg, N.C., Mandt, B.H., Obermeyer, W.H., Winsauer, P.J., Huber, R., Wikelski, M., Benca, R.M. (2004). Migratory sleeplessness in the White-Crowned Sparrow (*Zonotrichia leucophrys gambelii*). *PLoS Biol.* 2, 0924-0936.

Reiner, A., Perkel, D.J., Bruce, J.J., Butler, A.B., Csillag, A., Kuenzel, W., Medina, L., Paxinos, G., Shimuzu, T., Striedter, G., Wild, M., Ball, G.F., Durand, S., Gunturkun, O., Lee, D.W., Mello, C.V., Powers, A., White, S.A., Hough, G., Kubikova, L., Smulders, T.V., Wada, K., Dugas-Ford, J., Husband, S., Yamamoto, K., Yu, J., Siang, C., Jarvis, E.D. (2004). Avian Brain Nomenclature Forum. Revised nomenclature for avian telencephalon and some related brainstem nuclei. *J. Comp. Neurol.* 473, 377-414.

Reiner, A., Yamamoto, K., Karten, H.J. (2005). Organization and evolution of the avian forebrain. *Anat. Rec. A. Discov. Mol. Cell Evol. Biol.* 287, 1080-102. Review.

Reti, I.M., Reddy, R., Worley, P.F., Baraban, J.M. (2002). Selective expression of Narp, a secreted neuronal pentraxin, in orexin neurons. *J. Neurochem.* 82: 1561-1565.

Richardson, R.D., Boswell, T., Raffety, B.D., Seeley, R.J., Wingfield, J.C., Woods, S.C.. (1995). NPY increases food intake in white-crowned sparrows: effect in short and long photoperiods. *Am. J. Physiol.* 268(6 Pt 2):R1418-22

Rosin, D.L., Weston, M.C., Sevigny, C.P., Stornetta, R.L., Guyenet, P.G. (2003). Hypothalamic orexin(hypocretin) neurons express vesicular glutamate transporters VGLUT1 or VGLUT2. *J. Comp. Neurol.* 465, 593-603.

Sakurai, T., Mameiya, A., Ishii, M., Matsuzaki, I., Chemelli, R.M., Tanaka, H., Williams, S.C., Richardson, J.A., Kozlowski, G.P., Wilson, S., Arch, J.R.S., Buckingham, R.E., Haynes, A.C., Carr, S.A., Annan, R.S., McNulty, D.E., Liu, W.S., Terret, J.A., Elshourbagy, N.A., Bergsma, D.J., Yanagisawa, M. (1998). Orexins and orexin receptors: a family of hypothalamic neuropeptides and G protein-coupled receptors that regulate feeding behavior. *Cell* 92, 573-585.

Saldanha, C.J., Deviche, P.J., Silver, R. (1994). Increased VIP and decreased GnRH expression in photorefractory dark-eyed juncos (*Junco hyemalis*). *Gen. Comp. Endocrinol.* 93(1):128-36.

Saper, C.B., Chou, T.C., Scammell, T.E. (2001). The sleep switch: hypothalamic control of sleep and wakefulness. *Trends Neurosci.* 24(12):726-731.

Sartin, J.L., Dyer, C., Matteri, R., Buxton, D., Buonomo, F., Shores, M., Baker, J., Osborne, J.A., Braden, T., Steele, B. (2001). Effect of intracerebroventricular orexin-B on food intake in sheep. *J. Anim. Sci.* 79:1573-1577.

Shibahara, M., Sakurai, T., Nambu, T., Takenouchi, T., Iwaasa, H., Egashira, S.I., Ihara, M., Goto, K. (1999). Structure, tissue distribution, and pharmacological characterization of Xenopus orexins. *Peptides* 20, 1169-1176.

Silveyra, P., Lux-Lantos, V., Libertun, C. (2007). Both orexin receptors are expressed in rat ovaries and fluctuate with the estrous cycle: effects of orexin receptor antagonists on gonadotropins and ovulation. *Am. J. Physiol. Met.* 293, 977-985.

Smeets, W.J., Sevensma, J.J., Jonker, A.J. (1990). Comparative analysis of vasotocin-like immunoreactivity in the brain of the turtle *Pseudemys scripta elegans* and the snake *Python regius. Brain Behav. Evol.* 35, 65-84.

Smeets, W.J.A.J., González, A. (2001). Vasotocin and mesotocin in the brains of amphibians: state of the art. *Microsc. Res. Tech.* 54, 125-136.

Simao da Silva, E., Vicoso dos Santos, T., Hoeller, A.A., Souza dos Santos, T., Pereira, G.V., Meneghelli, C., Pezlin, A.I., Marcos dos Santos, M., Faria, M.S., Paschoalini, M.A., Marino-Neto, J. (2008). Behavioral and metabolic effects of central injections of orexins/hypocretins in pigeons. *Regul. Pept.* 147, 9-18.

Singletary, K.G., Delville, Y., Farrell, W.J., Wilczynski, W. (2005). Distribution of orexin/hypocretin immunoreactivity in the nervous system of the green treefrog, *Hyla cinerea. Brain Res.* 1041, 231-236.

Singletary, K.G., Deviche, P., Strand, C., Delville, Y. (2006). Distribution of orexin/hypocretin immunoreactivity in the brain of a male songbird, the house finch, *Carpodacus mexicanus. J. Chem. Neuroanat.* 32(2-4), 81-89.

Singletary, K.G., Simpson, L., Sagum, C., Delville, Y. (2009). A dual orexin receptor antagonist modulates the sleep/wake cycle in white-crowned sparrows. *SLEEP* 32, *Abstr. Suppl.,* 0097.

Stokes, T.M., Leonard, C.M., Nottebohm, F. (1974). The telencephalon, diencephalon, and mesencephalon of the canary, *Serinus canaria,* in stereotaxic coordinates. *J. Comp. Neurol.* 156, 337-374.

Su, J., Lei, Z., Zhang, W., Ning, H., Ping, J. (2008). Distribution of orexin B and its relationship with GnRH in the pig hypothalamus. *Res. Vet. Sci.* 85, 315-323.

Suzuki, H., Kubo, Y., Yamamoto, T. (2008). Orexin-A immunoreactive cells and fibers in the central nervous system of the axolotl brain and their association with tyrosine hydroxylase and serotonin immunoreactive somata. *J. Chem. Neuroanat.* 35, 295-305.

Taheri, S., Sunter, D., Dakin, C., Moyes, S., Seal, L., Gardiner, J., Rossi, M., Ghatei, M., Bloom, S. (2000). Diurnal variation in orexin A immunoreactivity and prepro-orexin mRNA in the rat central nervous system. *Neurosci. Lett.* 279(2), 109-12.

Takakusaki, K., Saitoh, K., Harada, H., Okumura, T., Sakamoto, T. (2004). Evidence for a role of basal ganglia in the regulation of rapid eye movement sleep by electrical and chemical stimulation for the pedunculopontine tegmental nucleus and the substantia nigra pars reticulata in decerebrate cats. *Neuroscience* 124, 207-220.

Takakusaki, K., Takahashi, K., Saitoh, K., Harada, H., Okumura, T., Kayama, Y., Koyama, Y. (2005). Orexinergic projections to the cat midbrain mediate alternation of emotional behavioural states from locomotion to cataplexy. *J. Physiol.* 568, 1003-1120.

Thannickal, T.C., Moore, R.Y., Nienhuis, R., Ramanathan, L., Gulyani, S., Aldrich, M., Cornford, M., Siegel, J.M. (2000). Reduced number of hypocretin neurons in human narcolepsy. *Neuron* 27(3):469-474.

Torrealba, F., Yanagisawa, M., Saper, C.B. (2003). Colocalization of orexin–A and glutamate immunoreactivity in axon terminals in the tuberomammillary nucleus in rats. *Neuroscience* 119, 1033-1044.

van der Leeuw, A.H., Bout, R.G., Zweers, G.A. (2001). Control of the cranio-cervical system during feeding in birds. *Amer. Zool.* 41 : 1352-1363.

van den Pol, A. (1999). Hypothalamic hypocretin (orexin): robust innervation of the spinal cord. *J. Neurosci.* 19(8), 3171-82.

Volkoff, H., Bjorklund, J.M., Peter, R.E., (1999). Stimulation of feeding behavior and food consumption in the goldfish, *Carassius auratus*, by orexin-A and orexin-B, *Brain Res.* 846, 204-209.

Watson, R.E., Weigand, S.J., Clough, J.A., Hoffman, G.E. (1986). Use of cryoprotectant to maintain long-term peptide immunoreactivity and tissue morphology. *Peptides* 7, 155–159.

Wilczynski, W., Northcutt, R.G. (1983). Connections of the bullfrog striatum: efferent projections, *J. Comp. Neurol.* 214, 333-343.

Willie, J.T., Chemelli, R.M., Sinton, C.M., Tokita, S., Williams, S.C., Kisanuki, Y.Y., Marcus, J.N., Lee, C., Elmquist, J.K,, Kohlmeier, K.A., Leonard, C.S., Richardson, J.A., Hammer, R.E., Yanagisawa, M. (2003). Distinct narcolepsy syndromes in orexin receptor-2 and orexin null mice: molecular genetic dissection of non-REM and REM sleep regulatory processes. *Neuron* 38(5), 715-730.

Wommack, J.C., Delville, Y. (2002). Chronic social stress during puberty enhances tyrosine hydroxylase immunoreactivity within the limbic system in golden hamsters. *Brain Res.* 933, 139–143.

Yokogawa, T., Marin, W., Faraco, J., Pezeron, G., Appelbaum, L., Zhang, J., Rosa, F., Mourrain, P., Mignot, E. (2007). Characterization of sleep in zebrafish and insomnia in hypocretin receptor mutants. *PLoS Biol.* 5, 2379-2397.

In: Neuroanatomy Research Advances
Editors: C. E. Flynn and B. R. Callaghan, pp.145-164

ISBN: 978-60741-610-4
©2010 Nova Science Publishers, Inc.

Chapter V

Visual Cortex: Crosstalk and Concomitant Communications between Extrastriate Visual Areas

Hiroyuki Nakamura[*] and Kazuo Itoh

Department of Morphological Neuroscience, Gifu University Graduate School of
Medicine, Gifu 501-1194, Japan

Abstract

Extrastriate visual cortex has been divided into the dorsal and ventral stream visual
areas. The dorsal stream visual areas are located in the occipito-parietal pathway directed
to the superior temporal sulcus and inferior parietal lobule visual areas, underlying motion
and spatial vision. These areas have been considered to receive visual information from
magnocellular retinal ganglion cells through layer 4Cα and layer 4B of the primary visual
area V1 (striate cortex), and then the cytochrome oxidase (CO)-rich thick stripes of the
secondary visual area V2. On the other hand, the ventral stream visual areas are located in
the occipito-temporal pathway directed to the inferior temporal cortex, underlying object
vision. These areas have been considered to receive visual information from the
parvocellular retinal ganglion cells through layer 4Cβ and layers 2-3 of V1, and then the
CO-rich thin stripes and the CO-poor interstripe regions of V2. This parallel visual
cortical information processing hypothesis is, however, too simple, and ignored abundant
connections between the dorsal and the ventral stream visual areas (Nakamura et al., *Soc.
Neurosci. Abstr., 18,* 294, 1992). In addition, recent analysis of the connections between
V1 and V2 CO-modules provided a line of evidence against the dorsal versus ventral
stream hypothesis (Sincich & Horton, *Science, 29,* 1734-1737, 2002; Nassi & Callaway,
J. Neurosci., 26, 12789-12798, 2006), and thus the whole story of visual cortical
information processing is now going to be reconstructed. We here describe the
connections between the extrastriate visual areas based on the previous reports, and our
publications and unpublished data to construct a graph scheme of visual cortical network.

---

[*]E-mail: hiron@gifu-u.ac.jp

The visual cortical network is hierarchically composed of several sets of visual areas and connections between them. Consider the areas as nodes and the connections as arcs, the network is a direct graph (Apollonio & Franciosa, *Descrete Math., 307,* 2598-2614, 2007). In this graph, functional groups of the areas and the connections are partial graphs. The partial graphs are dynamic in a sense that the nodes and arcs (the areas and connections) vary from time to time depending on what task or function is necessary. The dynamic partial graphs overlap each other to allow them common use of visual information.

Introduction

Vision provides us with detailed information about the world. The visual information from the retina is processed in our brain and enables us to recognize objects and events within the environment. In addition to pure recognition of the outer world, animals respond either consciously or unconsciously to the visual inputs. They also respond emotionally to the visual information of predators, food, or mate. These different activities of the visual areas are not isolated but are influencing each other. The question is how the brain creates such different outputs from vision. Our purpose of the present chapter is to demonstrate overlapping connections of the visual areas for different activities or outputs of the brain.

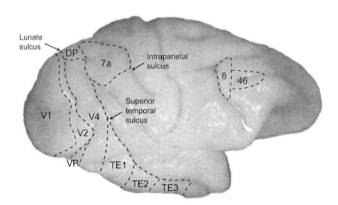

Figure 1. Visually related areas on the surface of right hemisphere in the Japanese macaque (*Macaca fuscata*). The right side of the figure is anterior and the top is dorsal. Abbreviations: 7a, posterior parietal area 7a; 8, prefrontal eye field area8; 46, prefrontal eye field area 46; DP, dorsal prelunate area; V1, primary visual area; V2, secondary visual area; V4, fourth visual area; VP, ventral posterior area; TE1-3, inferior temporal area 1-3. Original figure.

(1) Visual areas. Figure 1 shows the lateral surface view of the right hemisphere of a macaque monkey, illustrating the position of visual areas. The anatomy of the primate visual system has been studied in the macaque monkey, and we now recognize more than twenty-five visually related areas (Felleman & Van Essen, 1991; Van Essen et al., 1992). Most but not all of them are identified in the human brain using functional MRI (Wandell et al., 2007). Thus it is acceptable to consider that the visual cortex of macaques is similar to that of humans. In addition to the visual areas shown in Figure 1, several areas are hidden in the

sulci. Figure 2 shows other visual areas that lay in the lunate, intrapareital, superior temporal, inferior occipital, arcuate, and principal sulci. In this chapter, we focus on the connections of the extrastriate visual cortex explored in the macaque monkeys, because these are the only available concrete data so far on the connections of visual areas of the primate including the human being.

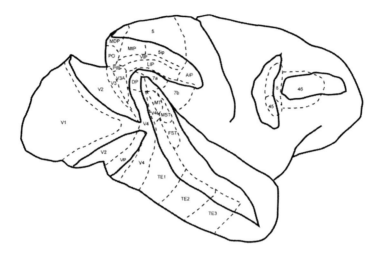

Figure 2. Visually related areas in the right hemisphere. Scheme with opened sulci (lunate, inferior occipital, intraparietal, superior temporal, arcuate, and principle sulci). The right side of the figure is anterior and the top is dorsal. Abbreviations: 5, parietal area 5; 5ip, intraparietal part of the area 5; 7a, posterior parietal area 7a; 7b, posterior parietal area 7b; 8, prefrontal eye field area8; 46, prefrontal eye field area 46; AIP, anterior intraparietal area; DP, dorsal prelunate area; FST, floor of superior temporal sulcal area; LIP, lateral intraparietal area; MIP, medial intraparietal area; MDP, medial dorsal parietal area; MST, medial superior temporal area; MT, middle temporal area; PIP, posterior intraparietal area; PO, parieto-occipital area, or V6/V6A; V1, primary visual area; V2, secondary visual area; V3, dorsal part of third visual area, or V3d; V3A, V3 accessory; V4, fourth visual area; V4t, V4 transitional; VIP, ventral intraparietal area; VP, ventral posterior area; TE1-3, inferior temporal area 1-3. Original figure.

(2) Parallel processing pathways. The visual information is sent from the primary visual area V1 to the extrastriate visual areas through cortico-cortical connections. Lesion studies of the posterior parietal and the inferior temporal cortex showed that object recognition is selectively impaired by lesions of inferior temporal areas, whereas judgments of spatial relations are impaired by lesions of area 7a and other posterior parietal areas (Ungerleider & Mishkin, 1982). Based on these results, Mishkin and colleagues proposed a parallel model of information processing in the visual cortex (Ungerleider & Mishkin, 1982; Mishkin et al., 1983). Figure 3 shows the anatomical correlate of the parallel processing hypothesis: The cortical connections from the occipital cortex V1 and V2 to the posterior parietal cortex via the middle temporal area (MT) compose the dorsal visual cortical stream for space vision, whereas the connections from V1 and V2 to the inferior temporal visual cortex via the fourth visual area V4 comprise the ventral cortical visual stream for object vision.

The hypothesis seemed to show good correspondence with the earlier bipartite model based on the findings of parvo- and magno-cellular retinal ganglion cells that project to the parvo- and magno-cellular layers of the lateral geniculate nucleus, respectively (Dreher et al, 1976; Sherman et al., 1976). Physiological and anatomical segregation of parvo- and magno-pathways in V1 further gave support for the hypothesis (Hubel & Wiesel, 1972; Hendrickson et al., 1978; Fitzpatrick et al., 1983; Blasdel & Fitzpatrick, 1984; Blasdel et al., 1985; Fitzpatrick et al., 1985). The magnocellular retinal ganglion cells respond to motion visual stimuli, and project to the magnocellular layers of the lateral geniculate nucleus. Information of motion vision is transmitted to layer 4Cα of V1, and then to layer 4B. From layer 4B, the information is sent to MT directly and indirectly via V2. This is called magnocellular or M-pathway. On the other hand, the parvocellular retinal ganglion cells process location and orientation of visual stimuli, and project to the parvocellular layers of the lateral geniculate nucleus. The visual information is transmitted to layer 4Cβ of V1. Neurons of layer 4Cβ project to layers 2-3, and those of layers 2-3 then project to V2. This is called parvocellular pathway or P-pathway. Apparently, the visual information processed in the P-pathway is necessary to analyze not only object shape but also space.

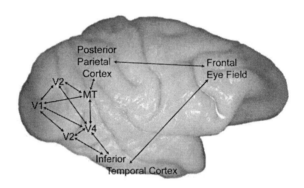

Figure 3. Dorsal versus ventral stream of the cortical visual processing drawn on the right hemisphere of macaque. The right side of the figure is anterior and the top is dorsal. MT, middle temporal area. Original figure.

The parallel processing or "bipartite" hypothesis was also supported by the finding of mostly segregated projections from cytochrome oxidase (CO)-rich thick stripes of V2 to MT and from CO-rich thin stripes and CO-poor interstripe regions to V4 (DeYoe & Van Essen, 1985). Further support came from a finding of segregation of neurons that are selective for color, form, and stereopsis in macaque V2. In addition, the distribution of color responsive neurons corresponds to the CO-rich thin stripes; that of form responsive neurons, to the CO-poor interstripe regions; and that of motion sensitive neurons, to the CO-rich thick stripes (Hubel & Livingstone, 1987). Because neurons in MT are selective to motion stimuli and those in V4 are selective to color and orientation, the parallel hypothesis seemed to well explain cortical visual processing (Livingstone & Hubel, 1988). It was thus hypothesized that the dorsal or occipito-parietal pathway is specialized for spatial perception locating *where* an object is, whereas the ventral or or occipito-temporal pathway is specialized for object perception identifying *what* an object is (Ungerleider & Misckin, 1982; also see Van Essen & Gallant, 1994).

The bipartite hypothesis is easy to understand, however, it is too simplified based on several assumptions and incorporates some problems. First, it is based on the assumption that the visual pathways originated from the magno- and parvo-cellular retinal ganglion cells are segregated throughout the visual cortical connections. Second, it is based on a hypothesis that topographically matched regions of the visual areas have connections each other, and visual information is processed consecutively and topographically. Third, the hypothesis does not account for the existence of robust cortico-cortical connections between the dorsal and ventral stream visual areas. Apparently, the visual processing of "*where* the object is" needs information of stimulus position that is processed in parvo-cellular system. Thus the connections should be incorporated into the visual cortical processing scheme. Van Essen and colleagues revised the hypothesis and created an idea of distributed network hypothesis (Felleman & Van Essen, 1991; Van Essen et al., 1992; Van Essen & Gallant, 1994). The new hypothesis incorporated hierarchy, parallel pathways, and abundant cross-connections, but the figure is too complicated to understand the features of cortical connections of the visual system.

We here describe our data on the connections between the extrastriate visual areas. The results do not support the parallel cortical visual processing hypothesis. We will illustrate a directed graph of distributed networks with areas as nodes and connections as arcs (Apollonio & Franciosa, 2007). The partial network for each function or task is described as overlapping dynamic partial graphs.

Materials and Methods

All animals were cared for in accordance with the National Institute Guide for the Care and Use of Laboratory Animals and the Guide for the Care, European Community Guidelines for the Care and Use of Animals in Scientific Experiments, and Use of the Laboratory Primates of the Primate Research Institute of Kyoto University. The results of Japanese monkey and those of Rhesus monkey were similar and we could not find any difference between these two species. We here describe the data without discrimination of these species.

(1) Tracer studies using macacque monkeys. A total of thirty-one adult macaque monkeys (*Macaca fuscata* and *Macaca mulatta*) of both sexes were used in this study. Under deep anesthesia with sodium pentobarbital (30 mg/kg, i.v.), animals were placed stereotaxic frame, and small amount of tracers (biotinylated dextran amine, WGA-HRP, fast blue, diamidino yellow, and nuclear yellow) were stereotaxically injected into the third tier visual areas (V3, V3A, VP), V4, posterior part of inferior temporal area (TE1, TEO, or PIT), lateral intraparietal area (LIP), and the anterior intraparietal area (AIT). After 2-14 days, the animals were transcardially perfused with a paraformaldehyde fixative solution. In most of the animals, the brain were cut into coronal sections; in some animals, white matter of the brain was taken out and the sulci were opened to prepare flatmount sections cut tangential to the cortical surface. Sections were mounted on gelatinized glass slides directly for fluorescent analysis, or were processed for histochemistry to visualize the tracers.

(2) Voltage sensitive dye experiments. To examine if the visual information be processed consecutive, point-to-pint activation through the visual areas, we used voltage sensitive dye imaging to elucidate the activation pattern of the visual cortex. Twenty-eight adult female ferrets (*Mustela putorius*) were used because they only have shallow sulci over the visual areas 17-21. In addition, it is able to cover the entire areas using current optical imaging

system. The animals were anesthetized with 1% isoflurane in 50:50 $N_2O:O_2$ gas, and were paralyzed with pancronium bromide (0.6mg/kg/h, i.v.). The animals were artificially ventilated so that expiratory CO_2 was kept between 3.3% and 4%, and the body temperature was maintained at 37 degrees Celsius. The exposed visual cortex was stained for 2 hrs with the voltage-sensitive dye RH795 (Molecular Probes). The pupil was dilated with 1% atropine sulfate eye drops and a contact lens was placed over one eye; the other eye was occluded.

The visual stimulus was shown on a computer display with refreshing rate at 120 Hz placed at a distance of 57 cm from the animal. The stimulus of a white square of 2 degrees width was flashed during 50 ms at 120 cd/m^2. The stimulus presentation was synchronized with the ECG signal and respiration was stopped during recording. A camera with an array of hexagonally arranged 464 photodiode detectors (WuTech Instruments H469-IV) and a Red Shirt Imaging macroscope were used for optical imaging over the visual areas 17, 18, 19, and 21. After the recordings, the brain was sectioned and cytoarchitectonic areal borders were identified.

Results

We here present our results that illustrate (1) concomitant projections from the CO-modules of V2 to the third tier visual areas, (2) incomplete segregation between magno- and parvo-cellular processing pathway in the visual cortex, (3) the existence of spreading wave of activation within and between visual areas, in addition to the retinotopically adjusted point to point activation, (4) the existence of robust connections between the dorsal and ventral stream visual areas, (5) the connections of parietal visual areas, and (6) the interpretation of these results using graph theory.

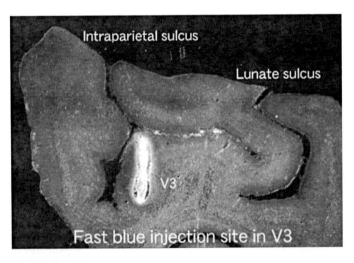

Figure 4. Injection of fast blue in V3 or V3d in macaque. Coronal section from the right hemisphere. The left side of the photo is medial, and the right side is lateral. The top is dorsal. Unpublished data.

(1) Concomitant processing. The third tier visual areas were first reported by Zeki (1978) as a dorso-ventrally elongated tier of cortex in front of V2 having the third retinotopical

representation. The cortical complex was initially proposed to have two areas: the third visual area V3 and the area V3 accessory. The third visual area is discontinuous at the foveal representation, and thus named V3d and V3v (Gattass et al., 1988). Based on the connectional and myeloarchitectonic differences between dorsal and ventral part of V3, Van Essen and colleagues named V3d as V3, and V3v as the ventral posterior area VP (Felleman et al., 1997). The areas including V3A are now considered as the third tier visual complex (Rosa & Tweedale, 2005).

We inject different tracers into the third tier visual areas, V3 (V3d), VP (V3v), and V3A to evaluate if these areas receive projections from neurons of which CO-modules of V2 (Nakamura et al., 2004, 2008b). Figure 4 shows one of the restricted injection sites of a retrograde tracer fast blue into V3 (V3d). Retrogradely labeled cells are found in V1, V2, parieto-occipital area PO, V3A, medial intraparietal area MIP, lateral intraparietal area LIP, ventral intraparietal area VIP, and the area 7a (Figure 5). Labeled cells are continuously distributed in V1 and V2, without any clustering as patches or bands. The distribution of labeled cells in V2 sometimes showed narrow gaps or slit of un-labeled region, but these are not wide enough to fit any of CO-modules. Labeled cells are localized in both supra- and infra-granular layers of V2; slightly more labeled cells are localized in the supra-granular layers than in the infra-granular layers. In V1, labeled cells are localized mainly in the supra-granular layers, and a few labeled cells are found in the infra-granular layers. The results thus showed that neurons in all the CO-modules of V2 project to V3 (V3d).

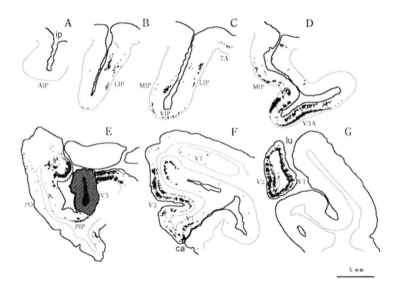

Figure 5. Distribution of labeled cells in the intraparietal areas after injection of fast blue in V3 shown in Figure 4. **A** is anterior, and **G** is posterior sections of right hemisphere. The left side is medial, and the top is dorsal. Dark and shaded region in E is the injection site. Labeled neurons were distributed continuously without clear patch or band structure in V2, indicating V3-projecting cells were distributed without correlation to the cytochrome oxidase modules. Unpublished data.

Figure 6 shows the relationship between the CO-modules and the distribution of retrogradely labeled cells in V2 after an injection of fast blue into VP (V3v). Like V3-projecting cells, retrogradely labeled cells are distributed continuously without any relationship to CO-rich stripes or CO-poor interstripe regions. Labeled cells are mostly distributed in the supragranular layers with a small amount of scattered labeled cells in the infragranular layers. Thus neurons in all the CO-modules of V2 project to VP (V3v) as well. Our preliminary experiments of tracer injections into V3A also support the existence of concomitant connections between the CO-modules of V2 and the third tier visual areas (Nakamura et al., 2008).

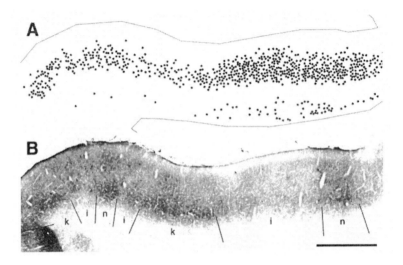

Figure 6. Distribution of labeled cells after an injection of fast blue into the ventral posterior area (VP or V3v). Dots in A shows labeled cells. B shows cytochrome oxidase-rich thick (k) and thin (n) stripes, and cytochrome oxidase-poor interstripe regions (i). Labeled cells were continuously localized without any correlation to the cytochrome oxidase modules in V2. Adopted from Nakamura et al. (2004).

Figure 7 illustrates our scheme on the concomitant communications between the CO-modules of V2 and the V3 (V3d) and VP (V3v). The scheme is incorporated with a tripartite model of object, motion, and spatial vision pathways. The tripartite scheme is a revised version of parallel pathway hypothesis. We only show the areas having robust connections here. The arrows in Figure 7 illustrate the feed-forward projections. The hierarchical levels of the areas are also shown in the figure: The areas located in the lower part of the figure are hierarchically low, and those located in higher part are hierarchically high (also see Maunsell & Van Essen, 1983; Felleman & Van Essen, 1991).

(2) Incomplete segregation of magno- and parvo-cellular visual cortical pathways based on CO-modules in V2. Even in the original paper of segregated dorsal versus ventral visual cortical projections, DeYoe and Van Essen pointed out that the segregation is incomplete. In their original paper, the V4-projecting cells are mostly localized in the CO-rich thin stripes and CO-poor interstripe regions of V2, but are also invaded into the CO-rich thick stripes and sometimes V4-projecting cells are located in the middle of the CO-rich thick stripes. The MT-projecting cells are not restricted in any of the CO-modules: those are distributed in all the modules and only tend to locate robustly in the CO-rich thick stripes. Our results confirmed the relationship between the CO-modules of V2 and the distribution of V4-projecting cells, and further illustrated the relationship between the CO-modules and the cells projecting to the

posterior part of inferior temporal visual area TE1 (Figure 8, adopted from Nakamura et al., 1993).

In addition to the incomplete segregation of dorsal and ventral pathway, researchers also recognized the difficulty in differentiating thick and thin CO-rich stripes. Even in some animals, only patchy or beaded CO pattern is observed instead of CO-rich stripes (Wong-Riley & Carroll, 1984; Tootell & Hamilton, 1989). The ambiguity of CO-pattern may reflect the varying neuronal activation that changes from time to time, which indicates that the CO-pattern is a task-flexible structure and so the function of connections as well. Moreover, recent analysis of the connections between V1 and V2 CO-modules provided evidences against the dorsal versus ventral stream hypothesis (Sincich & Horton, 2002a, 2002b; Nassi & Callaway, J Neurosci 2006). The whole story of visual cortical information processing is now going to be reconstructed and we need a new framework to understand the connections of the extrastriate visual areas.

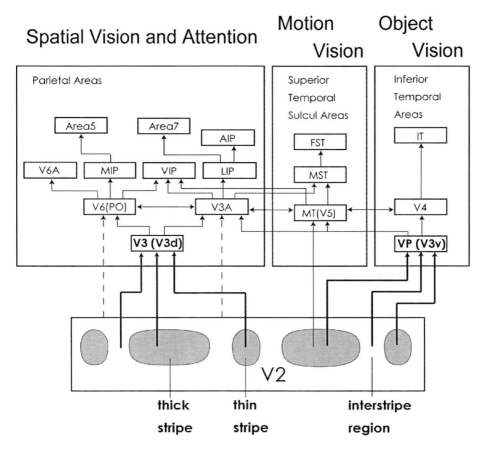

Figure 7. A scheme showing cells in all the cytochrome oxidase (CO) modules, i.e., CO-rich thick and thin stripes and CO-poor interstripe regions, of V2 project to the dorsal and ventral part of V3 (V3 or V3d, and VP or V3v). Extrastriate visual areas are arranged so as to show tripartite model of visual cortical processing. Abbreviations are as in Figure 2. Arrows only show feed-forward and intermediate projections. Original figure.

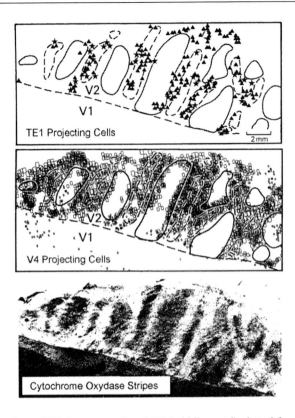

Figure 8. V2 cells projecting to TE1 (upper panel) and V4 (middle panel) plotted from adjacent flat-mount sections. Filled triangles in the upper panel indicate neurons that project to only TE1, whereas stars indicate neurons projecting to both TE1 and V4. Photograph of an adjacent section shows cytochrome oxidase-rich thick and thin stripes (lower panel). Adopted from Nakamura et al. (1993).

(3) Cortical activation wave. The parallel pathway hypothesis *a priori* assumes the point-to-point connections between the retinotopically identical regions of different visual areas, and the consecutive information flow from hierarchically lower to higher areas. The point-to-point communication idea is true so far as we explore the connections anatomically, however, activation across the whole area or cortex provide data against the topographic processing scheme. Recent studies using voltage sensitive dye imaging illustrate the existence of another information processing in addition to retinotopically adjusted consecutive activation of lower to higher visual areas (Roland et al., 2006; Nakamura et al., 2008a).

Figure 9 shows our recent data showing spreading wave of visual cortical activation in the ferret visual cortex (adopted from Nakamura et al., 2008). Soon after starting the presentation of visual stimuli placed at the center of visual field, a spot of the cortex at the border between the areas 17 and 18 (V1 and V2 in monkey) is activated, corresponding to the retinotopy of the visual stimuli (200-240ms, an arrow in 220ms indicates the spot). About 50ms later, the second spot of activation appears at the border of areas 19 and 21, corresponding to the retinotopy again (an arrow at 260ms). At that time, activation of the first spot spreads into the surrounding cortex. The spreading activation wave reaches the border of areas 18 and 19 during 100ms (260-360ms). The cortex around the second spot is also activated and the activation spreads to the 18-19 border (280-380ms). The spreading wave of activation includes all the areas we recorded, i.e., areas 17-21. The activation then shrinks and finally remains along the border of areas 18 and 19. The results thus suggest, in addition to the point-to-point topographical activation of areas, visual stimuli activate wide field of the visual areas across the vertical meridian representation to the cortical regions of lateral periphery representation. Therefore, the visual cortical information processing is not only consecutive over the areas, but also at the same time it is transmitted laterally over the area to reach the border. The wave of activity could be produced either by local lateral connections or by top-down connections that have wider termination field than bottom-up connections. The nature and functional importance of the traveling wave processing are not clear, but it is apparent that we have to consider some other neuronal processing than the traditional consecutive hierarchical parallel processing.

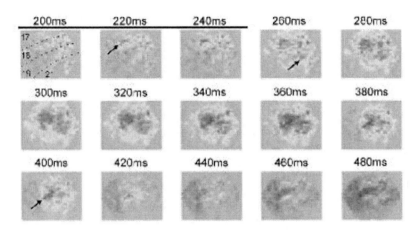

Figure 9. Expanding visual cortical activation illustrated using voltage sensitive dye in the ferret. Each panel represents the two-dimensional activation of the cortex after the start of recording on the timing indicated at the top of each panel. Visual stimulus is presented on the vertical meridian near the fovea during 200-250 ms of each recording. The areas 17-21 and the borders of these areas are indicated in the top-left panel. An arrow in the second panel at 220 ms indicates the first focal activation responding to the visual stimulus that appears 20 ms after the onset of the stimulus at the border between areas 17 and 18. Another arrow in the panel of 260 ms shows the second focal activation at the border of areas 19 and 21. Both focal activations expand to reach the areal borders. The expanded activation of the cortex shrinks to a linear activation region at the border of areas 18 and 19. Adopted from Nakamura et al. (2008a).

The spreading wave of cortical activation remind us the arguments between Ramon y Cajal and Cemillo Golgi on the neuronal structure: neuron doctrine versus reticular theory (Maurizio, 1975; Glickstein, 2006). The argument is between reductionism versus holism. In this chapter we rather favor holistic standpoint based on our recent results of connections in the visual cortex.

(4) Crosstalk or connections between the dorsal and ventral stream areas. We here address connectional data showing crosstalk between so-called dorsal and ventral visual areas. Figure 10 shows the lateral and medial view of the macaque monkey (*Macaca mulatta*) and a flattened view of the cortex by opening the sulci. Insets indicate the positions of cortex we are going to describe here.

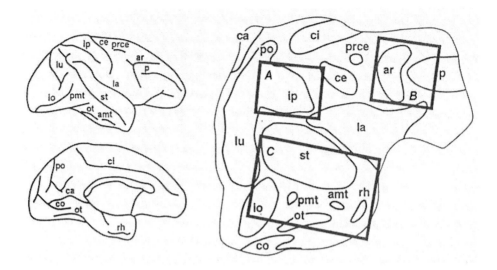

Figure 10. Lateral (left top) and medial (left bottom) view, and a scheme of flattened cortex (right). The right side of the figure is anterior and the top is dorsal in the right figures. Insets indicate position of Figures 11 (*A*), 12 (*B*), and 13(*C*). Abbreviations: amt, anterior middle temporal sulcus; ar, arcuate sulcus; ca, calcaline sulcus; ce, central suclus; ci, cingulated sulcus; co, collateral sulcus; io, inferior occipital sulcus; ip, intraparietal sulcus; la, lateral sulcus; lu, lunate sulcus; ot, occipito-temporal sulcus; p, principal sulcus; pmt, posterior middle temporal sulcus; po, parieto-occipital sulcus; prce, precentral sulcus; rh, rhinal sulcus; st, superior temporal sulcus. Unpublished data.

Figure 11 shows the distribution of labeled cells in the intraparietal visual areas after injections of retrograde tracers into the ventral stream visual areas V4 and TE1. The cells projecting to V4 and TE1 are located in the V3A, PIP, and LIP: V4-projecting cells are more densely distributed in the posterior areas V3A and PIP, whereas TE1-projecting cells are more densely distributed in the anterior area LIP. The results thus indicate that even the areas near the end-point of dorsal stream have abundant connections with the ventral stream visual areas.

As shown in Figure 8, V4 has robust connections with the occipital, hierarchically lower level visual areas. Ungerleider and colleagues described that the neurons in the foveal representation of V4 project to the ventral stream areas whereas those in the peripheral visual field representation of V4 project to the dorsal stream areas (Baizer et al., 1991; Ungerleider et al., 2008). Figure 11 shows that TE1 has more robust connections with the inferior temporal areas than with the occipital areas shown in Figure 8. Thus the pattern of connections with occipital and temporal areas is different between V4 and TE1. This suggest that V4 is part of occipital visual areas supplying visual information both to the dorsal and ventral stream visual areas.

Figure 12 shows the distribution of V4- and TE1-projecting cells in the frontal eye field (areas 8, 45, and 46) and an orbito-frontal area (area 12). The TE1-projecting cells outnumber the V4-projecting cells in these areas. Thus, both the hierarchically lower area (V4) and the higher area (TE1) in the ventral stream have robust connections with the frontal eye fields.

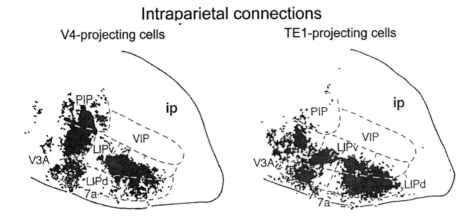

Figure 11. Plotting of V4- and TE1-projecting cells in the intraparietal sulcal areas. Dots indicate individual neurons. The right side of the figure is anterior and the top is medial. The lateral intraparietal areas (LIPd and LIPv) are further divided into posterior, medial, and anterior regions based on the distribution of labeled cells. Abbreviations: 7a, area 7a; ip, intraparietal sulcus; LIPd, dorsal part of the lateral intraparietal area; LIPv, ventral part of the lateral intraparietal area; PIP, posterior intraparietal area; V3A, accessory third visual area; VIP, ventral intraparietal area. Unpublished data.

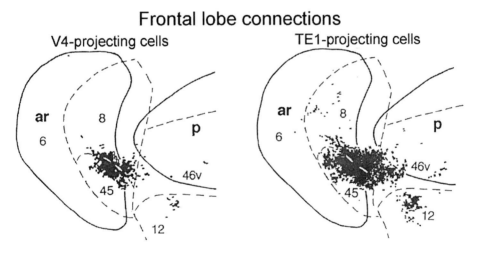

Figure 12. Plotting of V4- and TE1-projecting cells in the frontal eye field areas 8, 45, and 46, and an orbitofrontal area 12. Dots indicate individual neurons. The right side of the figure is anterior and the top is dorsal. Labeled cells are more abundant in TE1-projecting cells than V4-projecting cells. Unpublished data.

Figure 13 illustrates the distribution of V4- and TE1-projecting cells in the dorsal stream visual areas MT and FST. Hierarchically lower area V4 has more robust connections with lower dorsal stream area MT, whereas higher area TE1 has more robust connections with higher dorsal stream area FST. Overall, most of the dorsal stream areas have massive connections with the ventral stream areas.

Temporal lobe connections

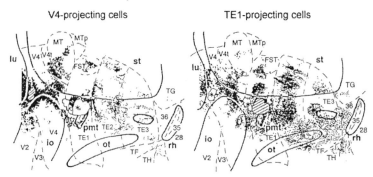

Figure 13. Plotting of V4- and TE1-projecting cells in the areas of the inferior temporal lobule and the superior temporal sulcus. The right side of the figure is anterior and the top is dorsal. Abbreviations: 28, area 28; 35, area 35; 36, area 36; FST, fundus of the superior temporal area; io, inferior occipital sulcus; lu, lunate suclus; MT, middle temporal area; ot, orbito-temporal sulcus; pmt, posterior middle temporal sulcus; rh, rhinal sulcus; st, superior temporal sulcus; TE1-3, temporal area 1-3. Unpublished data.

Figure 14 shows very few V4-projecting cells also projects to TE1. Out of 949 V4-projecting cells and 3539 TE1-projecting cells in TE2, only 17 project to both V4 and TE1 (1.8% of V4-projecting cells and 0.5% of TE1-projecting cells). The situation is similar in labeled cells in TE3: out of 405 V4-rojecting cells and 1014 TE1-projecting cells in TE3, only 11 project to both (2.7% of V4-projecting cells and 1% of TE1-projecting cells). The very small percentage is surprising because almost 15 % of TE1-projecting cells in V2 also project to V4 (Nakamura et al., 1993). We thus suggest that the connections from TE2-3 to V4 and TE1 are somewhat different in nature than those from V2 to V4 and TE1. Thus the relationship between areas TE1-3 is different from that between the area V2 and the areas V4 and TE1.

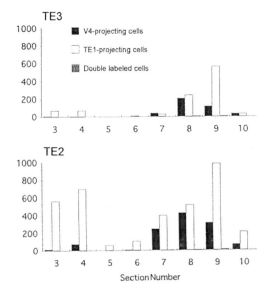

Figure 14. Number of single and double labeled cells in sections from the surface (3) to the bottom (10) in areas TE2 and TE3 after injections of retrograde tracer into V4 and TE1. Unpublished data.

(5) Connections of the intraparietal areas. Figure 15 illustrates our results showing the existence of direct, consecutive connections between the occipito-parietal area V3A to the parietal area LIP, and from LIP to the anterior intraparietal area AIP (Nakamura et al., 2001). The connections are the anatomical correlate of three-dimensional shape analysis in space.

(6) A graph to show connections and functions of the visual system. Parallel stream hypothesis emphasized consecutive projections from hierarchically lower to higher visual areas in the two distinct sets of visual areas. The hypothesis is easy to understand if our brain is like the ganglion chains of insects; on the contrary, primates have two-dimensional cortical sheets in which the areas are located as a mosaic. The areas are wired three-dimensionally to make a graph rather than the parallel chains. Figure 16 illustrates a simplified network that only shows major areas and robust connections between visual areas based on the previous reports (Seltzer & Pandya, 1978, 1980, 1986; Barbas & Mesulam, 1981; Rockland & Pandya, 1981; Maunsell & Van Essen, 1983; Ungerleider & Desimone, 1986; Huerta et al., 1987; Cavada & Goldman-Rakic, 1989; Andersen et al., 1990; Boussaoud et al., 1990; Morel & Bullier, 1990; Preuss & Goldman-Rakic, 1991; Barbas, 1993; Schall et al., 1995; Galletti et al., 2001; Nakamura et al., 2001; Ungerleider et al., 2008). We here apply graph theory to understand the connections (Apollonio & Franciosa, 2007). In Figure 16, in addition to preserving the hierarchical and parallel features of the cortical visual system, we illustrate the network as a graph with the areas as nodes and the connections as arcs. It is a direct graph since the visual information flow has directions, i.e., feed-forward, feedback, and intermediate connections. Apparently another anti-flow graph is overlapped because the information flow is usually bidirectional. The anti-flow graph consists of the same nodes as the original graph, and different direction arcs that are not necessarily trace the same trajectory.

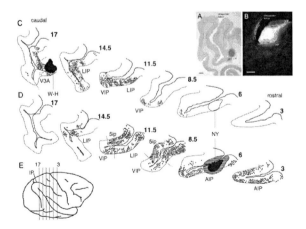

Figure 15. Distribution of labeling after injections of an anterograde and retrograde tracer WGA-HRP into the accessory third visual area V3A (**A**) and a retrograde tracer diamidino yellow into the anterior intraparietal area AIP (**B**). The sections show the intraparietal sulcal areas of the right hemisphere. The right side of the figure is anterior and the top is dorsal. Anterogradely labeled terminals and fibers and retrogradely labeled cells are distributed in the lateral intraparietal area (LIP) and the ventral intraparietal area (VIP) after an injection of WGA-HRP into V3A (**C**), whereas retrogradely labeled cells are distributed in the LIP, VIP, and the intraparietal part of area 5 (5ip). Distribution of terminals from V3A and that of labeled cells projecting to AIP overlapped at the posterior part of LIP where 3-dimensional visual response is recorded. **E** shows the levels of coronal sections in **C** and **D**. Adopted from Nakamura et al., 2001.

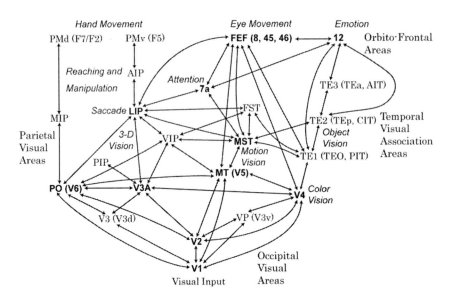

Figure 16. A graph of visual cortical network, showing the areas as nodes and the connections as arcs. Italicized letters indicate approximate functions of partial graphs without clear border. Original figure.

We tag visual functions such as cognition, motor, and emotion not on any specialized areas but over part of the network between several areas. Thus, each function is understood as activity of a partial graph. The partial graphs for different functions overlap each other, and moreover, the border of each partial graph is not clear. The partial graphs of neural network thus share the same visual areas as a common source of visual information. In addition, areas that participated in the graph vary according to the task and attention. We here suggest that the nodes and the arcs (the areas and the connections) of the partial graphs change dynamically according to what task is required and how is the attentional state of the animal. Thus we suggest that the dynamic partial graph, i.e., changing weight of connections and varying number of areas, is the basic feature of the neuronal network.

The dynamic partial graph hypothesis is not against the classical view of the functional specialization of areas. For example, V4 is considered to be the area for color perception (Zeki, 1983), but it is apparent that the other areas sending the wavelength information to V4 and the connections in between are *a priori* necessary for color perception (Gegenfurtner & Kiper, 2003). Other areas like TE1-3 that receive V4 outputs also respond to color information as well (Hanazawa et al., 2000; Koida & Komatsu, 2007). Another example is three-dimensional vision that is basically processed in LIP (Nakamura et al., 2003), but is also processed in the ventral superior temporal sulcal areas (Janssen et al., 2001).

Multiple representations of visual cortical functions was first documented by von Monakow (Polyak, 1957). His idea is based on the holistic understanding of the cortical fuction, like the reticular theory on which Golgi insisted. The idea is very attractive to consider how the brain works. The hypothesis of a dynamic partial graph as a functional unit is one of the holistic ideas to explain how the brain works.

Conclusions

Crosstalk and concomitant processing are gradually unveiled in the visual cortical connections. In this chapter, we showed evidence that the projections from V2 to V3 are not segregated by the CO-modules. In addition, we illustrated the existence of robust crosstalk or connections between the dorsal and ventral stream areas. The network between visual areas consists of a graph, and each function is based on the dynamic partial graph of cortical connections.

Acknowledgments

The experiments in the present chapter were conducted at the National Institute of Health (Bethesda, U.S.A.), Kyoto University Primate Research Institute (Inuyama, Japan), and the Karolinska Institute (Stockholm, Sweden). This study was supported by the Ministry of Education, Culture, Sports, Science and Technology of Japan (Grants-in-Aid for Scientific Research 18591912 to H. N. and 20592171 to H. N. and K. I.) and by the Cooperative Research Program of Primate Research Institute, Kyoto University (H. N. and K. I.).

References

Andersen, R. A., Asanuma, C., Essick, G., & Siegel, R. M. (1990). Cortico-cortical connections of anatomically and physiologically defined subdivisions within the inferior parietal lobule. *J. Comp. Neurol., 296,* 65-113.

Apollonio, N., & Franciosa, P. G. (2007). A characterization of partial directed line graphs. *Descrete Math., 307,* 2598-2614.

Baizer, J. S., Ungerleider, L. G., & Desimone, R. (1991). Organization of visual inputs to the inferior temporal and posterior parietal cortex in macaques. *J. Neurosci., 11,* 168-190.

Barbas, H. (1993). Organization of cortical afferent input to orbitofrontal areas in the rhesus monkey. *Neuroscience, 56,* 841-864.

Barbas, H., & Mesulam, M.-M. (1981). Organization of afferent input to subdivisions of area 8 in the rhesus monkey. *J. Comp. Neurol., 200,* 407-431.

Blasdel, G. G., & Lund, J. S. (1983). Termination of afferent axons in macaque striate cortex. *J. Neurosci., 7,* 1389-1413.

Blasdel, G. G., & Fitzpatrick, D. (1984). Physiological organization of layer 4 in macaque striate cortex. *J. Neurosci., 4,* 880-895.

Blasdel, G. G., Lund, J. S., & Fitzpatrick, D. (1985). Intrinsic connections of macaque striate cortex: Axonal projections of cells outside lamina 4C. *J. Neurosci., 5,* 3350-3369.

Boussaoud, D., Ungerleider, L. G., & Desimone, R. (1990. Pathways for motion analysis: Cortical connections of the medial superior temporal and fundus of the superior temporal visual areas in the macaque. *J. Comp. Neurol., 296,* 462-495.

Cavada, C., & Goldman-Rakic, P. S. (1989). Posterior parietal cortex in rhesus monkey: II. Evidence for segregated corticocortical networks linking sensory and limbic areas with the frontal lobe. *J. Comp. Neurol., 287*, 422-445.

DeYoe, E. A., & Van Essen, D. C. (1985). Segregation of efferent connections and receptive field properties in visual area V2 of the macaque. *Nature, 317*, 58-61.

Dreher, B., Fukada, Y., & Rodieck, R. W. (1976). Identification, classification and anatomical segregation of cells with X-like and Y-like properties in the lateral geniculate nucleus of old-world primates. *J. Physiol. (Lond.), 258*, 433-452.

Felleman, D. J., & Van Essen, D. C. (1991). Distributed hierarchical processing in the primate cerebral cortex. *Cereb. Cortex, 1*, 1-47.

Fitspatrick, D., Itoh, K., & Diamond, I. T. (1983). The laminar organization of the lateral geniculate body and the striate cortex in the squirrel monkey (*Saimiri sciureus*). *J. Neurosci., 3*, 673-702.

Fitzpatrick, D., Lund, J. S., & Blasdel, G. G. (1985). Intrinsic connections of macaque striate cortex: afferent and efferent connections of lamina 4C. *J. Neurosci., 5*, 3329-3349.

Galletti, C., Gamberini, M., Kutz, D. F., Fattori, P., Luppino, G., & Matelli, M. (2001). The cortical connections of area V6: an occipito-parietal network processing visual information. *Eur. J. Neurosci., 13*, 1572-1588.

Gattass, R., Sousa, A. P. B., & Gross, C. G. (1988). Visuotopic organization and extent of V3 and V4 of the macaque. *J. Neurosci., 8*, 1831-1845.

Gegenfurtner, K. R., & Kiper, D. C. (2003). Color vision. *Annu. Rev. Neurosci., 26*, 181-206.

Glickstein, M. (2006). Golgi and Cajal: The neuron doctrine and the 100th anniversary of the 1906 Nobel Prize. *Curr. Biol. 16*, R147-R151.

Hanazawa, A., Komatsu, H., & Murakami, I. (2000). Neural selectivity for hue and saturation of colour in the primary visual cortex of the monkey. *Eur. J. Neurosci., 12*, 1753-1763.

Hendrickson, A. E., Wilson, J. R., & Ogren, M. P. (1978). The neuroanatomical organization of pathways between the dorsal lateral geniculate nucleus and visual cortex in old world and new world primates. *J. Comp. Neurol., 182*, 123-136.

Hubel, D. H., & Wiesel, T. N. (1972). Laminar and columnar distribution of geniculo-cortical fibers in the macaque monkey. *J. Comp. Neurol., 146*, 421-450.

Hubel, D. H., & Livingstone, M. S. (1987). Segregation of form, color, and stereopsis in primate area 18. *J. Neurosci., 7*, 3378-3415.

Huerta, M. F., Kruibitzer, L. A., & Kaas, J. H. (1987). Frontal eye field as defined by intracortical microstimulation in squirrel monkeys, owl monkeys, and macaque monkeys II. Cortical connections. *J. Comp. Neurol., 265*, 332-361.

Koida, K., & Komatsu, H. (2007). Effects of task demands on the responses of color selective neurons in the inferior temporal cortex. *Nat. Neurosci., 10*, 108-116.

Livingstone, M., & Hubel, D. (1988). Segregation of form, color, movement, and depth: anatomy, physiology, and perception. *Science, 240*, 740-749.

Mishkin, M., Ungerleider, L. G., & Macko, K. A. (1983). Object vision and spatial vision: two cortical pathways. *Trends Neurosci., 6*, 414-417.

Maunsell, J. H. R., & Van Essen, D. C. (1983). The connections of the middle temporal visual area (MT) and their relationship to a cortical hierarchy in the macaque monkey. *J. Neurosci., 3*, 2563-2586.

Maurizio, S. (1975). *Golgi Centennial Symposium: perspectives in neurobiology.* New York, NY: Raven Press.

Morel, A., & Bullier, J. (1990). Anatomical segregation of two cortical visual pathways in the macaque monkey. *Visual Neurosci., 5,* 555-578.

Nakamura, H., Gattass, R., Desimone, R., & Ungerleider, L. G. (1992). Projections to visual areas V4 and TEO from temporal, parietal, and frontal lobes in macaques. *Soc. Neurosci. Abstr., 18,* 294.

Nakamura, H., Gattass, R., Desimone, R., & Ungerleider, L. G. (1993). The modular organization of projections from areas V1 and V2 to areas V4 and TEO in macaques. *J. Neurosci., 13,* 3681-3691.

Nakamura, H., Kuroda, T., Wakita, M., Kusunoki, M., Kato, A., Mikami, A., Sakata, H., Itoh, K. (2001). From three-dimensional space vision to prehensile hand movements: The lateral intraparietal area links the area V3A and the anterior intraparietal area in macaques. *J. Neurosci., 21,* 8174-8187.

Nakamura, H., Le, W. R., Wakita, M., Mikami, A., Itoh, K. (2004) Projections from the cytochrome oxidase modules of visual area V2 to the ventral posterior area in the macaque. *Exp. Brain Res., 155,* 102-110.

Nakamura, H., Chaumon, M., Klijn, F., & Innocenti, G. M. (2008a). Dynamic properties of the representation of the visual field midline in the visual areas 17 and 18 of the ferret (*Mustela putorius*). *Cereb. Cortex, 18,* 1941-1950.

Nakamura, H., Koketsu, D., Shirasu, M., Takahashi, T., Shirasu, M., Mikami, A., Itoh, K. (2008b). Cortical connections of visual area V3A in the macaque. *6th Forum Eur. Neurosci. (Abstr.), July 12-16,* 179, Geneva: Switzerland.

Polyak, S. (1957). *The vertebrate visual system.* Chicago, IL: Univ. Chicago Press.

Preuss, T. M., & Goldman-Rakic, P. S. (1991). Ipsilateral cortical connections of granular frontal cortex in the strepsirhine primate *Galago,* with comparative comments on anthropoid primates. *J. Comp. Neurol., 310,* 507-549.

Rockland, K. S., & Pandya, D. N. (1981). Cortical connections of the occipital lobe in the rhesus monkey: Interconnections between areas 17, 18, 19 and the superior temporal sulcus. *Brain Res., 212,* 249-270.

Roland, P. E., Hanazawa, A., Undeman, C., Eriksson, D., Tompa, T., Nakamura, H., Valentiniene, S., Ahmed, B. (2006). Cortical feedback depolarizarion waves: A mechanism of top-down influence on early visual areas. *Proc. Natl. Acad. Sci. U.S.A., 103,* 12586-12591.

Rosa, M. G., & Tweedale, R. (2005). Brain maps, great and small: lessons from comparative studies of primate visual cortical organization. *Philos. Trans. R. Soc. Lond. B Biol. Sci., 360,* 665-691.

Schall, J. D., Morel, A., King, D. J., & Bullier, J. (1995). Topography of visual cortex connections with frontal eye field in macaque: Convergence and segregation of processing streams. *J. Neurosci., 15,* 4464-4487.

Seltzer, B., & Pandya, D. N. (1978). Afferent cortical connections and architectonics of the superior temporal sulcus and surrounding cortex in the rhesus monkey. *Brain Res., 149,* 1-24.

Seltzer, B., & Pandya, D. N. (1980). Converging visual and somatic sensory cortical input to the intraparietal sulcus in the rhesus monkey. *Brain Res., 192,* 339-351.

Seltzer, B., & Pandya, D. N. (1986). Posterior parietal projections to the intraparietal sulcus of the rhesus monkey. *Exp. Brain Res., 62,* 459-469.

Sherman, S. M., Wilson, J. R., Kaas, J. H., Webb, S. V. (1976). X- and Y-cells in the dorsal lateral geniculate nucleus of the owl monkey (*Aotus trivirgatus*). *Science, 192,* 475-477.

Sincich, L. C., & Horton, J.C. (2002a). Divided by cytochrome oxidase: a map of the projections from V1 to V2 in macaques. *Science, 295,* 1734-1737.

Sincich, L. C., & Horton, J.C. (2002b). Pale cytochrome oxidase stripes in V2 receive the richest projection from macaque striate cortex. *J. Comp. Neurol., 447,* 18-33.

Tootell, R. B. H., & Hamilton, S. L. (1989). Functional anatomy of the second visual area (V2) in the macaque. *J. Neurosci., 9,* 2620-2644.

Ungerleider, L. G., & Mishkin, M. (1982). Two cortical visual systems. In: D. J. Ingle, M. A. Goodale, & R. J. W. Mansfield (Eds.), *The Analysis of Visual Behavior.* (pp. 549-586). Cambridge, MA: MIT Press.

Ungerleider, L. G., & Desimone, R. (1986) Cortical connections of visual area MT in the macaque. *J. Comp. Neurol., 248,* 190-222.

Ungerleider, L. G., Galkin, T. W., Desimone, R., & Gattass, R. (2008). Cortical connections of area V4 in the macaque. *Cereb. Cortex, 18,* 477-499.

Van Essen, D. C., Anderson, C. H., & Felleman, D. J. (1992). Information processing in the primate visual system: An integrated systems perspective. *Science, 255,* 419-423.

Wandell B.A., Dumoulin, S. O., & Brewer, A. A. (2007). Visual field maps in human cortex. *Neuron, 56,* 366-383.

Wong-Riley, M. T. T., & Carroll, E. W. (1984). Quantitative light and electron microscopic analysis of cytochrome oxidase-rich zones in V II prestriate cortex of the squirrel monkey. *J. Comp. Neurol., 222,* 18-37.

Zeki, S. M. (1978). The third visual complex of rhesus monkey prestriate cortex. *J. Physiol., 277,* 245-272.

Zeki, S. (1983). Colour coding in the cerebral cortex: the reaction of cells in monkey visual cortex to wavelengths and colours. *Neuroscience, 9,* 741-765.

In: Neuroanatomy Research Advances
Editors: C. E. Flynn and B. R. Callaghan, pp.165-169

ISBN: 978-60741-610-4
©2010 Nova Science Publishers, Inc.

Chapter VI

Final Publications of Christfried Jakob: On the Frontal Lobe and the Limbic Region

Lazaros C. Triarhou[*]
Economo–Koskinas Wing for Integrative and Evolutionary Neuroscience,
University of Macedonia, Thessaloniki, Greece

Abstract

One of the foremost neuroanatomists of the twentieth century, Christfried (Christofredo) Jakob (1866–1956) left a legacy of over 30 monographs and 200 papers, now becoming appreciated in the English biomedical literature. Born in Germany, he was summoned in 1899 to Buenos Aires by the Argentinian psychiatric academia. He spent the rest of his professional life (save for a brief return to Germany between 1910–1912) in affiliation with the National Universities of La Plata and Buenos Aires. The writings of Jakob cover a wide spectrum of topics, from the pathology of neuropsychiatric disorders to the phylogeny, ontogeny and dynamics of the cerebral cortex and their mental corollaries, and ultimately some of the most fundamental neurophilosophical questions. Although in many respects his innovative ideas opened up new ways of thinking in brain and behavior research, they still remain largely unheeded, most likely owing to their exclusive appearance in German or Spanish. The present study revisits Jakob's last two formal publications, dating to 1949. These are entitled 'The task of the frontal lobe in connection with a synthetic quantification of its constitutive elements' and 'The neuronal quantification of the limbic region in its relation to the endogenous affective sphere' (co-authored with his pupils Eduardo A. Pedace and Andrés R. Copello, respectively), and represent the culmination of Jakob's thought, integrating morphofunctional concepts in his quest for understanding the neuroanatomical fundamentals of the human mind. Cognitive function and emotional processing are at the core of current neurobiological research, and Jakob's pioneering concepts remain worthy of consideration six decades later.

[*] E-mail address: triarhou@uom.gr, phone +30 2310 891-387, fax +30 2310 891-388

Introduction

Christfried (Christofredo) Jakob (1866–1956) was a German-born neuropathologist, neurobiologist and neurophilosopher, who spent most of his professional life in Argentina. Having worked under Friedrich Albert von Zenker (1825–1898) and Adolf von Strümpell (1853–1925) at Erlangen and Bamberg, Germany, Jakob subsequently became affiliated with the Universities of La Plata and Buenos Aires, and established one of the most important neuropathological laboratories in South America. Jakob is considered the father of Argentinian neurobiology [Orlando, 1966; Outes, 2006; Triarhou & del Cerro, 2006a, 2006b].

Brief Exposé of Jakob's Work

Jakob has left an invaluable treasure of over 30 monographs and 200 articles, written in German or Spanish, spanning over a wide range of diverse scientific topics [Orlando, 1966; Outes, 2006; Triarhou & del Cerro, 2006a, 2006b; Triarhou, 2007]. He had already reached international renown through early successful atlases of human [Jakob, 1911a] and comparative neuroanatomy [Jakob & Onelli, 1911, 1913]. He later produced landmark works on cortical and evolutionary neurobiology, studying in detail the normal and pathological human nervous system, as well as dozens of the autochthonous species – some extinct today – found in the Patagonian fauna, including the broad-snouted 'yacaré' (*Caiman latirostris*), a reptile of the Alligatoridae family [Jakob, 1945], and the 'pichiciego' or fairy armadillo (*Chlamyphorus truncatus*), a mammal of the Dasypodidae family [Jakob, 1943a].

On a coarse recounting, Jakob beginnings have a positivistic Virchowian view, mixed with Herbertian philosophy. His positivism is refined until 1912, when some general ideas of his mentor Theodor Ziehen are provisorily adopted; these, in turn, become gradually rejected around 1930, when a mystic, yet positivistic, *Weltanschauung* from his travels gives him a less Kantian, more admirative stance in front of the cosmos. Such a dominant *leitmotiv* leads him to a more Pythagorean worldview, introducing even proportions such as the *section aurea* in neuronal counting, which becomes very clear in his articles of the late 1940s. From 1949 to 1953 Jakob sketched his interests in unpublished anthropological notes [Crocco, 2008].

Jakob's Final Publications

Among Jakob's strongest interests were the human frontal lobes [Pedace, 1949] and the limbic system, particularly the anatomical bases of emotion [Orlando, 1964; Triarhou, 2008a, 2008b].

The two articles that follow are the first English translations of Jakob's last two published papers [Jakob & Pedace, 1949; Jakob & Copello, 1949]. This endeavour forms part of an ongoing effort to make available select landmark works by Jakob not hitherto available in the English biomedical literature. Besides their historical interest, these documents contain valuable scientific information, especially in view of the current interest in the frontal lobe and the limbic region, as well their structure and function under normal and pathological circumstances.

Reflecting a life's culmination in the thought of the 83-year-old neurobiologist, the papers were presented at the Third South American Congress of Neurosurgery in Buenos Aires, on April 3–9, 1949, with Professor Ramón Carrillo (1906–1956), the great Argentinian neurosurgeon and social policy officer – and a Jakob alumnus [Crocco, 2006; Ordóñez, 2004] – as General Secretary of the Congress.

The two papers give a summary of mostly quantitative neuroanatomical data on the cellular and axonal components of the human frontal lobe, cingulate (supracallosal) and hippocampal (inferior limbic) gyrus. For the sake of numerical comparisons, it is herein reiterated that Economo & Koskinas [1925] had estimated the total number of neurons in the cerebral cortex of both hemispheres at about 14×10^9 (6×10^9 being the smaller granule cells and 8×10^9 all the remaining larger neurons); the current estimate of the number of nerve cells in the human cerebral cortex stands at 20×10^9 [Pakkenberg & Gundersen, 1997].

Conclusion

Jakob's views on frontal lobe function evolved over half a century, from his early anatomical and neuropsychological papers [Jakob, 1906a, 1906b, 1910, 1911b], through the 'middle period' [Jakob, 1913a, 1913b, 1921, 1923], all the way to the late neurobiological [Jakob, 1939a, 1939b, 1941a, 1941b, 1941c, 1943b] and neurophilosophical [Jakob, 1946] synthetic treatises.

A detailed discussion of the older views and the current state of affairs regarding the anatomical components of the 'visceral brain' has been given elsewhere [Triarhou, 2008a], as has the evolutionary context of Jakob's ideas [Triarhou, 2008b].

Acknowledgments

The author gratefully acknowledges the courtesy of the National Library of Medicine, Bethesda, MD, and Staatsbibliothek Berlin, Germany.

References

Crocco, M. (2006). Breve biografía de Ramón Carrillo (1906–1956). *Electroneurobiología (Buenos Aires),* **14**, 173–186.

Crocco, M. (2008). Personal communication, December 17, 2008.

Economo, C. von, & Koskinas, G.N. (1925). *Die Cytoarchitektonik der Hirnrinde des Erwachsenen Menschen.* Wien–Berlin: Julius Springer.

Jakob, C. (1906a). Estudios biológicos sobre los lóbulos frontales cerebrales. *La Semana Médica (Buenos Aires)*, **13**, 1375–1381.

Jakob, C. (1906b). La leyenda de los lóbulos frontales cerebrales como centros supremos psíquicos del hombre. *Archivos de Psiquiatría y Criminología (Buenos Aires)*, **5**, 678–699.

Jakob, C. (1910). La significación de la histoarquitectura comparada para la psicología moderna. *Revista del Jardín Zoológico de Buenos Aires*, **6**, 159–162.

Jakob, C. (1911a). *Das Menschenhirn: Eine Studie über den Aufbau und die Bedeutung seiner Grauen Kerne und Rinde. I. Teil. Tafelwerk nebst Einführung in den Organisationsplan der Menschlichen Zentralnervensystems.* München: J. F. Lehmann's Verlag.

Jakob, C. (1911b). La histoarquitectura comparada de la corteza cerebral y su significación para la psicología moderna. *Archivos de Psiquiatría y Criminología (Buenos Aires)*, **10**, 385–387.

Jakob, C. (1913a). La biología en el sistema de las ciencias filosóficas y naturales. *Anales de la Academia de Filosofía y Letras*, **2**, 55–67.

Jakob, C. (1913b). La psicología orgánica y su relación con la biología cortical. *Archivos de Psiquiatría y Criminología (Buenos Aires)*, **12**, 680–698.

Jakob, C. (1921). La teoría actual de las gnosias y praxias como factores fundamentales en el dinamismo de la corteza cerebral. *Crónica Médica (Lima)*, **38**, 17–24.

Jakob, C. (1923). *Elementos de Neurobiología, vol. I: Parte Teórica.* La Plata, Argentina: Facultad de Humanidades y Ciencias de la Educación de la Universidad Nacional de La Plata.

Jakob, C. (1939a). *Folia Neurobiológica Argentina, Atlas I – El Cerebro Humano: Su Anatomía Sistemática y Topográfica.* Buenos Aires: Aniceto López.

Jakob, C. (1939b). *Folia Neurobiológica Argentina, Atlas II – El Cerebro Humano: Su Anatomía Patológica en Relación a la Clínica.* Buenos Aires: Aniceto López.

Jakob, C. (1941a). *Folia Neurobiológica Argentina, Atlas III – El Cerebro Humano: Su Ontogenía y Filogenía.* Buenos Aires: Aniceto López.

Jakob, C. (1941b). *Folia Neurobiológica Argentina, Tomo I. Neurobiología General.* Buenos Aires: Aniceto López.

Jakob, C. (1941c). La función psicogenética de la corteza cerebral y su posible localización. *Anales del Instituto de Psicología de la Facultad de Filosofía y Letras de la Universidad de Buenos Aires*, **3**, 63–80.

Jakob, C. (1943a). *Folia Neurobiológica Argentina, Tomo II. El Pichiciego (Chlamydophorus Truncatus): Estudios Neurobiológicos de un Mamífero Misterioso de la Argentina.* Buenos Aires: Aniceto López.

Jakob, C. (1943b). *Folia Neurobiológica Argentina, Tomo III. El Lóbulo Frontal: Un Estudio Monográfico Anatomoclínico sobre Base Neurobiológica.* Buenos Aires: Aniceto López.

Jakob, C. (1945). *Folia Neurobiológica Argentina, Tomo IV. El Yacaré (Caimán latirostris) y el Origen del Neocortex: Estudios Neurobiológicos y Folklóricos del Reptil más Grande de la Argentina.* Buenos Aires: Aniceto López.

Jakob, C. (1946). *Folia Neurobiológica Argentina, Tomo V. Documenta Biofilosófica, Folleto I. Biología y Filosofía.* Buenos Aires: López y Etchegoyen.

Jakob, C., & Copello, A.R. (1949). La cuantificación neuronal de la región limbica en su relación con la esfera introyental afectiva. *Archivos de Neurocirugía,* **6**, 475–481.

Jakob, C., & Onelli, C. (1911). *Vom Tierhirn zum Menschenhirn: Vergleichend Morphologische, Histologische und Biologische Studien zur Entwicklung der Grosshirnhemisphären und ihrer Rinde.* München: J. F. Lehmann's Verlag.

Jakob, C., & Onelli, C. (1913). *Atlas del Cerebro de los Mamíferos de la República Argentina: Estudios Anatómicos, Histológicos y Biológicos Comparados sobre la Evolución de los Hemisferios y de la Corteza Cerebral.* Buenos Aires: Guillermo Kraft.

Jakob, C., & Pedace, E.A. (1949). La misión del lóbulo frontal frente a una cuantificación sintética de sus elementos productores. *Archivos de Neurocirugía,* **6**, 467–474.

Ordóñez, M.A. (2004). Ramón Carrillo, el gran sanitarista Argentino. *Electroneurobiología (Buenos Aires),* **12**, 144–147.

Orlando, J.C. (1964). Sobre el cerebro visceral. Documentación histórica de una prioridad científica. *Revista Argentina de Neurología y Psiquiatría,* **1**, 197–201.

Orlando, J.C. (1966). *Christofredo Jakob: Su Vida y Obra.* Buenos Aires: Editorial Mundi.

Outes, D.L. (2006). A medio siglo de la muerte de Christofredo Jakob, 1956–2006: Fuentes de la concepción biológica de la doble corteza. *Revista Electroneurobiología (Buenos Aires),* **14**, 3–35.

Pakkenberg, B., & Gundersen, H.J.G. (1997). Neocortical neuron number in humans: effect of sex and age. *Journal of Comparative Neurology,* **384**, 312–320.

Pedace, E.A. (1949). Contribución de la Escuela Neurobiológica Argentina del Profesor Chr. Jakob en el estudio del lóbulo frontal. *Archivos de Neurocirugía,* **6**, 464–466.

Triarhou, L.C. (2007). Christofredo Jakob as a naturalist: the 1923 scientific voyage aboard HSDG *Cap Polonio* to La Tierra del Fuego. *Electroneurobiología (Buenos Aires),* **15**, 61–116.

Triarhou, L.C. (2008a). Centenary of Christfried Jakob's discovery of the visceral brain: an unheeded precedence in affective neuroscience. *Neuroscience and Biobehavioral Reviews,* **32**, 984–1000.

Triarhou, L.C. (2008b). Tripartite concepts of mind and brain, with special emphasis on the neuroevolutionary postulates of Christfried Jakob and Paul MacLean. In: S. P. Weingarten, & H. O. Penat (Eds.), *Cognitive Psychology Research Developments.* Hauppauge, NY: Nova Science Publishers (in press).

Triarhou, L.C., & del Cerro, M. (2006a). Semicentennial tribute to the ingenious neurobiologist Christfried Jakob (1866–1956). 1. Works from Germany and the first Argentina period, 1891–1913. *European Neurology,* **56**, 176–188.

Triarhou, L.C., & del Cerro, M. (2006b). Semicentennial tribute to the ingenious neurobiologist Christfried Jakob (1866–1956). 2. Publications from the second Argentina period, 1913–1949. *European Neurology,* **56**, 189–198.

In: Neuroanatomy Research Advances
Editors: C. E. Flynn and B. R. Callaghan, pp.171-182

ISBN: 978-60741-610-4
©2010 Nova Science Publishers, Inc.

Chapter VII

The Human Olfactory System: An Anatomical and Cytoarchitectonic Study of the Anterior Olfactory Nucleus

Daniel Saiz Sánchez[1], Isabel Úbeda Bañón[1], Carlos de la Rosa Prieto[1], Lucía Argandoña Palacios[2], Susana García Muñozguren[2], Ricardo Insausti[1] and Alino Martínez Marcos[1]

Laboratorio Neuroanatomía Humana, Fac. Medicina/CRIB, Univ. Castilla-La Mancha, Albacete, Spain[1]
Servicio de Neurología, Complejo Hospitalario Universitario de Albacete, Albacete, Spain[2]

Abstract

The sense of smell is only poorly-developed in humans and neuroanatomical studies have therefore often neglected the olfactory system. Recent data have shown that the olfactory system is affected early in neurodegenerative conditions such as Alzheimer's and Parkinson's disease, where hyposmia appears before other symptoms. Such findings emphasize the importance of understanding olfactory system structure and function. The present work revisits the anatomic and cytoarchitectonic structure of the human olfactory system, with particular emphasis on poorly-characterized regions affected in neurodegenerative diseases such as the anterior olfactory nucleus. The anterior olfactory nucleus, the first relay in the olfactory pathway after the olfactory bulb, projects to the olfactory cortex as well as to the ipsi- and contralateral olfactory bulbs. Histologic studies have revealed that α-synuclein and tau proteins, markers of neurodegenerative diseases, accumulate in this nucleus in Parkinson's and Alzheimer's disease respectively. However, literature descriptions of the nucleus remain controversial, particularly regarding its extent and the classification of its different subdivisions. This study reevaluates the structure of the human anterior olfactory nucleus and provides an updated description of this structure in the normal human.

Introduction

The olfactory system is relatively under-developed in human compared to other mammalian species, and humans are considered to be 'microsmatic' (Price, 1990). Because anosmia is often regarded as a minor handicap of little clinic relevance, detailed neuroanatomical studies have only rarely addressed the human olfactory system (Humphrey and Crosby, 1938; Crosby and Humphrey, 1941; Liss, 1956; Nakashima et al., 1985; Ohm et al., 1988a; Ohm et al., 1988b; Price, 1990; Smith et al., 1991; Smith et al., 1993). Indeed, rostral structures of the olfactory system such as the anterior olfactory nucleus have only been poorly characterized (Mai et al., 2008).

Hodologically, the anterior olfactory nucleus is a key structure in the olfactory pathway. The anterior olfactory nucleus is the first structure that receives projections from the olfactory bulbs. The nucleus projects both back to the bulbs and onwards to the olfactory cortices (Price, 1990). Reciprocal connections linking the nucleus to the fundus and to the upper lip of the rostral superior temporal sulcus provide a neural substrate for the integration of olfactory inputs with other sensory modalities prior to memory formation (Mohedano-Moriano et al., 2005).

The anterior olfactory nucleus is becoming increasingly relevant in a clinical context. Olfactory deficits (hyposmia and anosmia) are early symptoms of 2 important neurodegenerative disorders: Parkinson's disease (Korten and Meulstee, 1980; Hawkes et al., 1999; Muller et al., 2002; Doty, 2003; Ponsen et al., 2004; Stiasny-Kolster et al., 2005; Tolosa et al., 2007; Lerner and Bagic, 2008; Ross et al., 2008) and Alzheimer's disease (Serby, 1987; Burns, 2000; Doty, 2003; Peters et al., 2003; Hawkes, 2006). Sensory dysfunction correlates with neuropathological changes in the olfactory system. The olfactory bulb and anterior olfactory nucleus are deposition sites for Lewy bodies (α-synuclein) (Daniel and Hawkes, 1992; Pearce et al., 1995; Del Tredici et al., 2002; Braak et al., 2003; Smutzer et al., 2003; Kranick and Duda, 2008; Lerner and Bagic, 2008; Úbeda-Bañón et al., 2009) and neurofibrillary tangles (protein tau) (Esiri and Wilcock, 1984; Struble and Clark, 1992; Kovacs et al., 1999; 2001; Smutzer et al., 2003; Kovacs, 2004) in the early stages of Parkinson's and Alzheimer's diseases respectively.

The aim of the present work is to extend the characterization of the human anterior olfactory nucleus. In the following we first analyze the macroscopic structure of the human olfactory system. We then review the cytoarchitectonic characterization of the olfactory nucleus based on literature reports and from our own investigations. Finally, we discuss the main conclusions of this work and their hodologic and clinical significance.

The Macroscopic Organization of the Human Olfactory System

The olfactory mucosa is located in the nasal cavity above the superior concha. Olfactory receptor cells are embedded in the mucosa along with supporting cells (Ding and Dahl, 2003; Menco and Morrison, 2003). Olfactory receptors cells are bipolar, with a ciliated apical dendrite with cilia and a basal axon that passes through the foramina in the cribriform plate of the ethmoid bone to reach the olfactory bulb (Clerico et al., 2003).

The olfactory system within the cranium includes the olfactory bulb and the olfactory peduncle; this bifurcates in the anterior perforated substance into the medial and lateral olfactory striae (Fig. 1). The lateral olfactory stria reach a number of secondary olfactory structures including the anterior olfactory nucleus (AON), the olfactory tubercle (OT), the piriform cortex (PC), the anterior cortical amygdaloid nucleus (ACO), the periamgydaoloid cortex (PAC), and part of the entorhinal cortex (EC) (Price, 1990; Insausti et al., 2002).

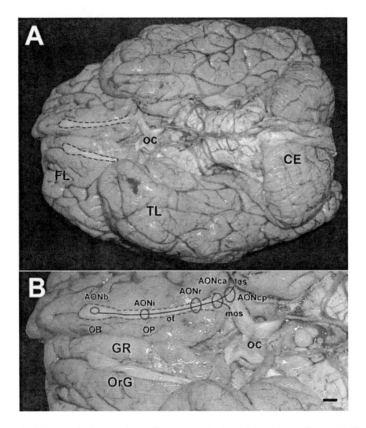

Figure 1. (A) Ventral vision of the human brain illustrating the location of the olfactory bulbs. (B) Detail of olfactory structures. Abbreviations: AON: anterior olfactory nucleus; AONb: bulbar; AONca: cortical anterior, AONcp: cortical posterior; AONi: intrapeduncular; AONr: retrobulbar; CE: cerebellum; FL: frontal lobe; GR: gyrus rectus; los: lateral olfactory stria; mos: medial olfactory stria; OB: olfactory bulb; oc: optic chiasm; OP: olfactory peduncle; OrG: orbital gyrus; ot: olfactory tract; TL: temporal lobe. Scale bar for A, 1cm; for B, 1,3cm.

Microscopic Organization of the Human Olfactory System

The human olfactory system is divided into different sub-regions, of which one is the anterior olfactory nucleus. In turn, the anterior olfactory nucleus is sub-divided along its rostro-caudal axis. In the following we describe the olfactory bulb and the olfactory peduncle before discussing the subdivisions of the anterior olfactory nucleus as revealed by both horizontal and coronal sections.

The Olfactory Bulb

The laminated structure of human olfactory bulb includes six principal layers: the outer nerve layer (ONL), the glomerular layer (GL), the external plexiform layer (EPL), the mitral cell layer (MCL), the internal plexiform layer (IPL) and the granule cell layer (GCL) (Smith et al., 1991; Smith et al., 1993) (Fig. 2A, B).

The ONL corresponds to the axons of the olfactory receptor neurons. The GL is characterized by spheres of neuropil termed glomeruli (indicated by asterisks in Fig. 2B) surrounded by periglomerular cells. The EPL and IPL contain few cell bodies, while the MCL comprises the principal projecting cells (the mitral and tufted cells). The GCL is composed of several strata of granule cells. Some authors have included an additional deeper layer termed the stratum album (Crosby and Humphrey, 1941; Hoogland and Huisman, 1999). Periglomerular and granule cells are the major types of interneurons. Axons from the olfactory mucosa synapse onto mitral and tufted cell dendrites within the glomeruli. These incoming axons are positive for olfactory marker protein (Hoogland et al., 2003). In turn, axons from the mitral and tufted cells make up the olfactory tract that extends to the olfactory penduncle and the olfactory cortex. Lewy bodies have been found in different layers of the olfactory bulb in Parkinson's disease (Del Tredici et al., 2002; Braak et al., 2003; Úbeda-Bañón et al., 2009) and deposits of β-amyloid in the olfactory bulb are also found in Alzheimer's disease (Kovacs et al., 1999; Kovacs, 2004). Diffusion weighted imaging (DWI) has revealed disruption of the olfactory tract in Parkinson's disease; this may provide a method for the identification of individuals at risk of developing the disease (Scherfler et al., 2006).

The Olfactory Peduncle

The olfactory penduncle in the human brain is quite long, extending for several centimeters (Fig. 1). It lies along the ventral surface of the frontal lobe from the olfactory bulb to the anterior perforated substance, and extends into the olfactory sulcus parallel to the gyrus rectus (Mai et al., 2008). Nissl-staining has revealed sublayers within the human olfactory penduncle (Crosby and Humphrey, 1941) (Fig. 2C, 2D); an external layer has been described that predominantly contains dopaminergic cells (Hoogland and Huisman, 1999). A rostral extension of the lateral ventricle has recently been reported in the peduncle to extend to the immediate vicinity of the bulb; this may provide a pathway by which newly-generated cells in the ventricle can access the bulb (Curtis et al., 2007). However, this finding has been debated (Sanai et al., 2007) and remains to be confirmed in human.

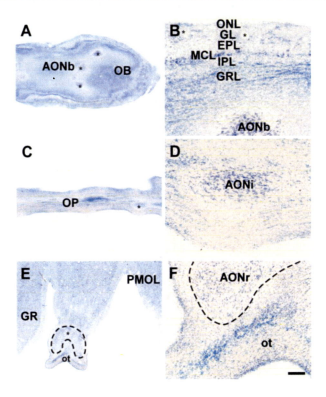

Figure 2. Horizontal (A-D) and coronal (E, F) sections of the human brain. (A, B) Olfactory bulb. (C, D) Olfactory peduncle. (E, F) Anterior olfactory nucleus retrobulbar. Asterisks in A, C, E correspond to portions of anterior olfactory nucleus. Asterisks in B correspond to glomeruli. Abbreviations: AON: anterior olfactory nucleus; AONb: bulbar; AONi: intrapeduncular; AONr: retrobulbar; EPL: external plexiform layer; GL: glomerular layer; GR: gyrus rectus; GRL: granule cell layer; IPL: internal plexiform layer; MCL: mitral cell layer; OB: olfactory bulb; ONL: outer nerve layer; OP: olfactory peduncle; ot: olfactory tract; PMOL: posteromedial orbital lobe. Calibration bar for A, C, E, 1000 μm; for B, D, F, 160μm.

The Anterior Olfactory Nucleus

A primary goal of this chapter is to provide a detailed characterization of the substructure of the human anterior olfactory nucleus. However, different subdivisions have been proposed in the literature. Crosby and Humprey considered four divisions: the anterior olfactory nucleus, dorsalis, lateralis and medialis (Crosby and Humphrey, 1941). Price, in a comparative analysis of monkey and human, included the bulbar (comprising the olfactory bulb and olfactory penduncle), medial, and lateral portions (Price, 1990). Hoogland and Huisman included the intrapeduncular portion (Hoogland and Huisman, 1999). Mai, in a recent edition of a respected human brain atlas, divides the anterior olfactory nucleus into one portion located in the retrobulbar region and a posterior part (Mai et al., 2008). The posterior portion is located medial to the olfactory tract, while an 'olfactory area' is designated in the lateral and dorsal vicinity of the olfactory tract. The area extends rostro-caudally from the retrobulbar level to the olfactory tubercle (Mai et al., 2008), and may correspond to other proposed subdivisions of the anterior olfactory nucleus.

Having carefully considered these earlier subdivisions, we propose that the anterior olfactory nucleus (AON) is best represented by 7 divisions along the rostro-caudal axis. These subregions are: bulbar (AONb), intrapeduncular (AONi), retrobulbar (AONr), cortical anterior lateral (AONcal), cortical anterior medial (AONcam), cortical posterior, lateral (AONcpl) and cortical posterior medial (AONcpm) (Figs. 2, 3).

The Anterior Olfactory Nucleus Bulbar

The anterior olfactory nucleus bulbar (AONb) comprises a number of discrete clusters of morphologically distinguishable groups of cell bodies embedded into the stratum album (indicated by asterisks in Fig. 2A; Fig. 2B). In our studies the number of such clusters has ranged from 1 to 4, as previously described (Crosby and Humphrey, 1941; Price, 1990). The AONb is a site where Lewy bodies are particularly abundant during the early stages of **Parkinson's disease** (Del Tredici et al., 2002; Braak et al., 2003; Úbeda-Bañón et al., 2009) **while, in Alzheimer's disease, both** β-amyloid (Struble and Clark, 1992; Kovacs et al., 1999; Kovacs, 2004) and tau (Esiri and Wilcock, 1984; Ohm and Braak, 1987; ter Laak et al., 1994; Kovacs et al., 1996; Kovacs et al., 2001; Tsuboi et al., 2003) deposits have been reported within the AONb.

The Anterior Olfactory Nucleus Intrapeduncular

As noted earlier, the olfactory peduncle in the human brain is a structure several centimeters in length that links the olfactory bulb to the orbitofrontal cortex. This includes olfactory tract that comprises the axons of mitral and tufted cells (Fig. 2C). The anterior olfactory nucleus intrapeduncular (AONi) comprises several clusters of cell bodies contained within the olfactory peduncle (indicated by asterisks in Fig. 2C; Fig. 2D). This nucleus is **affected by** α-synucleinopathy (Lewy bodies and neurites) in Parkinson's disease (Del Tredici et al., 2002; Braak et al., 2003; Úbeda-Bañón et al., 2009).

The Anterior Olfactory Nucleus Retrobulbar

The olfactory peduncle joins the ventral surface of the brain at the level of the anterior perforated substance (Fig. 2E). At this point the anterior olfactory nucleus retrobulbar (AONr) is located immediately above the olfactory tract. The AONr comprises a cluster of cell bodies that typically adopt a horseshoe-like form around the olfactory tract (Fig. 2E, F). Immediately above this horseshoe structure fibers extend dorsally to connect with the cortex in a region that others consider to be part of the olfactory area (Mai et al., 2008). However, it is not yet known whether this cortical area receives olfactory axons and therefore properly constitutes an olfactory structure. **In Parkinson's disease, Lewy bodies are particularly** abundant in the AONr (Úbeda-Bañón et al., 2009).

The Anterior Olfactory Nucleus Cortical Anterior Medial (Aoncam) and Lateral (Aoncal)

Caudally, the olfactory tract becomes progressively closer to the cortical surface although it still protrudes (Fig. 3A). The AON cortical anterior medial (AONcam) and lateral (AONcal) are found in this area (Fig. 3B). The AONcam corresponds to part of the anterior olfactory nucleus medial of Price (Price, 1990) and to part of the anterior olfactory nucleus posterior of Mai (Mai et al., 2008), and is flanked medially by the gyrus rectus. The AONcal corresponds to part of the anterior olfactory nucleus lateral of Price (Price, 1990) and to part of the olfactory area of Mai (Mai et al., 2008), and is flanked laterally by the area piriformis insulae. **In Parkinson's disease, Lewy bodies are found in both AONcam and AONcal** (Úbeda-Bañón et al., 2008a; Úbeda-Bañón et al., 2009) while, **in Alzheimer's disease,** neurofibrillary tangles of tau protein are also found in both areas (Argandoña-Palacios et al., 2008; Saiz-Sánchez et al., 2008).

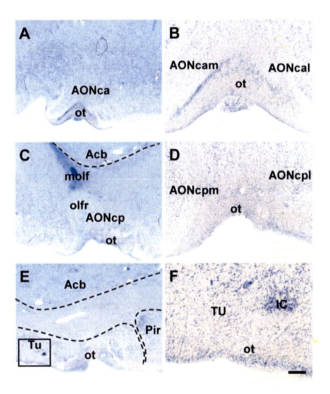

Figure 3. Coronal sections of the human brain. (A, B) Anterior olfactory nucleus, cortical anterior. (C, D) Anteior olfactory nucleus, cortical posterior. (E, F) Olfactory tubercle and piriform cortex. Asterisk in E correspond to one Island of Calleja. Frame in E corresponds to F. Abbreviations: Acb: nucleus accumbens; AON: anterior olfactory nucleus; AONca: cortical anterior; AONcam: cortical anterior medial; AONcal: cortical anterior lateral; AONcp: cortical posterior; AONcpm: cortical posterior medial; AONcpl: cortical posterior lateral; IC: islands of Calleja; molf: medial olfactory radiation; olfr: olfactory radiation; ot: olfactory tract; Pir: piriform cortex; Tu: olfactory tubercle. Calibration bar for A, C, E, 1000 µm; for B, D, 320 µm; for F, 160µm.

The Anterior Olfactory Nucleus Cortical Posterior Medial (Aoncpm) and Lateral (Aoncpl)

. Moving more caudally, the olfactory tract now becomes fully incorporated into the orbitofrontal cortex (Fig. 3C). The AONcpm and AONcpl can be recognized at this level (Fig. 3D). Both portions are separated by the olfactory radiation that splits off under the nucleus accumbens into the medial olfactory radiation and the olfactory radiation proper. The fibers of the medial olfactory radiation are directed to the anterior commissure where contacts are eventually made on the contralateral side. It appears that the contralateral fibers of the medial olfactory radiation originate in the AON. The AONcpm corresponds to the anterior olfactory nucleus medialis of Price (Price, 1990) and to the posterior part of the AON as defined by Mai (Mai et al., 2008) and is delimited medially by the precommissural archicortex. The AONcpl corresponds to the anterior olfactory nucleus lateralis of Price (Price, 1990) and to part of the olfactory area of Mai (Mai et al., 2008) and is delimited laterally by the piriform cortex.

The AON disappears approximately at the level of the limen insulae, to be replaced by other olfactory structures including the olfactory tubercle and the Islands of Calleja (Meyer et al., 1989) (Fig. 3E, F). Both the AONcpm and the AONcpl are reported to contain Lewy bodies in Parkinson's disease (Pearce et al., 1995; Úbeda-Bañón et al., 2008a; Úbeda-Bañón et al., 2009) and tau neurofibrillary tangles in Alzheimer's disease (Argandoña-Palacios et al., 2008; Saiz-Sánchez et al., 2008). Together, these subdivisions correspond to what had previously been identified as the anterior olfactory nucleus (Pearce et al., 1995) that displays dopaminergic (Ikemoto et al., 1998) and calbindinergic (Úbeda-Bañón et al., 2008b) cells. No data are available regarding the neuronal connectivity of these regions in the human brain, but in macaque monkeys the AON cortical posterior is the first structure that receives direct projections from the olfactory bulbs. This region projects to the fundus and to the upper lip of the rostral superior temporal sulcus, so providing a neural substrate for olfactory memory formation (Mohedano-Moriano et al., 2005).

Conclusion

The human anterior olfactory nucleus can be partitioned along its rostro-caudal axis into 7 divisions. These subdivisions are: bulbar (AONb), intrapeduncular (AONi), retrobulbar (AONr), cortical anterior lateral (AONcal), cortical anterior medial (AONcam), cortical posterior lateral (AONcpl) and cortical posterior medial (AONcpm).

Hodologically, the AON is a key structure in the olfactory system. The AON is the first structure that receives efferents from the olfactory bulb. AON projections both return to the bulb and extend onward to the rest of the olfactory cortex; the nucleus is therefore in a pivotal position to influence all aspects of olfactory information processing. Although no data are available regarding neuronal connectivities of AON subregions in human, it seems likely that the different AON divisions will show different afferent and efferent connections, as already demonstrated in other mammals.

The human olfactory system, and particularly the olfactory bulb and the AON, are major targets for the deposition of Lewy bodies in Parkinson's disease and of neurofibrillary tangles and β-amyloid in Alzheimer's disease. Neuronal dysfunction and loss in the olfactory bulb and AON are likely to underlie the hyposmia reported among the first symptoms of both diseases. Detailed understanding of the substructure and cytoarchitecture of the olfactory system will assist investigations into the early pathoetiology of these disorders.

Acknowledgments

This work was supported by the Autonomous Government of Castilla-La Mancha/Fondo Europeo de Desarrollo Regional (FEDER) Councils of Health (grant numbers GCS-2006_E/03, PI-2006/15); and Education and Science (PCC08-0064). The material used in this work was obtained from the following brain banks: *Banc de Teixits Neuròlogics, Universistat deBarcelona-Hospital Clínic* and from the *Banco de Tejidos/Fundación para investigaciones neurológicas, Universidad Complutense de Madrid*. Their donations made this work possible. The authors thank members of LNH. The assistance of International Science Editing in revising the English version of the manuscript is also acknowledged. This work is part of the Doctoral Thesis of Daniel Saiz Sánchez.

References

Argandoña-Palacios L., Saiz-Sánchez D., Úbeda-Bañón I., De la Rosa-Prieto C., García-Muñozguren S., Villanueva P., Insausti R., Martinez-Marcos A.(2008). Somatostatin- and TAU protein immunoreactivities in the anterior olfactory nucleus in Alzheimer disease *Society for Neuroscience.* Washington. 739.735/O731

Braak H., Del Tredici K., Rub U., de Vos R. A., Jansen Steur E. N., Braak E. (2003). Staging of brain pathology related to sporadic Parkinson's disease. *Neurobiology of aging* 24(2):197-211.

Burns A. (2000). Might olfactory dysfunction be a marker of early Alzheimer's disease? *Lancet* 355(9198):84-85.

Clerico D. M., W.C. T., Lanza D. C. 2003. Anatomy of the human nasal passages. In: Doty RL, editor. *Handbook of Olfaction and Gustation.* New York: Marcel Dekker. pp. 1-16.

Crosby C. E., Humphrey T. (1941). Studies of the vertebrate telencephalon. II. The nuclear pattern of the anterior olfactory nucleus, tuberculum olfactorium and the amygdaloid complex in adult man. T*he Journal or Comparative Neurology* 74(2):309-353.

Curtis M. A., Kam M., Nannmark U., Anderson M. F., Axell M. Z., Wikkelso C., Holtas S., van Roon-Mom W. M., Bjork-Eriksson T., Nordborg C., Frisen J., Dragunow M., Faull R. L., Eriksson P. S. (2007). Human neuroblasts migrate to the olfactory bulb via a lateral ventricular extension. *Science* (New York, NY 315(5816):1243-1249.

Daniel S. E., Hawkes C. H. (1992). Preliminary diagnosis of Parkinson's disease by olfactory bulb pathology. *Lancet* 340(8812):186.

Del Tredici K., Rub U., De Vos R. A., Bohl J. R., Braak H. (2002). Where does parkinson disease pathology begin in the brain? *Journal of neuropathology and experimental neurology* 61(5):413-426.

Ding X., Dahl A. R. 2003. Olfactory Mucosa: Composition, Enzymatic localization, and Metabolism. In: Doty RL, editor. *Handbook of Olfaction and Gustation.* New York: Marcel Dekker. pp. 51-73.

Doty R. L. 2003. Odor Perception in Neurodegenerative Diseases. In: Doty RL, editor. *Handbook of Olfaction and Gustation.* New York: Marcel Dekker. pp. 479-501.

Esiri M. M., Wilcock G. K. (1984). The olfactory bulbs in Alzheimer's disease. *Journal of neurology, neurosurgery, and psychiatry* 47(1):56-60.

Hawkes C. (2006). Olfaction in neurodegenerative disorder. A*dvances in oto-rhino-laryngology* 63:133-151.

Hawkes C. H., Shephard B. C., Daniel S. E. (1999). Is Parkinson's disease a primary olfactory disorder? *Qjm* 92(8):473-480.

Hoogland P. V., Huisman E. (1999). Tyrosine hydroxylase immunoreactive structures in the aged human olfactory bulb and olfactory peduncle. *Journal of chemical neuroanatomy* 17(3):153-161.

Hoogland P. V., van den Berg R., Huisman E. (2003). Misrouted olfactory fibres and ectopic olfactory glomeruli in normal humans and in Parkinson and Alzheimer patients. *Neuropathology and applied neurobiology* 29(3):303-311.

Humphrey T., Crosby C. E. (1938). The human olfactory bulb. *Hosp Bull Univ Mich* 4:61-62.

Ikemoto K., Nagatsu I., Kitahama K., Jouvet A., Nishimura A., Nishi K., Maeda T., Arai R. (1998). A dopamine-synthesizing cell group demonstrated in the human basal forebrain by dual labeling immunohistochemical technique of tyrosine hydroxylase and aromatic L-amino acid decarboxylase. *Neuroscience letters* 243(1-3):129-132.

Insausti R., Marcos P., Arroyo-Jimenez M. M., Blaizot X., Martinez-Marcos A. (2002). Comparative aspects of the olfactory portion of the entorhinal cortex and its projection to the hippocampus in rodents, nonhuman primates, and the human brain. *Brain research bulletin* 57(3-4):557-560.

Korten J. J., Meulstee J. (1980). Olfactory disturbances in Parkinsonism. *Clinical neurology and neurosurgery* 82(2):113-118.

Kovacs I., Torok I., Zombori J., Kasa P. (1996). Neuropathologic changes in the olfactory bulb in Alzheimer's disease. *Neurobiology* (Budapest, Hungary) 4(1-2):123-126.

Kovacs T. (2004). Mechanisms of olfactory dysfunction in aging and neurodegenerative disorders. *Ageing research reviews* 3(2):215-232.

Kovacs T., Cairns N. J., Lantos P. L. (1999). beta-amyloid deposition and neurofibrillary tangle formation in the olfactory bulb in ageing and Alzheimer's disease. *Neuropathology and applied neurobiology* 25(6):481-491.

Kovacs T., Cairns N. J., Lantos P. L. (2001). Olfactory centres in Alzheimer's disease: olfactory bulb is involved in early Braak's stages. *Neuroreport* 12(2):285-288.

Kranick S. M., Duda J. E. (2008). Olfactory dysfunction in Parkinson's disease. *Neuro-Signals* 16(1):35-40.

Lerner A., Bagic A. (2008). Olfactory pathogenesis of idiopathic Parkinson disease revisited. *Mov Disord* 23(8):1076-1084.

Liss L. (1956). The histology of the human olfactory bulb and the extracerebral part of the tract; a study with silver-carbonate. *The Annals of otology, rhinology, and laryngology* 65(3):680-691.

Mai J. K., Paxinos G., Voss T. (2008). Atlas of the Human Brain. New York: *Elsevier.*

Menco B. P. M., Morrison E. D. 2003. Morphology of the mammalian olfactory epithelium: form, fine structure, function, and pathology. In: Doty RL, editor. Handbook of Olfaction and Gustation. New York: *Marcel Dekker.* pp. 17-49.

Meyer G., Gonzalez-Hernandez T., Carrillo-Padilla F., Ferres-Torres R. (1989). Aggregations of granule cells in the basal forebrain (islands of Calleja): Golgi and cytoarchitectonic study in different mammals, including man. *The Journal of comparative neurology* 284(3):405-428.

Mohedano-Moriano A., Martinez-Marcos A., Munoz M., Arroyo-Jimenez M. M., Marcos P., Artacho-Perula E., Blaizot X., Insausti R. (2005). Reciprocal connections between olfactory structures and the cortex of the rostral superior temporal sulcus in the Macaca fascicularis monkey. *The European journal of neuroscience* 22(10):2503-2518.

Muller A., Mungersdorf M., Reichmann H., Strehle G., Hummel T. (2002). Olfactory function in Parkinsonian syndromes. *J Clin Neurosci* 9(5):521-524.

Nakashima T., Kimmelman C. P., Snow J. B., Jr. (1985). Olfactory marker protein in the human olfactory pathway. *Arch Otolaryngol* 111(5):294-297.

Ohm T. G., Braak E., Probst A. (1988a). Somatostatin-14-like immunoreactive neurons and fibres in the human olfactory bulb. *Anatomy and embryology* 179(2):165-171.

Ohm T. G., Braak E., Probst A., Weindl A. (1988b). Neuropeptide Y-like immunoreactive neurons in the human olfactory bulb. *Brain research* 451(1-2):295-300.

Ohm T. G., Braak H. (1987). Olfactory bulb changes in Alzheimer's disease. *Acta neuropathologica* 73(4):365-369.

Pearce R. K., Hawkes C. H., Daniel S. E. (1995). The anterior olfactory nucleus in Parkinson's disease. *Mov Disord* 10(3):283-287.

Peters J. M., Hummel T., Kratzsch T., Lotsch J., Skarke C., Frolich L. (2003). Olfactory function in mild cognitive impairment and Alzheimer's disease: an investigation using psychophysical and electrophysiological techniques. *The American journal of psychiatry* 160(11):1995-2002.

Ponsen M. M., Stoffers D., Booij J., van Eck-Smit B. L., Wolters E., Berendse H. W. (2004). Idiopathic hyposmia as a preclinical sign of Parkinson's disease. *Annals of neurology* 56(2):173-181.

Price J. L. 1990. Olactory System. In: Paxinos G, editor. The Human Nervous System. San Diego: *Academic Press.* pp. 979-998.

Ross G. W., Petrovitch H., Abbott R. D., Tanner C. M., Popper J., Masaki K., Launer L., White L. R. (2008). Association of olfactory dysfunction with risk for future Parkinson's disease. *Annals of neurology* 63(2):167-173.

Saiz-Sánchez D., Úbeda-Bañón I., De la Rosa-Prieto C., García-Muñozguren S., Argandoña-Palacios L., Insausti R., Martinez-Marcos A.(2008). Distribution of calbindin and TAU protein immunoreactivity in the anterior olfactory nucleus in Alzheimer disease *Society for Neurscience.* Washington. 739.734/N712.

Sanai N., Berger M. S., Garcia-Verdugo J. M., Alvarez-Buylla A. (2007). Comment on "Human neuroblasts migrate to the olfactory bulb via a lateral ventricular extension". *Science* (New York, NY 318(5849):393; author reply 393.

Scherfler C., Schocke M. F., Seppi K., Esterhammer R., Brenneis C., Jaschke W., Wenning G. K., Poewe W. (2006). Voxel-wise analysis of diffusion weighted imaging reveals disruption of the olfactory tract in Parkinson's disease. *Brain* 129(Pt 2):538-542.

Serby M. (1987). Olfactory deficits in Alzheimer's disease. *Journal of neural transmission* 24:69-77.

Smith R. L., Baker H., Greer C. A. (1993). Immunohistochemical analyses of the human olfactory bulb. T*he Journal of comparative neurology* 333(4):519-530.

Smith R. L., Baker H., Kolstad K., Spencer D. D., Greer C. A. (1991). Localization of tyrosine hydroxylase and olfactory marker protein immunoreactivities in the human and macaque olfactory bulb. *Brain research* 548(1-2):140-148.

Smutzer G. S., Doty R. L., Arnold S. E., Trojanowski J. Q. 2003. Olfactory system neuropathology in Alzheimer's Disease, Parkinson's Disease, and Schizophrenia. In: Doty RL, editor. Handbook of Olfaction and Taste. New York: *Marcel Dekker*. pp. 503-523.

Stiasny-Kolster K., Doerr Y., Moller J. C., Hoffken H., Behr T. M., Oertel W. H., Mayer G. (2005). Combination of 'idiopathic' REM sleep behaviour disorder and olfactory dysfunction as possible indicator for alpha-synucleinopathy demonstrated by dopamine transporter FP-CIT-SPECT. *Brain* 128(Pt 1):126-137.

Struble R. G., Clark H. B. (1992). Olfactory bulb lesions in Alzheimer's disease. *Neurobiology of aging* 13(4):469-473.

ter Laak H. J., Renkawek K., van Workum F. P. (1994). The olfactory bulb in Alzheimer disease: a morphologic study of neuron loss, tangles, and senile plaques in relation to olfaction. *Alzheimer disease and associated disorders* 8(1):38-48.

Tolosa E., Compta Y., Gaig C. (2007). The premotor phase of Parkinson's disease. Parkinsonism & related disorders 13 *Suppl*:S2-7.

Tsuboi Y., Wszolek Z. K., Graff-Radford N. R., Cookson N., Dickson D. W. (2003). Tau pathology in the olfactory bulb correlates with Braak stage, Lewy body pathology and apolipoprotein epsilon4. *Neuropathology and applied neurobiology* 29(5):503-510.

Úbeda-Bañón I., Saiz-Sánchez D., de la Rosa-Prieto C., Argandoña-Palacios L., García-Muñozguren S., Martinez-Marcos A. (2009). Lewy bodies affect non-dopaminegic cells in the human olfactory system in Parkinson's disease. *under review.*

Úbeda-Bañón I., Saiz-Sánchez D., De la Rosa-Prieto C., García-Muñozguren S., Argandoña-Palacios L., Martinez-Marcos A.(2008a). Anosmia as early predictor of parkinson disease: aTyrosine hydroxylase immunoreactivity in the human olfactory bulb and anterior olfactory nucleus.*International Symposium on Olfaction and Taste*. San Francisco. P52.

Úbeda-Bañón I., Saiz-Sánchez D., De la Rosa-Prieto C., García-Muñozguren S., Argandoña-Palacios L., Martinez-Marcos A.(2008b). Anosmia as early predictor of parkinson disease: Calbindin immunoreactivity in the human olfactory bulb and anterior olfactory nucleus.*Novel Advances in Parkinson's Disease (Fundación Ramón Areces)*. Salamanca. P-20.

In: Neuroanatomy Research Advances
Editors: C. E. Flynn and B. R. Callaghan, pp.183-196

ISBN: 978-60741-610-4
©2010 Nova Science Publishers, Inc.

Chapter VIII

Caudata (Amphibia) Brains and Telencephalon: Volumetric Organization and Hyperspatial Interpretations (CFA Projections)

*Michel Thireau**

Muséum national d'Histoire naturelle (MNHN), Département: "Régulations développement et diversité moléculaire" (RDDM), Case postale n° 30, 57 rue Cuvier 75231 Paris cedex 05, France

Abstract

Studies on vertebrate brain evolution commonly use either qualitative or quantitative methods [1]. The latter require cytological examination of tiny brains, to recognize various neurons populations and obtain their reliable volumetric data. Before the discovery of allometry [2], brain size was an obstacle to the interpretation of ratios [3,4].

Allometric analysis itself raises obstacles: a necessary use of an average rate for the calculation of indices and, moreover, a restriction to uni- or bi- dimensional comparisons [5].

With the use of Correspondence Factor Analysis (CFA), novel interpretations of the volumetric values of the different brain divisions are derived from a hyperspace in which the barycentric juxtaposition allows multidimensional comparisons (phi1phiN) between species and volumes projected on biplots [6].

Choosing to work on Caudata Order (newts and salamanders) allows us to understand the role of all the telencephalon neurons populations in a Vertebrate radiation, as well as the impact of neoteny on Caudata brain organization [7].

The main results obtained during the last ten years show that the brain of each species is taxonomically characteristic (= neurotaxonomy [8-10]) under a general tendency to scale invariance (fractality).

---

* thireau@mnhn.fr

Neurotaxonomy proposes support and possible arbitration in a wide variety of systematic questions (such as polymorphism and polytypy [11]); and finally provide a key to understanding the brain and species hyperspaces links [12-14].

Introduction

For about two centuries, neurobiologists, such as the pioneering Cuvier [3] and Serres [4], have attempted to understand the biological significance of volumetric variations among vertebrate brains *in toto* or divided into sections of various sizes. Following Brandt [2], and his revolutionary quantitative method of analysis, the results of somato-encephalic allometries were studied in terms of growth rates and derived encephalization indices (for a review see [15]).

We use CFA (Correspondence Factor Analysis , cf [6]) for a global treatment of Caudata (newts and salamanders) by crossing data between brain volumes and species. Using N-dimensional hyperspaces we generate various factorial combination mappings (phi1-phiN) and direct comparisons between "species points" and "brain structural volumes points" in Caudata. In other words, hyperspatial organization of all these "points" is interpreted according to, mainly, their projections through phi1ph2 factorial maps.

During the last 10 years (1997-2007), we have studied a wide variety of factorial maps obtained from matrixes of Caudata species crossed with volumes of brain divisions (5 parts, 3 telencephalic areas, 16 telencephalic structures cf [5]). The most important results obtained concern the form of monotypy (and not polytypy) in *Speleomantes strinatii* distribution area, neurotaxonomy, neoteny and a scale invariance tendency (fractal process) within the volumetric brain organization of Caudata.

Neuroanatomy

In all Amphibia Caudata (see their general aspect with a *Mesotriton alpestris* [Fig.1] lateral view) the brain is narrow, elongated and not curved. While brain's general morphology is preserved among Amphibia Caudata species, the telencephalon varies, either with families belonging (cf. examples in Fig.1: Hynobiidae = D1, Salamandridae = D2) or according to a special adaptation (such as the skull shape of a burrowing species, *Batrachoseps attenatus* [Fig. 1, D3 = Plethodontidae]). Brains of Caudata have an internal organization building up morphogenetic fields. Their various neurons populations are determined according to qualitative or quantitative changes of nuclei nature. Transverse sections for 44 Caudata species where studied from this analysis angle [16, 17, 18, 5].

Figure 2 represent three transverse sections, cut at regular intervals (a, b and c), of the right cerebral hemisphere of *Lissotriton montandoni*. The different populations of neurons (cf Fig. 2 legend) are a set of gray matter and white matter. Tiny black points symbolize the gray matter (neurons nuclei) while white matter (tractus), at side, is lacking of. Any population of neurons (which may be call also "nuclear mass" or "structure") is distinct because limited by the ventricular wall, the outside of the brain, and some breaking off of neurons nuclei size and density. Such boundaries are marked as black lines on Figure 2 and they are, generally, related to sulci of the ventricular wall (I or II). The olfactive area (AO) is especially important in evolution of the Caudata brain and its main areas -Bulbus olfactorius accessorius (BOA), Nucleus olfactorius anterior (NOA) and some divisions of the Bulbus olfactorius principalis (BOP)- are illustrated (Fig. 2 a, b). Behind AO, a dorsal part -the Pallium- is divided in four structures and, three of them, the Archipallium (Arc), the Pallium dorsal (Pd), the Pallium lateral (Pl), appear in Figure 2 b, c. Always behind AO, but ventrally, the subpallium is divided in six structures, whose three are present in Figure 2 b, c: the septum (Sep), the striatum (St) and the nucleus inter-striato-septalis (NISS). Complete list of structures identified inside Caudata telencephalon is drawn up in publications [5 or 8].

General organization of the Caudata telencephalon is expressed with Figure 3 where Olfactive area (hatched obliquely and with BOA and NOA located), Pallium (hatched vertically) and Subpallium (chequered) expanse is delimited. Finally, Figures 4 and 5 suggest some three-dimensional wire drawing and possible removals of Caudata telencephalon areas by the way of infography technical [7].

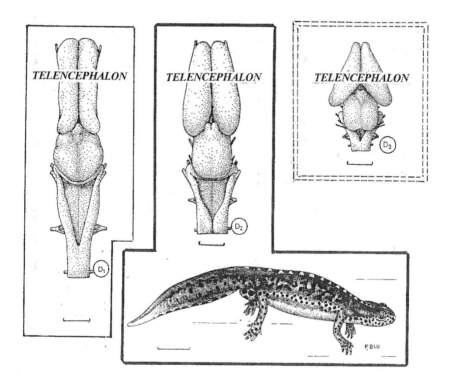

Figure 1. Dorsal views of brains from different species of Amphibia Caudata : *Onychodactylus japonicus* (Hynobiidae) = D1 ; *Mesotriton alpestris* (Salamandridae) = D2 ; *Batrachoseps attenuatus* (Plethodontidae) = D3. A lateral view of *Mesotriton alpestris* show the Caudata external morphology of this Vertebrate order. Shape of the brain differs among newts and salamanders (= Caudata), particularly for the telencephalon. The scale length for the three brains is equivalent to 1 millimeter. The scale under *M. alpestris* is 1 centimeter length..

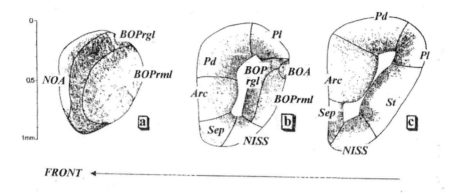

Figure 2. Three transverse sections of the right cerebral hemisphere of *Lissotriton montandoni* : front (a), middle (b) and caudal (c). Cytoarchitectonic organization of the telencephalon is based on various characteristics. Neurons populations are identified, well defined, isolated and differently named. The bounding between these nuclear masses appears by means of black lines crossing the ventricular wall. Arc = archipallium, BOA = Bulbus olfactorius accessorius, BOPrgl = Bulbus olfactorius principalis rostral granular cell layer, BOPrml = Bulbus olfactorius principalis rostral mitral cell layer, NISS = Nucleus inter-striato-septalis, NOA = Nucleus olfactorius anterior, Pd = Dorsal Pallium, Pl = Lateral pallium, Sep = Septum, St = Striatum.

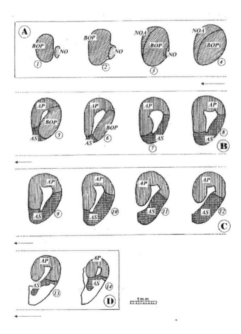

Figure 3. Organization of three main nuclear masses (AO, AP, AS) in the caudata telencephalon (A,B,C,D). Forteen transversal sections at regular intervals are diagramed from frontal (1) to caudal (14) parts of Caudata right cerebral hemisphere, not involving the Bulbus olfactorius anterior. Inside sections 5 to 14, the ventricular light (II) is present. Firstly absent (1-4) the ventricular light II opens in the third ventricule (III) by means of Monro foramen (11 to 13). The olfactory area (AO = 1 to 6) is hatched obliquely (BOP = Bulbus olfactorius principalis, NOA = Nucleus olfactorius anterior). The pallial area (AP = 5 to 14) is hatched vertically and the subpallial area (AS = 5 to 14) is chequered. The rostro-telencephalic region is invaded by structures of the olfactory area (AO) whereas the mid- and posterior telencephalon are divided between a dorsal pallial area (AP) and a ventral subpallial area (AS). The nervus olfactorius (NO) was not included in the measurements.

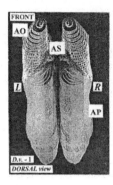 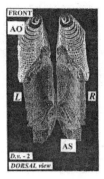 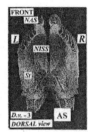

Figure 4. Three *Salamandra salamandra fastuosa* telencephalic dorsal views (D.v.- 1, 2, 3 ; R = right hemisphere, L = left hemisphere) are retained. They were obtained in using photogramms for a computer reconstruction program. The whole telencephalon (D.v.- 1) is divided in three parts : the olfactory area (AO) in front, the subpallial area (AS) ventrally, and the pallial area (AP) dorsally. After computer removal (D.v.- 2) of the pallium (AP), it remains the olfactory area (AO) and the subpallium (AS). After additional computer removal (D.v.- 3) of the olfactory area (AO), the subpallium (AS) stay alone and some of its parts are pointed out : NAS (Nucleus antero-septalis), NISS (Nucleus inter-striato-septalis) and St (Striatum).

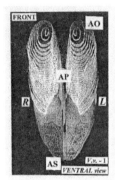 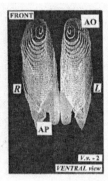 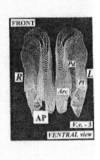

Figure 5. Three *Salamandra salamandra fastuosa* telencephalic ventral views (V.v.- 1, 2, 3 ; R = right hemisphere, L = left hemisphere) are retained. In the whole telencephalon (V.v.- 1), the olfactory area (AO) invaded the the rostro-ventral hemispheric region continued ventrally with the subpallial area (AS) while the pallial area dorsally situated (AP), appears hardly. After computer removal (V.v.- 2) of the subpallium (AS), it remains the olfactory area (AO) and the pallium (AP). After additional computer removal (V.v.- 3), the pallium (AP) stay alone and its structuration in arch give evidence to Pallium dorsal (Pd) at the arch vault with archipallium (Arc) medially and Pallium lateral (Pl) laterally.

Monotypy and Polymorphism

During half a century, *Speleomantes strinatii* (Plethodontidae) was recognized to be a polytypic species by researchers, ie as including two subspecies : *Speleomantes s. strinatii* in the south part of the distribution area and *Speleomantes s. gormani* at north. However, recently, [19] and [20] have given a classic demonstration that *S. strinatii* is monotypic and do not show any subspecific process, but simply a classic polymorphism.

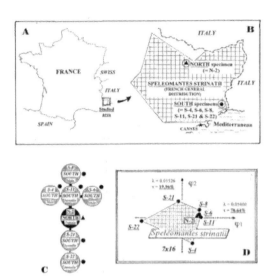

Figure 6. We collected in France (A) seven specimens (B) of *Speleomantes strinatii*. We measured 16 telencephalisation indices for the north specimen (N-2) and the south specimens (S-4, S-6, S-8, S-11, S-21, S-22). Although the south specimens were different in size and sexe (males and juvenile), the north specimen (a female) is always present among the six south specimens analysed through as well a minimum spanning tree (C) as a main (phi1phi2) factorial projection D (7x16). These convergent results highlight a polymorphism among the seven specimens of *S. strinatii* and reject a supposed polytypy (*S. s. strinatii* versus *S.s. gormani*).

We have been able to confirm the *Speleomantes strinatii* monotypy from study of seven specimens : one coming from the north and six from the south of french distribution area (Fig. 6-A-B [11]). Minimum spanning tree (Fig. 6-C) and CFA projection (phi1phi2) of species against brain volumes (Fig. 6-D), do not authorize any distinction between specimens coming from the north (N-2) or the south (S-4, S-6, S-8, S-11, S-21, S-22). In other words, the whole (7 specimens) form an integrated group because the intratelencephalic patterns are similar among specimens coming from distant parts (north and south) of the distribution area extent of *Speleomantes strinatii*. Its monotypy is confirm, for the first time, by the way of brain neuroanatomy [21].

Neurotaxonomy

According to current research, Caudata species are distinguished by various characters coming from morphology, anatomy, eco-ethology, molecular sequences fields, mtDNA but never relating to the brain architectony [22, 23]. However, variations in volumetric brain organization provide a taxonomic characterization, allowing the confirmation of certain established taxonomic levels, or providing arguments useful for resolving continuing taxonomic problems [1].

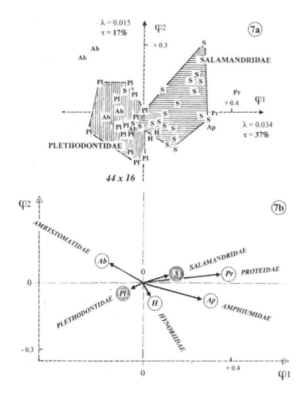

Figure 7a. Main factorial projection (phi1phi2, 44x16) of all the studied caudata species (N = 44) on basis of their telencephalic structures volumes (N = 16). The species families belonging are only relevant: 5 species Ab (Ambystomatidae), 1 species Ap (Amphiumidae), 2 species H (Hynobiidae), 14 species Pl (Plethodontidae), 2 species Pr (Proteidae), 20 species S (Salamandridae). Distribution of the telencephalic profiles of the species points (Ab, Ap, H, Pl, Pr, S), differs according to their family belonging and, for example, the convex hulls for Plethodontidae (vertical lines) or Salamandridae (horizontal lines) are emerging separately. Figure 7b. The distribution of the 6 Caudata families studied is obtained by introducing the mean telencephalic profiles of each family into panel used for the figure 7a, as a supplementary variable. Mean differences between families are projected circles separately, near (Pl, H, S) or far (Pr, Ap, Ab) from the 0 barycenter.

The term neurotaxonomy appears with comments, in a founding work ([8]: 393 and 408). Multifactorial analysis of brain nuclear masses volumes for a diversified lot of Amphibia Caudata species and subspecies (Fig. 7-A) helps to identify the relationships between taxonomy and volumetric organisation of the forebrain [9]. The creation of the concept of neurotaxonomy aim for start, on a new basis, systematics and neurosciences as practised on amphibians, because a certain telencephalic speciation sign the new concept of neurotaxonomy. A representation of neurotaxonomy at the level of families in Urodela (Fig. 7-B) was proposed [10].

Today, it appears than neurotaxonomy can be expressed without the use allometric indices of volumetric nuclear masses, but with CFA direct use on raw data matrixes [24].

Neurotaxonomy offers to neurobiologists a new and potentially useful analytical grid for a variety of studies. A bridge is established between brains as a set of morphogenetic fields and brains as a result of genomic expression [14].

Neoteny (Figures 8 A, B, C)

Caudata manifest a more or less important neotenic process in Ambystomatidae, Amphiumidae, Cryptobranchidae, Dicamptodontidae, Hynobiidae, Plethodontidae, Proteidae, Salamandridae and Sirenidae families [25]. The question of qualitative relationships between brain organization and neoteny had been qualitatively [26 and 27] and quantitatively [7] considered.

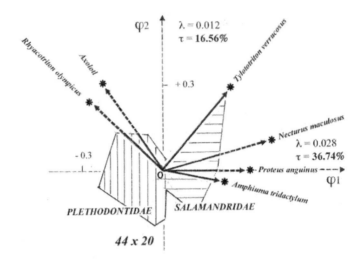

Figure 8a. Main (phi1phi2) factorial projection (44x20) of all Caudata species (N = 44) on basis of their telencephalic structures volumes (N = 16). Separated convex hulls are highlighted for Plethodontidae (vertical lines) and Salamandridae (horizontal lines). Further these convex hulls, the neotenic species (N = 4+2) studied – either obligate (*Amphiuma tridactylum*, *Necturus maculosus* and *Proteus anguinus*), or facultative (Axolotl) or being supposed [cf 23:501; 26:225] (*Rhyacotriton olympicus* and *Tylototriton verrucosus*) - are projected far from point 0, barycentre of the distribution. In short, driving forces materialised with arrows going from 0 to neotenic species, are operating among Caudata species (N = 44) and particularly in the distribution of Proteidae (*Necturus maculosus* and *Proteus anguinus*) or Amphiumidae (*Amphiuma tridactylum*) families. So, neurotaxonomy and neoteny are associated, specially in the evolutive radiation of these two neotenic families.

The projection of all species of Caudata (N = 44) and all telencephalic structures or areas and brain itself -ie finally 20 items (=16+3+1)- give evidence to a driving force associated to neoteny, it overlap neurotaxonomy phi1phi2 factorial projection extant, and goes beyond (Fig. 8a). In some typical neotenic species (facultative or obligates), the bulbus olfactorius accessorius is either developed (Axolotl) or reduced (*Amphiuma tridactylum*) or absent (*Necturus maculosus*, *Proteus anguinus*) (Fig. 8b). Multidimensional analysis of their various brains volumes provides evidence that, in Caudata, neoteny is a driving force associated with the expression of neurotaxonomy (Fig. 8a and b). It is mainly the Area olfactoria (Fig. 8c) which bear the emergence of the organizing tandem : neurotaxonomy-neoteny [7].

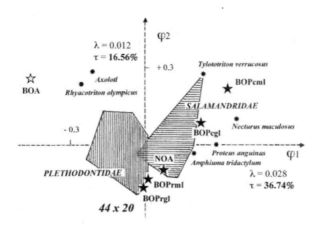

Figure 8b. Same correspondance factor analysis (44x20) and projection (phi1phi2) that in the figure 8a. Plethodontidae (N = 14) and Salamandridae (N = 20) convex hulls, neotenic species (N = 4+2) projections are associated to the projections of the six structures constituting the olfactory area : BOA = Bulbus olfactorius accessorius, BOPcgl = Bulbus olfactorius principalis caudal granular cell layer, BOPcml = Bulbus olfactorius principalis caudal mitral cell layer, BOPrgl = Bulbus olfactorius principalis rostral granular cell layer, BOPrml = Bulbus olfactorius principalis rostral mitral cell layer, NOA = Nucleus olfactorius anterior.

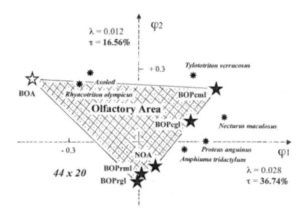

Figure 8c. Same correspondance factor analysis (44x20) and projection (phi1phi2) than in the figure 8a. A convex hull of the olfactory area (N = 6) shows two main volumetric see-saws : .- one along phi1 which concern the BOA (Bulbus olfactorius accessorius) opposite to the BOP (Bulbus olfactorius principalis), and another along phi2 concerning the BOP, rostral *versus* caudal parts. Finaly the volumetric variations inside the olfactory area govern the neurotaxonomic and neotenic processes in the Caudata (Amphibia), take as a panel large (N = 44) or restricted to neotenic species (N = 4-6/44).

Fractal Organization Tendency

In Amphibia Caudata (a taxon no so complex than Mammals), divisions of the brain are numerous with a maximum inside the telencephalon. Neurotaxonomy is well expressed on basis of all intratelencephalic divisions (cf. Fig 7, 8). But what about neurotaxonomy expression when only a part of all intratelencephalic divisions is studied? In other words, what role may eventually play the differences in number, position, size of the studied structures, about the emergence of neurotaxonomy? Hyperspatial organization of the brain five parts as the various divisions of the telencephalon, are a result of hazard under the classical control of natural selection, but also, the expression of a special geometric conservation that the Figure 9 analyse suggest in looking at consistently convex hulls of Plethodontidae and Salamandridae families. While the matrix studied is changing in extant (3 to 6 brains divisions) in quality and size (whole brain [Fig. 9-1], whole telencephalon [Fig. 9-2], areas in telencephalon [Fig. 9-3, Fig. 9-4, Fig. 9-5]) the "mistaken" projected species are not very numerous: one in Fig. 9-3 to six in Fig. 9-4 for a total of 34 (32).

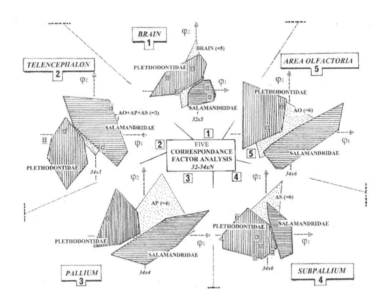

Figure 9. Five Correspondance Factor Analysis (CFA) between 34(32) species of caudata (14 -or 12- Plethodontidae and 20 Salamandridae) and volumes of various parts of their brains. Structures and species points in hyperspaces are projected on phi1phi2 from: CFA n°1 (32x5) for brain five main divisions, CFA n°2 (34x3) for telencephalon three large areas, CFA n°3 (34x4) for pallial for structures, CFA n°4 (34x6) for subpallial six structures, CFA n°5 (34x6) for six divisions of area olfactoria. Convex hulls of Plethodontidae (*vertical lines*) and Salamandridae (*horizontal lines*) are highlighted in each CFA analysis (n° 1, 2, 3, 4 ou 5). Limits for five convex hulls (*points enclosed*) from various volumes projected on phi1phi2 (brain five main divisions, telencephalon three large areas, pallium for structures, subpallium six structures, area olfactoria six divisions) are only suggested. Despite differences in nature, number and size of parts in the brains, neurotaxonomy (Plethodontidae *versus* Salamandridae) tend to be preserved. However, it happens some misplaced projections (Plethodontid species among convex hull of Salamandridae or Salamandrid species among convex of Plethodontidae). The tendency of brain scale invariance (fractal process) is specialy pronounced for the pallium, which is recognize to bring a special contribution in phylogenetic evolution of the vertebrate brains.

So, there is a tendency to invariance in result – ie neurotaxonomy largely preserved– while the brain size vary in volumes from the whole (Fig. 9-1) to telencephalon alone (Fig. 9-2) to each telencephalic area in the end (Fig. 9-3, Fig. 9-4, Fig. 9-5).

Such results highlight a scale invariance tendency, ie a tendency to fractal organization of the brain. This tendency is discrete for the most conservative structures (five brain parts and subpallium), but clearly expressed in the Area olfactoria and, above all, inside the Pallium.

Conclusion

Attempt to understand the Vertebrate brain complexity take as a whole, and through set of data, need to use some modelisations. Cytoarchitectony of the brain is above all the outcome of various and numerous factors at work. With species phylogenetically closed together (Amphibia Caudata, N=44), identification and volumes researches for all intratelencephalic structures (N=16) then correspondance factor analysis (CFA) achievements, offer main factorial maps (phi1phi2) subject of interpretations. Looking on species or structures projected points, the observant may suggest some dominating interpretations correlated to points dispersal patterns. This is specially true for species points accepted according to their families belonging. Convex hulls can be discerned – Salamandridae and Plethodontidae families emergence- from sets of Caudata brain volumes. This discrepancy between volumetric organization of Caudata brain divisions and species taxonomy had been named neurotaxonomy [8]. Neurotaxonomy bear the hallmarks of Caudata brains ways of speciation. Neurotaxonomy has been improved with polymorphism of *Speleomantes strinatii* (Plethodontidae) [11], neotenic species of Caudata [7], intratelencephalic and brain fractal organization in Caudata. But we have also opened some voices contributing to a research program.

1. Caudata neurotaxonomy depends mainly of Area Olfactoria and more generally of telencephalic organization. Similar to Caudata, the Mammals phylogeny (Tenrecinae, Insectivores, Prosimii, non-human Simiiformes, Man and Bats) depends also of their brain volumetric organization and especially through Telencephalon (in Man) opposite to Myelencephalon (in Tenrecinae), as inside the telencephalon, Neocortex (in Man) opposite to Main Olfactory Bulb (in Tenrecinae) [12].
2. Neurotaxonomy can be used after experiments on intratelencephalic redevelopment in transgenic *Xenopus laevis* expressing antiapoptotic factors. The cytoarchitectonic redistributions resulting from the genetic regulation of apoptosis provide evidence to Area Olfactoria neurotaxonomic process and phylogenetic perspective to Pallial Area [14].
3. Caudata neurotaxonomy appears obviously on phi1phi2 (but also on phi1phi3) factorial maps for a 34x16 hyperspace (34 Plethodontidae and Salamandridae species, 16 intratelencephalic structures without any redundancy) [29]. Structural particularisms of species to this hyperspace area revealed onto factorial axes of lower inertia (phi3, phi4, phi5) [10]. The Plethodontidae family present adapted but representative species, so neurotaxonomy is more expressed on phi3phi4 factorial map [11].

These examples just above indicate that neurotaxonomy complete understanding, sometimes need a review of lower inertia axis. The structural organization complexity of the Caudata brain is preserved through Correspondance Factor Analysis (CFA) use, continued in argumented expertise relied on factorial axis combinated or alone.

But overall, neurotaxonomy require intellectual travels associating neuroanatomy, taxonomy and modelisations, the whole generating large range of improvments but at the price of developments as rich as difficult [30].

References

[1] Butler, A., Hodos, W. (2005). *Comparative vertebrate neuroanatomy: evolution and adaptation* (2nd ed.). New-York: Wiley.

[2] Brandt, A. (1867). Sur le rapport du poids du cerveau à celui du corps chez différents animaux. *Bull. Soc. Impér. Natur., Moscou, 4*, 525-543.

[3] Cuvier, G. (1800-1805). *Leçons d'anatomie comparée*. Paris: Baudoin.

[4] Serres, E.R.A. (1824-1828). *Anatomie comparée du cerveau, dans les quatre classes des animaux vertébrés, appliquée à la physiologie et à la pathologie du système nerveux*. Paris & Montpellier: Gabon.

[5] Thireau, M. (1977). *Analyse volumétrique comparée de l'encéphale, et en particulier du télencéphale, des Amphibiens Urodèles*. Ph.D. Thesis Paris7 & MNHN. Paris: Muséum national d'Histoire naturelle.

[6] Escoffier, B., & Pagès J. (2008). *Analyses factorielles simples et multiples: objectifs, méhodes et interprétation* (4th ed.). Paris: Dunod.

[7] Thireau, M., Salomon, M., & Doré, J.-C. (2002). Relations entre la néoténie des Amphibiens Urodèles et les hétérochronies volumétriques multidimensionnelles des étages encéphaliques ou des structures intratélencéphaliques. *Bull. Soc. Zool. Fr., 127, 2*, 149-180.

[8] Thireau, M., & Doré, J.-C., Viel, C. (1997). Neurotaxonomie (*N. novum*) et représentation du genre *Triturus* au sein des Amphibiens Urodèles, à partir de l'analyse multivariée du volume des structures intratélencéphaliques. *Bull. Soc. Zool. Fr., 122, 4*, 393-411.

[9] Thireau, M. & Doré, J.-C. (1998). An introduction to neurotaxonomy: multidimensional analysis of the volumetric organisation of the telencephalon in Amphibia Urodela. In C. Miaud & R. Guyétant (Eds.), *Current Studies in Herpetology* (425-433). Le Bourget du Lac, France: Societas Europaea Herpetologica.

[10] Doré, J.-C., Ojasoo, T., Thireau, M. (2002). Using the Volumetric Indices of Telencephalic Structures to Distinguish *Salamandridae* and *Plethodontidae*: Comparison of Three Statistical Methods. *J. theor. Biol., 214*, 427-439.

[11] Thireau, M., & Doré, J.-C. (2000). Analyse multivariée du polymorphisme des volumes structuraux intratélencéphaliques chez *Speleomantes strinatii* (Aellen, 1958) de France. *Bull. Soc. Zool. Fr., 125, 3*, 251-267.

[12] Thireau, M., & Doré, J.-C. (2002). Liens phylogénétiques dégagés entre – Tenrécinés, Insectivores, Prosimiens, Homme – et Chiroptères (Méga- ou Micro-), au moyen

d'analyses multivariées du volume des étages encéphaliques et de quelques macro-structures télencéphaliques. *Bull. Soc. Zool. Fr.*, *127, 2,* 181-204.

[13] Thireau, M., & Doré, J.-C. (2003). Evolutionary Anatomy of the Primate Cerebral Cortex, 2001 et S.J. Gould: regards croisés. *C.R. Palevol.*, *2,* 373-381.

[14] Chaieb, S., Coen, L., Doré, J.-C. & Thireau, M. (2007). Neurotaxonomy and intratelencephalic redevelopment in transgenic *Xenopus laevis* expressing antiapoptotic factors. In CNRS & DEPSN (Eds.), *Fifth European Conference on Comparative Neurobiology:Evolution and the generation of novelties in the nervous system* (Poster 38, abstract). Orsay: Institut de neurobiologie.

[15] Jerison, H.J. (2001). The study of primate brain evolution: where do we go from here? In D. Falk & K.R. Gibson (Eds.), *Evolutionary Anatomy of the Primate Cerebral Cortex* (305-337). Cambridge: Cambridge University Press.

[16] Thireau, M. (1975a). L'allométrie pondérale encéphalo-somatique chez les Urodèles I. Relations intraspécifiques. *Bull. Mus. natn. Hist. nat., Paris, 3ème sér., n° 297, Zool. 207,* 467-482.

[17] Thireau, M. (1975b). L'allométrie pondérale encéphalo-somatique chez les Urodèles I. Relations interspécifiques. *Bull. Mus. natn. Hist. nat., Paris, 3ème sér., n° 297, Zool. 207,* 483-501.

[18] Thireau, M. (1975c). Etude cytoarchitecturale qualitative et quantitative du télencéphale de Salamandra salamandra (L.) (Amphibia, Caudatya, Salamandridae). *Bull. Mus. natn. Hist. nat., Paris, 3ème sér., n° 297, Zool. 207,* 503-535.

[19] Lanza, B.; Caputo, V.; Nascetti, G; Bullini, L. (1995). Morphologic and genetic studies of the European plethodontid salamanders: taxonomic inferences (genus Hydromantes). *Museo Regionale di Scienze naturali Monografie (Turin), 16,* 1-366;.

[20] Nascetti, G.; Cimmaruta, R.; Lanza, B.; Bullini, L. (2000). Molecular Taxonomy of European PLethodontid Salamanders (Genus Hydromantes). *Journal of Herpetology, 30, 2,* 161-183.

[21] Frost, D. R. (2008). Speleomantes italicus (Dunn, 1923) & Speleomantes strinatii (Aellen, 1958). Amphibian Species of the World: an Online Reference. Version 5.2 (15 July, 2008). Available from : URL : http://research.amnh.org/herpetology/ amphibia/ index.php. *American Museum of Natural History*, New York, USA

[22] Raffaëlli, J. (2007). *Les Urodèles du monde*. Condé-sur-Noireau: Pencle.

[23] Zhang, P.; Papenfuss, T.J.; Wake, M.H.; Qu, L.; Wake, D.B. (2008). Phylogeny and biogeography of the family Salamandridae (Amphibia: Caudata) inferred from complete mitochondrial genomes. *Molecular Phylogenetics and Evolution, 49,* 586-597.

[24] Thireau, M.; Doré, J-C. (2006). La correction allométrique n'est pas indispensable à la neurotaxonomie des Urodèles. *Bull. Soc. Zool. Fr., 131, 3,* 207-224.

[25] Duellman, W., Trueb L. (1986) [1994]. *Biology of Amphibians*. New-York: Mc Graw-Hill Book C°.

[26] Roth, G., Nishikawa, K.C., Naujoks-Manteuffel, C., Schmidt, A. & Wake D.B. (1993). Paedomorphosis and simplification in the nervous system of salamanders. *Brain Behav. Evol., 42,* 137-170.

[27] Eisthen H., Sengelaub, D., Schroeder, D., Albertts, J. (1994). Anatomy and forebrain projections of the olfactory and vomeronasal organ in Axolotls (*Ambystoma mexicanum*). *Brain Behav. Evol., 44,* 108-124.

[28] Thorn R., & Raffaëlli, J. (2001). *Les Salamandres de l'Ancien Monde*. Paris: Boubée.

[29] Thireau, M., & Doré, J.-C. (2007). Neurotaxonomie des Amphibiens Urodèles (Salamandridae/Plethodontidae), que choisir : l'analyse factorielle des correspondances ou des classifications ascendantes hiérarchiques plus ou moins optimisées?. *Bull. Soc. Zool. Fr., 132,1- 2,* 67-86.

[30] Thireau, M. (2003). Sciences au musée, sciences nomades. In B. Pellegrini (Ed), *La neurotaxonomie, discipline nouvelle en quête de mediation* (131-139). Genève & Paris: Georg.

In: Neuroanatomy Research Advances
Editors: C. E. Flynn and B. R. Callaghan, pp.197-206

ISBN: 978-60741-610-4
©2010 Nova Science Publishers, Inc.

Chapter IX

Vagal Tone: Neuroanatomy, Function, and Application

Vladimir Miskovic[1] and Louis A. Schmidt[1,2]

McMaster Integrative Neuroscience Discovery and Study, McMaster University,
Hamilton, Ontario, Canada[1]
Department of Psychology, Neuroscience & Behaviour, McMaster University,
Hamilton, Ontario, Canada[2]

Abstract

Reciprocal communication between the brain and the cardiovascular system is important in sustaining neurobehavioral states that allow organisms to cope with their environment. The vagal circuit is one of the key brain cardio-regulatory circuits implicated in emotion regulation and stress responsiveness. Here we briefly cover the neuroanatomy of the vagal circuit, the functional significance of tonic cardiac vagal function, and ways of quantifying this measure for research purposes. We also illustrate the application of the vagal tone construct for research on stress vulnerability in clinical and nonclinical populations.

Introduction

The importance of reciprocal brain-heart connections has long been recognized by physiologists (e.g., Bernard, 1867) especially during states of acute 'excitation' and emotional arousal (Darwin, 1999, originally published in 1872). In more recent years, psychophysiologists have emphasized the bidirectional communication between the brain and the cardiovascular system in theories of basic sensory orienting (Sokolov, 1963), cognitive

---

*Correspondence should be addressed to: Louis A. Schmidt, Department of Psychology, Neuroscience & Behaviour, McMaster University, Hamilton, Ontario L8S 4K1, Canada; email: schmidtl@mcmaster.ca

processing (Lacey & Lacey, 1978) and emotion regulation (Porges, Doussard-Rosevelt, & Maiti, 1994). The manner in which the brain regulates the internal viscera, including the heart, supports distinct neurobehavioral states that enable animals to respond adaptively to different environmental challenges. The vagal circuit in particular is a key cardio-regulatory circuit that has been proposed as a biological moderator for a broad range of dysfunctions that share in common an inability to effectively regulate stress (Thayer & Lane, 2009). Here we provide a brief overview of 1) the neuroanatomy of the cardiac vagal circuit 2) the functional significance of a resting cardiac vagal tonus, 3) the quantification of vagal tone and 4) the application of vagal tone to research on stress vulnerability in clinical and nonclinical populations.

Neuroanatomy of Vagal Cardiac Control

Retrograde viral labeling studies in rodents (Ter Horst & Postema, 1997) as well as pharmacological and neuroimaging studies in humans (Ahern et al., 2001; Gianoros et al., 2004; Lane et al., 2008) have shown that central regulation of cardiac function occurs at multiple levels of the neuraxis, ranging from brainstem nuclei to forebrain structures (ventral prefrontal cortex, anterior cingulate cortex, amygdala, hypothalamus) that have been implicated in complex psychological and homeostatic processes. The parasympathetic nervous system (PNS) and the sympathetic nervous system (SNS) represent a common final pathway for neural regulation of the heart. These two autonomic branches modulate the intrinsic depolarizing rate of pacemaker cells in the sinoatrial node (the heart's primary pacemaker) and thereby affect the time interval between successive heart beats (chronotropic control). In addition, the autonomic system affects the contractility of the ventricular myocardium, thereby changing the force with which blood is expelled into the periphery (inotropic control) and the velocity of atrioventricular bioelectrical conduction (dromotropic control).

Source nuclei for the PNS innervation of the heart originate from the 10th cranial nerve, the vagus. The literal translation of vagus is "wandering", referring to the nerve's wide ramification throughout the body, ranging from the cardiovascular to the alimentary systems. The vagus is bilateral, with a left and right branch. It is primarily the right vagus that is of interest to cardiovascular psychophysiologists, as the right vagus exerts principal control over the heart's pacemaker cells (Brodal, 1981). There are ipsilateral connections between the right vagus at the level of the brainstem and the right cerebral cortex. These anatomical connects are also presumed to have functional significance in the regulation of emotion (see Lane & Schwartz, 1987). Interestingly, lateralized neural organization in the regulation of emotion is also evident at more rostral levels of the neuraxis, such as the prefrontal cortex (Schmidt & Fox, 1999).

Vagal efferents originate from two separate medullary sources: the dorsal motor nucleus (unmyelinated vagus) and the nucleus ambiguus (myelinated vagus). In mammals, the unmyelinated vagus primarily innervates sub-diaphragmatic structures, such as the stomach, pancreas and colon. By contrast, the myelinated vagus provides primary control of the heart, releasing acetylcholine (ACh) onto the sinoatrial node and slowing heart rate. The myelinated vagal branch also contains special visceral efferents that permit social vocalization (via innervation of the larynx, pharynx and soft palate) and non-verbal signaling (via innervation of facial muscles). Given its neuroanatomical connectivity, the myelinated vagus is uniquely positioned to modulate neurobehavioral states associated with social engagement (see Porges, 2001, for a review). The evolution of vagal myelination in mammals marked a drastic, neurobehavioral shift from the non-social world of reptiles (see Porges, 1995, for a review).

Neurons responsible for sympathetic innervation of the heart originate from the intermediolateral cell column of the spinal cord. The sympathetic system increases the rate of depolarization in pacemaker cells of the sinoatrial node through release of norepinephrine and speeds up heart rate, in addition to potentiating muscle contractility. The metabolic adjustments associated with increased sympathetic drive are important in generating brief, energetic bursts of activity that sustain the so-called 'fight-flight' responses.

Functional Significance

Historically, the dominance of the PNS (vagotonia) or the SNS (sympathicotonia) in visceral regulation has been implicated in psychosomatic illness and affective-personality functioning. Eppinger and Hess (1910) were the first to suggest a link between the resting tonus of the vagus (its baseline level of activity) and clinical neuroses. They further suggested that vagotonia and sympathicotonia were associated with distinct personality traits. Subsequent work (Callaway & Thompson, 1953; Wenger, 1941) provided more robust empirical tests of the Eppinger-Hess hypotheses. For example, Wenger (1941) employed factor analytic techniques in order to derive an autonomic 'factor score' (indicative of autonomic balance). He demonstrated that this factor was continuously distributed about a central tendency of PNS-SNS balance and that a bias toward vagotonia was related to improved behavioral regulation.

More recent, and more sophisticated, models of autonomic control than those articulated in the early 20th century have called into question the existence of a single parasympathethic-sympathetic continuum (see e.g., Berntson, Cacioppo, & Quigley, 1991). Berntson et al. have described an autonomic space model in which autonomic control of visceral function is represented in a 2-dimensional space, with the possibility of reciprocal, synergistic or orthogonal modes of PNS and SNS activation.

The Eppinger-Hess construct of vagotonia has been re-formulated in more modern times, on the basis of recent findings in neuroanatomy and neurophysiology, into a vagal circuit of emotion regulation (see Porges et al., 1991, 1994a, for reviews). According to the vagal circuit of emotion regulation, the mammalian myelinated vagus exerts a 'brake' on central and peripheral stress activation (Porges, 2001). Individual differences in resting vagal function (or vagal "tonus") therefore represent a physiological index of stress vulnerability, where low vagal tone is associated with greater stress reactivity. Several decades of empirical research in typically developing infants, children, adults, as well as clinical populations, have supported the validity of vagal tone as a stress metric (see Beauchaine, 2001; Porges, 1992).

For example, Fox (1989) found that infants with higher vagal tone were more reactive than infants with lower vagal tone to positive and negative events at 5 months, and were more sociable at 14 months. By contrast, low resting vagal tone has been related to frustration, fear and distress in neonates (Gunnar, Porter, Wolf, Rigatuso & Larson, 1995), infants (Calkins & Fox, 1992; Stifter & Fox, 1990) and toddlers (Porges et al., 1994b). Low vagal tone has also been linked to deficits in emotion regulation skills in healthy pre-school (Calkins, 1997; Cole, Zahn-Waxler, Fox, Usher, & Welsh, 1996; Santucci et al., 2008) and school-age (Eisenberg et al., 1996; Jemerin & Boyce, 1990) children. Similarly, poor vagal regulation of cardiac function has been related to lower peer status (Graziano, Keane & Calkins, 2007) and increased social withdrawal (Kagan et al., 1988) in young children. Lower vagal tone predicts maladjustment in children exposed to stressors such as marital conflict (El-Sheikh, Harger & Whitson, 2001) and parental problem-drinking (El-Sheikh, 2005). Studies of adults have noted that a low resting vagal tone predicts slower cardiovascular recovery following stress (Lane, Adcock & Burnett, 1992; Souza et al., 2007), greater central reactivity to affective challenge (O'Connor et al., 2007), and shyness and low sociability (Schmidt & Fox, 1994). Among clinical populations, low vagal tone has been linked to panic disorder (e.g., McCraty et al., 2001), bipolar personality disorder (Austin et al., 2007), mood (Rechlin et al., 1994) and anxiety (Friedman, 2007; Thayer et al., 1996) disorders.

Quantification of Vagal Activity

Vagal tone can be indexed non-invasively in human populations by quantifying the amount of heart rate variability that is due to respiration. Heart rate exhibits substantial beat-to-beat variability, with the degree of variability linked to behavioral reactivity, attention, emotion expression and regulation (Porges, 1992, 1994). At resting baseline, heart rate variability oscillates at several different frequencies due to a combination of parasympathetic, sympathetic, thermoregulatory, humoral, and respiratory influences. The highest frequency of heart rate variability (0.12 to 0.40 Hz in adolescents and adults; 0.24 to 1.04 Hz in children) oscillates at the same rate as respiration. Heart rate varies in response to reflexive cardio-pulmonary rhythms driven by brainstem nuclei, and this source of variability is known as the respiratory sinus arrhythmia (RSA). Heart rate increases during periods of inspiration (due to an inhibition of vagal outflow and cholinergic blockade) and decreases during expiration (due to a disinhibition of vagal outflow and cholinergic stimulation). These respiratory-induced cardiac oscillations reflect primarily PNS influence and the amplitude of RSA is taken as an index of vagal efferent activity or vagal tone, though the two do not perfectly overlap under all conditions (Berntson, Cacioppo & Quigley, 1993; Berntson et al., 1997). Both time domain and frequency domain methods exist for the quantification of RSA (Berntson et al., 1997; Porges & Bohrer, 1990). Time domain methods rely on quantifying the amount of peak-to-trough amplitude in successive R-waves present in the electrocardiogram (ECG; Schechtman, Kluge, & Harper, 1988). An alternative time domain approach (Bohrer & Porges, 1982) involves first time sampling the interbeat intervals, and then applying two sets of filters: the moving polynomial filter (used to remove low frequency components of heart rate variability) and special bandpass filters (used to isolate respiratory periodicities in the cardiac series). Frequency domain methods most commonly rely on Fourier transform techniques to decompose heart rate variability into distinct frequency bands. Autoregressive methods and wavelet analyses are other frequency domain techniques that are sometimes used to quantify RSA. A pneumatic chest cuff is sometimes recommended for accurate estimates of RSA, since respiratory rate can fall outside of the fixed high frequency range (Berntson et al., 1997). However, in a method comparison study, Richards (1995) has demonstrated that recording respiratory rate in infants is not necessary for obtaining valid RSA estimates. Other researchers (e.g., Denver et al., 2007) have likewise argued that controlling for respiratory rate does not have a substantial influence on RSA quantification.

Application Issues

Given the ready availability of technological resources (both hardware and software-based) for the non-invasive recording of biological signals in human populations and the ease of quantifying vagal efferent activity, researchers have had increasing opportunity to assess stress sensitivity in typical development and in the most vulnerable populations. For example, evidence from a wide range of human and non-human animal studies is beginning to suggest that early developmental insults are linked to alterations in multiple stress-response systems (Coe & Lubach, 2008; Matthews, 2002; Philips, Jones & Goulden, 2006; Schneider, Moore, Kraemer, Roberts, & DeJesus, 2002). The experience of child maltreatment is one example of an early adverse life event that provides researchers with a window into how the developmental pathways of cognitive and socio-emotional systems are perturbed by environmental insults. Structural (anatomical) and functional (physiological) modifications of stress-regulatory systems represent a potential mechanism linking early adversity with later dysfunction, including psychopathology (Pollak, 2008). We (Miskovic, Schmidt, Georgiades, Boyle, & MacMillan, 2009) recently indexed resting vagal tone in a group of females exposed to child maltreatment (physical, sexual and emotional abuse and neglect) and their age-matched non-maltreated peers. Importantly, we also assessed the stability of this physiological stress vulnerability metric across a period of 6 months in the maltreated group in order to examine whether the neurobiological correlates of maltreatment persist over time or reflect dynamic, short-term changes. We found that maltreated females exhibited a lower vagal tone (low RSA amplitude) than their non-maltreated age-matched peers and that this between-group difference persisted over a 6-month time period. Moreover, there was modest stability in this neurophysiological measure within the maltreated group over the same time period. We interpreted these findings in terms of plasticity within brain regions that regulate vagal function and stress responsiveness. These neural circuits are especially sensitive during the early post-natal period, making them highly receptive to both positive and negative influences (e.g., Schore, 1994). Importantly, while genes make a significant contribution to the structure and function of the vagal emotion regulation circuit (e.g., Boomsma et al., 1990; Neumann et al., 2005; Thayer et al., 2003), this neural system is also sensitive to environmental input during particular developmental periods.

What does low vagal tone reflect in children exposed to environmental trauma? Given the well established link between vagal function and effective emotion regulation (Beauchaine, 2001), our findings suggest that child maltreatment may be associated with a compromised ability to handle stress, placing these children at increased risk for psychiatric disorders in the future. Furthermore, recent evidence from our laboratory links low vagal tone in healthy adults to biased attentional processing of pictures depicting social threat (angry faces). Thus, maltreated children may be cognitively hypervigilant to possible sources of threat in their environment (Pollak et al., 1997), as they inhabit a hostile psychological world that is replete with a constantly present potential for harm to self.

Future studies will need to address the ways in which pre-natal and peri-natal insults affect the function of the vagal circuit, especially in light of recent findings that adult survivors of prematurity and extremely low birth weight evidence patterns of increased timidity (Schmidt, Miskovic, Boyle, & Saigal, 2008) and delayed brain maturation (Miskovic, Schmidt, Boyle, & Saigal, 2009).

Conclusions

We have provided for the reader a brief outline of an important brain-heart-emotion circuit, tracing some of its neuroanatomy and function in social mammals. Tonic levels of arousal in this circuit can be readily quantified, in non-invasive ways, for research purposes. We focused on illustrating one of the ways in which such research can be applied, by tracking the influence of early life adversity (e.g., species-atypical caregiving experiences) on the function of vagal pathways and the establishment of maladaptive neurobehavioral states. Understanding the dynamics of brain-heart communication promises to continue providing insights into human sensory, cognitive and affective processing.

Acknowledgments

This research was supported by grants from the Natural Sciences and Engineering Research Council of Canada (NSERC) and the Social Science and Humanities Research Council of Canada (SSHRC) awarded to Louis Schmidt and a doctoral scholarship from NSERC awarded to Vladimir Miskovic under the direction of Louis Schmidt.

References

Ahern, G.L., Sollers, J.J., Lane, R.D., Labiner, D.M., Herring, A.M., Weinand, M.E. et al., (2001). Heart rate and heart rate variability changes in the intracarotid sodium amobarbital (ISA) test. *Epilepsia, 42,* 912–921.

Austin, M.A., Riniolo, T.C., & Porges, S.W. (2007). Borderline personality disorder and emotion regulation: Insights from the polyvagal theory. *Brain and Cognition, 65,* 69-76.

Beauchaine, T. P. (2001). Vagal tone, development and Gray's motivational theory: Toward an integrated model of autonomic nervous system functioning in psychopathology. *Development and Psychopathology, 13,* 183-214.

Bernard, C. (1867). *Lecture on the physiology of the heart and its connections with the brain, delivered at the Sorbonne*, the 27th March, 1865. Tr. By J.S. Morel, Savannah, Purse.

Berntson, G.G., Bigger, J.T., Cacioppo, J.T., Eckberg, D.L., Grossman, P., Kaufmann, P.G., et al. (1997). Heart rate variability: Origins, methods, and interpretive caveats. *Psychophysiology, 34*, 623-648.

Berntson, G.G., Cacioppo, J.T., Quigley, K.S., & Fabro, V.J. (1991). Autonomic determinism: The modes of autonomic control, the doctrine of autonomic space, and the laws of autonomic constraint. *Psychological Review, 98*, 459-487.

Bohrer, R.E., & Porges, S.W. (1982). The application of time-series statistics to psychological research: An introduction. In G. Keren (ed.), *Psychological Statistics*. Hillsdale, NJ: Erlbaum, 309-345.

Boomsma, D.I., van Baal, G.C., & Orlebeke, J.F. (1990). Genetic influences on respiratory sinus arrhythmia across different task conditions. *Acta Genetics Medical Gemellol (Roma), 39*, 181–191.

Brodal, A. (1981). *Neurological anatomy in relation to clinical medicine* (3rd ed.). New York: Oxford University Press.

Calkins, S. D. (1997). Cardiac vagal tone indices of temperamental reactivity and behavioral regulation in young children. *Developmental Psychobiology, 31*, 125-135.

Calkins, S. D., & Fox, N. A. (1992). The relations among infant temperament, security of attachment, and behavioral inhibition at twenty-four months. *Child Development, 63*, 1456-1472.

Callaway, E., & Thompson, S.V. (1953). Sympathetic activity and perception: An approach to the relationships between autonomic activity and personality. *Psychosomatic Medicine, 15*, 443-455.

Coe, C.L., & Lubach, G.R. (2008). Fetal programming: Prenatal origins of health and illness. *Current Directions in Psychological Science, 17*, 36-41.

Cole, P. M., Zahn-Waxler, C., Fox, N. A., Usher, B. A., & Welsh, J. D. (1996). Individual differences in emotion regulation and behavior problems in preschool children. *Journal of Abnormal Psychology, 105*, 518-529.

Darwin, C. (1872/1999). *The expression of the emotions in man and animals*. London: Harper Collins.

Denver, J.W., Reed, S.F., & Porges, S.W. (2007). Methodological issues in the quantification of respiratory sinus arrhythmia. *Biological Psychology, 74*, 286-294.

Eisenberg, N., Fabes, R. A., Karbon, M., Murphy, B. C., Carlo, G., & Wosinki, M. (1996). Relations of school children's comforting behaviour to empathy-related reactions and shyness. *Social Development, 5*, 330-351.

El-Sheikh, M. (2005). Does poor vagal tone exacerbate child maladjustment in the context of parental problem drinking? A longitudinal examination. *Journal of Abnormal Psychology, 114*, 735–741.

El-Sheikh, M., Harger, J., & Whitson, S. M. (2001). Exposure to interparental conflict and children's adjustment and physical health: The moderating role of vagal tone. *Child Development, 72*, 1617–1636.

Eppinger, H., & Hess, L. (1910). *Vagatonia*. New York: The Nervous and Mental Disease Publishing Company.

Fox, N. A. (1989). Psychophysiological correlates of emotional reactivity during the first year of life. *Developmental Psychology, 25*, 364-372.

Friedman, B.H. (2007). An autonomic flexibility-neurovisceral intregation model of anxiety and cardiac vagal tone. *Biological Psychology, 74*, 185-199.

Gianaros, P.J., Van Der Veen, F.M., & Jennings, J.R. (2004). Regional cerebral blood flow correlates with heart period and high-frequency heart period variability during working-memory tasks: Implications for the cortical and subcortical regulation of cardiac autonomic activity. *Psychophysiology, 41*, 521–530

Graziano, P. A., Keane, S. P., & Calkins, S. D. (2007). Cardiac vagal regulation and early peer status. *Child Development, 78*, 264–278.

Gunnar, M. R., Porter, F. L., Wolf, C. M., Rigatuso, J. & Larson, M. C. (1995). Neonatal stress reactivity: Predictions to later emotional temperament. *Child Development, 66*, 1-13.

Jemerin, J. M., & Boyce, W. T. (1990). Psychobiological differences in childhood stress response. II. Cardiovascular markers of vulnerability. *Journal of Developmental & Behavioral Pediatrics, 11*, 140-150.

Kagan, J., Reznick, J., & Snidman, N. (1988). Biological bases of childhood shyness. *Science, 240*, 167-171.

Lacey, B.C., & Lacey, J.I. (1978). Two way communication between the heart and the brain. *American Psychologist, 33*, 99–113.

Lane, J.D., Adcock, R. A., & Burnett, R. E. (1992). Respiratory sinus arrhythmia and cardiovascular responses to stress. *Psychophysiology, 29*, 461-470.

Lane, R.D., & Schwartz, G. (1987). Induction of lateralized sympathetic input to the heart by CNS during emotional arousal: A possible neurophysiologic trigger of sudden cardiac death. *Psychosomatic Medicine, 49*, 274-284.

Lane, R.D., Weidenbacher, H., Fort, C.L., Thayer, J.F., & Allen, J.J.B. (2008). Subgenual anterior cingulate (BA25) activity covaries with changes in cardiac vagal tone during affective set shifting in healthy adults. *Psychosomatic Medicine, 70*, A-42.

Matthews, S.G. (2002). Early programming of the hypothalamo-pituitary-adrenal axis. *Trends in Endocrinology and Metabolism, 13*, 373-380.

McCraty, R., Atkinson, M., Tomasino, D., & Stuppy, W. P. (2001). Analysis of twenty-four hour heart rate variability in patients with panic disorder. *Biological Psychology, 56*, 131-150.

Miskovic, V., Schmidt, L.A., Boyle, M., & Saigal, S. (2009). Regional electroencephalogram (EEG) spectral power and hemispheric coherence in young adults born at extremely low birth weight. *Clinical Neurophysiology, 120*, 231-238.

Miskovic, V., Schmidt, L.A., Georgiades, K., Boyle, M., & MacMillan, H.L. (2009). Stability of resting frontal electroencephalogram (EEG) asymmetry and cardiac vagal tone in adolescent females exposed to childhood maltreatment. *Developmental Psychobiology, 51*, 474-487.

Neumann, S.A., Lawrence, E.C., Jennings, J.R., Ferrell, R.E., & Manuck, S.B. (2005). Heart rate variability is associated with polymorphic variation in the choline transporter gene. *Psychosomatic Medicine, 67*, 168–171.

O'Connor, M.F., Harald, G., McRae, K., & Lane, R.D. (2007). Baseline vagal tone predicts BOLD response during elicitation of grief. *Neuropsychopharmacology, 32*, 2184-2189.

Philips, D.I., Jones, A., & Goulden, P.A. (2006). Birth weight, stress, and the metabolic syndrome in adult life. *Annals of the New York Academy of Sciences, 1083*, 28-36.

Pollak, S.D. (2008). Mechanisms linking early experience and the emergence of emotions: Illustrations from the study of maltreated children. *Current Directions in Psychological Science, 17*, 370-375.

Pollak, S.D., Cicchetti, D., Klorman, R., & Brumaghim, J.T. (1997). Cognitive brain event-related potentials and motion processing in maltreated children. *Child Development, 68*, 773-787.

Porges, S.W. (1991). Vagal tone: An autonomic mediator of affect. In J.A. Garber & K.A. Dodge (eds.), *The development of affect regulation and dysregulation.* (pp. 111-128). New York: Cambridge University Press.

Porges. S.W. (1992). Vagal Tone: A physiological marker of stress vulnerability. *Pediatrics, 90*, 498-504.

Porges, S.W. (1995). Orienting in a defensive world: Mammalian modifications of our evolutionary heritage. A Polyvagal Theory. *Psychophysiology, 32*, 301-318.

Porges, S.W. (2001). The polyvagal theory: Phylogenetic substrates of a social nervous system. *International Journal of Psychophysiology, 42*, 123-146.

Porges, S.W., & Bohrer, R.E. (1990). Analyses of periodic processes in psychophysiological research. In J.T. Cacioppo & L.G. Tassinary (eds.), *Principles of psychophysiology: Physical, social, and inferential elements* (pp.708-753). New York: Cambridge University Press.

Porges, S.W., Doussard-Roosevelt, J.A., & Maiti, A. K. (1994a). Vagal tone and the physiological regulation of emotion. In N.A. Fox (ed). *Emotion regulation: Behavioral and biological considerations.* Monograph of the Society for Research in Child Development, 59 (2-3, Serial No. 240), 167-186.

Porges, S.W., Doussard-Roosevelt, J.A., Portales, A.L., & Suess, P.E. (1994b). Cardiac vagal tone: Stability and relation to difficultness in infants and three-year-old children. *Developmental Psychobiology, 27*, 289-300.

Rechlin, T., Weis, M., Spitzer, A., & Kaschka, W.P. (1994). Are affective disorders associated with alterations of heart rate variability? *Journal of Affective Disorders, 32*, 271–275.

Richards, J.E. (1995). Reliability of respiratory sinus arrhythmia in R-R intervals, in 14-, 20-, and 26-week old infants. *Infant Behavior and Development, 18*, 155-161.

Santucci, A.K., Silk, J.S., Shaw, D.S., Gentzler, A., Fox, N.A., & Kovacs, M. (2008). Vagal tone and temperament as predictors of emotion regulation strategies in young children. *Developmental Psychobiology, 50*, 205-216.

Schechtman, V.L., Kluge, K.A., & Harper, R.M. (1988). Time-domain system for assessing variation in heart rate. *Medical and Biological Engineering and Computing, 26*, 367-373.

Schmidt, L.A., & Fox, N.A. (1994). Patterns of cortical electrophysiology and autonomic activity in adults' shyness and sociability. *Biological Psychology, 38*, 183-198.

Schmidt, L.A., & Fox, N.A. (1999). Conceptual, biological, and behavioral distinctions among different categories of shy children. In L.A. Schmidt & J. Schulkin (Eds.),

Extreme fear, shyness and social phobia: Origins, biological mechanisms and clinical outcomes (pp. 47-66). New York: Oxford University Press.

Schmidt, L.A., Miskovic, V., Boyle, M., & Saigal, S. (2008). Shyness and timidity in young adults who were born at extremely low birth weight. *Pediatrics, 122*, e181-187.

Schneider, M.L., Moore, C.F., Kraemer, G.W., Roberts, A.D., & DeJesus, O.T. (2002). The impact of prenatal stress, fetal alcohol exposure, or both on development: Perspectives from a primate model. *Psychoneuroendocrinology, 27*, 285-298.

Schore, A. (1994). *Affect regulation and the origin of the self: The neurobiology of emotional development*. Hillsdale, NJ : Lawrence Erlbaum Associates, Inc.

Sokolov, E. N. (1963). *Perception and the conditioned reflex*. Oxford: Pergamon Press.

Souza, G.G.L., Mendonça-de-Souza, A.C.F., Barrios, E.M., Coutinho, E.F.S., Oliveira, L., & Mendlowicz, M.V. (2007). Resilience and vagal tone predict cardiac recovery from acute social stress. *Stress: The International Journal on the Biology of Stress, 10*, 368-374.

Stifter, C.A., & Fox, N.A. (1990). Infant reactivity: Physiological correlates of newborn and 5-month temperament. *Developmental Psychology, 26*, 582-588.

Ter Horst, G.J., & Postema, F. (1997). Forebrain parasympathetic control of heart activity: Retrograde transneuronal viral labeling in rats. *American Journal of Physiology, 273*, H2926–H2930.

Thayer, J.F., Friedman, B.H., & Borkovec, T.D. (1996). Autonomic characteristics of generalized anxiety disorder and worry. *Biological Psychiatry, 39*, 255-266.

Thayer, J.F., & Lane, R.D. (2009). Claude Bernard and the heart-brain connection: Further elaboration of a model of neurovisceral integration. *Neuroscience and Biobehavioral Reviews, 33*, 81-88.

Thayer, J.F., Merritt, M.M., Sollers 3rd, J.J., Zonderman, A.B., Evans, M.K., Yie, S. et al. (2003). Effect of angiotensin-converting enzyme insertion/deletion polymorphism DD genotype on high-frequency heart rate variability in African Americans. *American Journal of Cardiology, 92*, 1487–1490

Wenger, M.A. (1941). The measurement of individual differences in autonomic balance. *Psychosomatic Medicine, 3*, 427-434.

In: Neuroanatomy Research Advances   ISBN 978-1-60741-610-4
Editors:C.E. Flynn and B.R. Callaghan, pp.207-265 © 2010 Nova Science Publishers, Inc.

Chapter X

QUANTITATIVE MICROSCOPIC ANALYSIS
OF MYELINATED NERVE FIBERS

Dimiter Prodanov[1,2,]*, *Hans K.P. Feirabend*[3] *and Enrico Marani*[4]
[1]Bioelectronic Systems Group, Interuniversity Microelectronics
Center (IMEC), Leuven, Belgium
[2]Laboratory for Experimental Functional Neurosurgery,
Catholic University of Leuven, Leuven, Belgium
[3]Department of Anatomy and Embryology, Leiden University
Medical Center (LUMC), Leiden, the Netherlands
[4]Biomedical Signals and Systems, Faculty Electrical Engineering,
Mathematics and Informatics, Twente University,
Enschede, the Netherlands

Abstract

A better understanding of the structure and function of peripheral nerve fibers could
facilitate the search for new treatments for demyelinating disorders and nerve regeneration and lead to further improvement of neural prostheses. The availability of quantitative anatomic (morphometric) data is, therefore, a crucial part of this process. Due to
the labor intensiveness of the conventional morphometric protocols, extensive morphometric studies are still only occasional. Therefore, many structures in the peripheral
and central nervous systems are still poorly described quantitatively. In this chapter,
we will give an account of the most important studies dealing with the fiber composition and topography of peripheral nerves and spinal roots.

Our research in this field was directed toward several objectives: to characterize
better the (i) fiber composition and (ii) functional topography of peripheral nerves, and
(iii) to devise innovative methodologies that facilitate measurements of nerve fibers.
Using the conventional morphometric approach, we have demonstrated that parametric population models could well describe the fiber composition of peripheral nerves.
These models could be used for objective classification of the myelinated nerve fibers
into $A\alpha$, $A\beta$, $A\gamma$ or $A\delta$ fiber classes. Anatomical and physiological criteria for such
classification are derived for the rat. By means of nonparametric spatial statistics, it

---

*Correspondence: Dr. Dimiter Prodanov, MD, PhD, Bioelectronics Systems group, NEXT-BIO, IMEC,
Kapeldreef 75, 3001 Leuven, Belgium
Note: See Glossary at the end of chapter.

has been shown that some muscle representations are topographically organized along their course in the peripheral nerves. Presented results are discussed in the perspective of the development of nerve-electrode interfaces.

Finally, a comprehensive account is given of the new statistical approaches for fiber classification and spatial statistical analysis. The applicability of presented approaches is discussed for other PNS studies — for example, in fiber regeneration and toxicology.

Acknowledgments

The authors would like to acknowledge Mr. Herman Choufoer and Ms. Inge Nieuwman for their excellent technical assistance, and Prof. Niko Nagelkerke for the critical reading and discussion of the statistical discourse. The figures are prepared with the help of the *LaPrint* script by Arno Linnemann. Symbolical computation was assisted by the computer algebra system *Maxima*. The authors declare no competing financial interests.

1. Introduction

Morphometry[1] can be defined as the quantitative study of anatomical structures. Morphometric data provide a counterpart for other types of quantitative data common in disciplines like biochemistry, molecular biology or physiology. In this manner, analysis of morphometric data could reveal the presence of various structural and functional relationships (see Sec. 2.2.).

Due to the labor intensiveness of the conventional microscopic morphometric protocols, extensive morphometric studies in the peripheral (PNS) and central (CNS) nervous systems are seldom performed. In particular, many of the fiber systems in the PNS and CNS are still poorly studied quantitatively. Our research in PNS was directed towards *three* major objectives: to improve the general understanding of the (i) fiber composition and (ii) functional topography of peripheral nerves, and (iii) to devise innovative methodologies that facilitate measurements and classification of the myelinated nerve fibers. This chapter aims to provide better understanding of two aspects of the myelinated nerve fiber systems:

1. **The classification of myelinated nerve fibers**

   Despite the extensive use of rat peripheral nerves as experimental models, there are few studies in the literature that explore the classification of myelinated nerve fibers in the rat. It is silently assumed that many of the obtained results from the early cat studies[2] can be transferred without adaptation to the rat. However, this belief is, in most cases, unsustainable (for some examples see [1]). The classification of the nerve fibers in the rat will be reexamined in Sec. 2..

2. **The functional topography of nerve fibers**

   The functional topography[3] of nerve fibers, and the fascicle geometry can have impact on the spatial selectivity of peripheral nerve stimulation [3, 4]. Historically,

---

[1] We will further narrow the meaning of the term to quantitative microscopic studies.

[2] Most of the "textbook" neurophysiological and neuroanatomical studies were performed in cats.

[3] Functional topography is defined as the topography of the nerve fibers with respect to their targets of innervation[2].

Quantitative Microscopic Analysis of Myelinated Nerve Fibers   209

two concepts about the spatial arrangement of the nerve fibers have been proposed: a cable-like structure or mesh-like (plexiform) arrangement (recent overview in [5]). While earlier anatomical studies kept to the opinion of Sunderland[6] that more proximal nerves were more plexiform in their structure, in Sec. 4. we will present some arguments in favor of the presence of proximal cable-like structure supported by more recent findings [2, 7, 8].

Finally, in Sec. 5. we will present some innovative methods that could facilitate future morphometric and topographic studies in the PNS and CNS. Further mathematical details about these methods are presented in a series of Appendices.

2.   Composition of Nerves

Nerve fibers originate from motor or sensory neurons, which belong to the somatic or autonomic parts of the central nervous system. Along their course, the nerve fibers assemble into fascicles, which in turn gather in nerve trunks. The fascicular organization of human peripheral nerves was recognized in the XVIIIth century by Van Leeuwenhoek but was lost and rediscovered later by Prochaska[9]. The fasciculation patterns originate from the arrangement of the mesenhymatous bulge during development [10]. The emergence of the fasciculation pattern was explained by the concept of a spatio-temporal correlation between the growth of the axons from the ventral horn and the order of innervation in proximo-distal sequence in the limbs (see also Sec. 4.4.).

The fascicular organization improves the nerve resistance to tension and preserves the nerve trunk against compression and stretching. It also functions as a metabolically-active diffusion barrier. Other essential components of the nerves are some specialized connective tissues and blood vessels (*vasa nervorum*). The structure of a peripheral nerve is schematically represented in Fig. 1.

The subdivision of the nerve constituents in the nerve was proposed originally in XIXth century [11]. Retzius defined the loose connective tissue surrounding the nerves as epineurium, the perifascicular lamellated sheath as perineurium and the intrafascicular tissue as endoneurium (Fig. 1). The *epineurium* is the outermost supportive layer of connective tissue. It keeps the fascicles together and is loosely attached to the surrounding tissue. Its main function is to assure and maintain the mobility of the nerve in its bed [12, 13]. The epineurium is composed mainly of flat collagen bundles, which take oblique courses and intersect each other at acute angles [14]. The *perineurium* encloses bundles of nerve fibers into individual fascicles. It is arranged in concentric sheets of collagen fibrils forming networks. The directions of collagen bundles in these networks vary with the size of the nerve fascicle; the ones enclosing larger fascicles take longitudinal and circular courses (e.g., in the tibial nerve), whereas those enclosing smaller fascicles (e.g., in the peroneal nerve) run spirally [14]. The *endoneurium* consists of collagen fibrils and occasional fibroblasts and blood vessels [15]. The collagen fibrils form tube-like structures that accommodate individual nerve fibers. These tubes follow undulating courses like the corresponding nerve fibers. The endoneurial sheath is composed of an *inner* and an *outer* collagen layer[14]. So-described structures protect the nerve fibers against external forces [12, 13, 16].

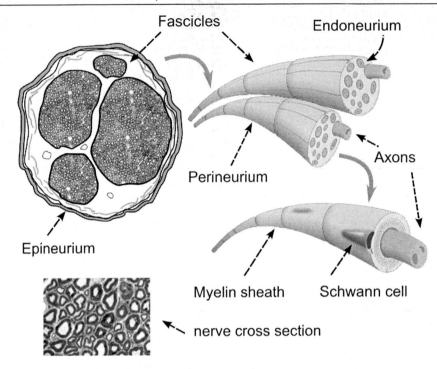

The nerve consists of nerve fibers, connective tissues (epineurium, perineurium and endoneurium) and blood vessels. The **epineurium** mainly consists of 10-20 μm thick bundles of collagen fibrils. Individual fascicles are enclosed by **perineuria**. The **endoneurium** consists of two layers: a mesh-like *inner* layer and an *outer* layer consisting of longitudinally oriented 1-3 μm thick bundles [14]. Myelinated nerve fibers are enclosed by the membranes of the **myelin sheath** formed by the *Schwann cells*. Only at the nodes of Ranvier the axonal membrane is exposed. The inset represents a microscopic preparation of a semi-thin sural nerve cross section colored by Toluidine blue [2; Ch. 4].

Figure 1. Microscopic anatomy of the peripheral nerve.

2.1. Nomenclature of the Nerve Fibers

The *anatomical* classification of nerve fibers can be based on morphological features, such as the size of the fiber profile, the presence of myelin or the relationship between the axon and the myelin sheath (e.g., the g-ratio) etc. The most common classification is in terms of size (e.g., fiber profile diameter $d[f]$ or fiber profile area $A[f]$): a fiber class comprises all fibers within a certain size range. Fibers can be classified as well by other criteria, such as myelin profile area, myelin profile thickness, number of myelin lamellae, or the value of the g-ratio.

Physiologically, nerve fibers can be classified on the basis of their conduction velocity, the electrical response toward specific stimuli, the shape of the compound action potential, etc. For example, there are slowly-conducting unmyelinated fibers and fast-conducting myelinated fibers. Erlanger and Gasser[17] demonstrated the existence of **three** main functional groups of nerve fibers, designated A, B, and C; the A-fibers are the fastest and thickest, while the C-fibers are the slowest and have the finest diameter [17]. The A-fibers are

Table 1. Physiological classification of the myelinated nerve fibers in PNS

Fiber class notation	Innervation	Conduction velocity in humans [m/s]
	Motor fibers	
$A\alpha$	extrafusal muscle fibers	72 – 120
$A\gamma$	intrafusal muscle fibers	12 – 36
	Sensory fibers	
$A\alpha$/ Ia	receptors of muscle spindle	72 – 120
$A\alpha$/ Ib	Golgi tendon organ	72 – 120
$A\beta$/ II	all cutaneous mechanoreceptors: muscle spindle flower spray; touch and pressure; some nociceptors [1]	36 – 72
$A\delta$/ III	free nerve endings of touch and pressure, cold thermoreceptors, nociceptors of neospinothalamic tract	6 – 30

The table is adapted from [18] and [19]. Notations for the fiber classes are given according to Erlanger and Gasser and alternatively according to Lloyd. The conduction velocities presented in Table 1 are considered by many researchers without proof to be the same for all mammal species, and in particular, for rats and mice (see Sec. 2.3.).

myelinated and the B fibers are thinly myelinated, while the C-fibers are unmyelinated.

We will further use mixed notations: large myelinated fibers will be designated as A-fibers. The class of fiber will be denoted by a small Greek letter and the eventual sub-class will be designated by an Arabic number and the function of the fiber (e.g., 'sensory' or 'motor'). The nomenclature of the A nerve fibers is concisely summarized in Table 1.

2.2. Relationship between Size and Conduction Velocity of the Nerve Fibers

Physiological studies show that there exists an empirical relationship between the nerve fiber size and its conduction velocity. The form of this relationship is affected strongly by the presence of myelin around the axon (review in [20]). Unmyelinated fibers follow a power low relationship between the fiber diameter and its conduction velocity (see for example [21, 22]).

In contrast, the pioneering work of Hursh [23] established a linear relationship between the size of a myelinated fiber (as determined *ex vivo*) and its conduction velocity (as determined *in vivo*). The factor determined experimentally for all myelinated fibers in the cat was 6 m/s/μm.

The form of the relationship between nerve fiber size and its conduction velocity has been disputed in the early physiological literature. While the initial studies of Gasser and Erlanger[24] showed evidence for a linear relationship, Blair and Erlanger[25] suggested a power law. Later measurements in cats [26, 23] and in frogs[4] [27, 28] ruled in favor of

---

[4]Interestingly, the factor for frogs is about 2.5 m/s/μm.

a **quasi-linear relationship** between the diameter of a myelinated fiber and its conduction velocity. The extensive electrophysiological and morphometric studies performed in 1970s by Arbuthnott, Boyd and Kalu yielded the coefficients for the different fiber classes used currently in literature [29, 30, 31]. Studies of Arbuthnott, Boyd and Kalu showed that the variation of the conduction velocity with the fiber diameter was approximately linear but with different slopes for the different fiber types:

$$CV_{class} = k_{class} \cdot d[f]_{class} \tag{1}$$

It was calculated that for large fibers (e.g., $A\alpha$ fibers) the factor was 5.7 m/s/μm, while for the smaller fibers ($A\beta$, $A\gamma$ and $A\delta$) the factor was 4.6 m/s/μm[31].

The presence of this relationship implies that the anatomical and physiological classifications at least partially correspond. Such correspondence is important because not all data are easily obtainable during one experiment.

Observations made in quail [32], pigeon [33], cat [26, 23], and human [34] nerves agree well with values of the factors in [29, 30, 31] and suggest a similar relationship between fiber morphology and its conduction velocity. Therefore, this relationship probably reflects actions of some structural laws optimizing the conduction in myelinated fibers, as also suggested by Rushton [35] by the principle of corresponding states.

Despite its obvious practical importance, the basis for this relationship has so far received little attention in theoretical neurophysiological studies. Besides the initial theoretical considerations in [35] there are only few modeling studies on myelinated fibers (see for example [36] and [37]).

2.3. Unresolved Issues

The nomenclature of the A-fibers remains ambiguous. *Muscle afferent* fibers were subdivided into groups I, II and III by Lloyd[38] based on the observation that afferent fiber-diameter histograms of muscle nerves frequently show three distinct peaks [31]. Erlanger and Gasser[17] designated the largest A fibers as $A\alpha$. On the other hand, *cutaneous afferent* fibers fall into two electrophysiological groups. Lloyd[38] designated these latter groups as II and III, since the mean diameter of the large cutaneous afferents is considerably less than that of group I muscle afferents. Some later works also followed this nomenclature (see for example [39, 40]). Alternatively, cutaneous afferents are designated $A\beta$ and $A\delta$ after Erlanger and Gasser[17]. *Efferent* fibers comprise 2 major groups: $A\alpha$ and $A\gamma$ designated after Erlanger and Gasser[17]. The $A\alpha$-fibers originate from the α-motor neurons, while the $A\gamma$-fibers originate from the γ-motor neurons. A historical overview about the nerve fiber classification can be found in [41].

Other unresolved issues in fiber classifications are the exact values of the cut-off borders between the fiber classes both in terms of fiber diameters and in terms of conduction velocities (see Sec. 3.4.). Even for human nerves different sources give somehow different cut-off borders between the fiber classes (see for example [18] and [19]).

The relationship described by Hursh [23] was used in virtually all reviews and textbooks providing tables with cut-off borders between the fiber classes in terms of fiber diameters. By doing so the authors made two silent assumptions: (i) that all classes of myelinated fibers obey the same relationship and (ii) that there are no species differences in terms of the specific fiber class conduction velocities. Such assumptions could be misleading due to two reasons. First, as demonstrated by Arbuthnott, Boyd and Kalu the relationship of Hursh is incomplete. Secondly, as it was demonstrated [42], for the rat unlike for the men, the fibers from homologous anatomical classes tend to be finer. Therefore, commonly-used reference values for the (human) anatomical fiber classification are not applicable for the rat PNS.

Interspecies differences in fiber class conduction velocities are sometimes neglected. For instance, the upper limits of 30 m/s for $A\delta$-fibers appropriate for adult cat peripheral nerve are sometimes erroneously applied to rat studies (review in [1]). As an alternative, in Sec. 3.3. we propose a modified classification of the A-fibers (Table 3).

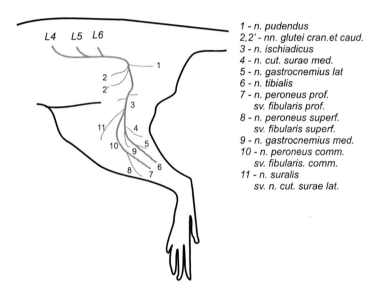

In the rat, the sciatic nerve (**3**) originates from the spinal nerve L4–L6 [43, 44]. At the middle of the thigh, it splits into several fascicles, which further distally give rise to the tibial (**6**), common peroneal (**10**) and sural nerves (**11**), and a cutaneous branch (**4**) [45, 44]. The nerves are drawn and named according to the atlas of Hebel and Stromberg [46].

Figure 2. Gross anatomy of the rat sciatic nerve and its founding spinal roots.

3. Fiber Analysis of the Nerves

3.1. Morphometry of the Sciatic Nerve System

The system of the sciatic nerve accounts for the sciatic nerve proper, its founding lumbar roots and its major branches. It should be noted that there are important species differences. For example, in the mouse, the sciatic nerve originates only from L4 and L5 [47]. The connectivity of the sciatic nerve system in the rat is presented in Fig. 2. The normal morphology of the sciatic nerve serves as a basis for quantitative comparisons in regeneration [48], developmental [49] and toxicological studies [50, 51]. Two of the most important parameters in those studies are considered to be the absolute fiber counts $N[f]_{total}$ and fiber densities $\lambda[f]$ [48].

General quantitative studies of the rat hind limb nerves have been published in [49] on the effect of undernourishment on the development of the L5 spinal roots and the sciatic nerve; in [45] on the effects of deafferentation in the sciatic, tibial, peroneal, and sural nerves; and in [42] on the myeinated fiber morphology of the sciatic nerve system. The most important morphometric parameters from different quantitative studies are summarized in Table 2. The table demonstrates a good agreement between the studies for the fiber counts in the sural and tibial nerves and the L4 dorsal root. On the other hand, the fiber counts of the sciatic nerve seem to be mode diverse. This could be attributed to differences in sampling or inter-animal variation. The packing of fibers in the spinal roots (expressed as the relative total fiber area $A[f]_{rel}$) was also found to be higher than in the peripheral nerves. The fiber density varied with the functional character of the nerve—it was higher in the dorsal roots compared to the ventral roots [42].

Variation of the fiber numbers (Table 2) and cross-sectional areas (not shown) in the dorsal roots could be explained by regression models [42]. In contrast, dependence on the segmental level was absent for the density of fibers and $A[f]_{rel}$. In a similar manner, analysis of the tabulated fiber counts published in [52] showed a negative correlation between the dorsal sacral root segment level and its number of fibers ($r = -0.96$; $p < 0.05$) [42]. Therefore, fiber counts for the dorsal roots should be reported per single root and not as averages of several root levels. In contrast to the dorsal roots, no dependence for the fiber number was found in the ventral roots [42]. Ventral roots turned out to be more uniform also with respect to their densities and areas. On the other hand, there were segmental differences in their composition, which were not present in the dorsal roots [42].

3.2. Fiber Population Modeling

In most of the studies on nerve regeneration, the authors limit their attention to simple comparisons of mean parameters, such as fiber diameter, number of fibers or g-ratio (see, for example, [56]). Since the nerves are composed of several morphologically and functionally different fiber populations, summarizing the nerve microscopic anatomy by a single sample mean/variance pair is unsustainable. Unfortunately, this is still the usual approach in assessing fiber regeneration (review in [48]). In this section we will present an alternative approach.

It was demonstrated that some essential information about nerve microscopic anatomy can be revealed by means of population mixture modeling [57, 58, 42]. The fiber size distributions could be separated in a number of components using a systematical statistical procedure rather than by setting arbitrary cut-off borders between fiber classes.

To our knowledge, population mixture modeling was first employed in fiber analysis by Kaar and Fraher[57] who studied the development of myelination in the rat ventral root L5. The nerve fiber population in the root was modeled using a two-component Gaussian model accounting for the presence of $A\alpha$ and $A\gamma$-fibers. The authors identified as $A\alpha$ fibers the population with a peak at 9.77 μm (spread 2.77 μm) and share of 65.2%; and as $A\gamma$ fibers the population with a peak at 3.69 μm (spread 1.24 μm) and share of 34.8%. The cut-off border between the fiber classes can be estimated at 5.67 μm (Eq. 46). As the authors used different models, it is difficult to compare their findings to later literature data.

Quantitative Microscopic Analysis of Myelinated Nerve Fibers 215

Table 2. Morphometric parameters of the hind limb nerves and roots

material	$N[f]_{total}$	$A[f]_{rel}$, %	$\lambda[f] \cdot 10^{-3} \; \mu m^{-2}$	Reference
		ventral roots		
L4	1163 ± 136	66.8 ± 2.1	10.901 ± 0.739	[42]
L5	1611 ± 240	67.2 ± 1.8	12.280 ± 0.880	[42]
L6	1400 ± 29	67.9 ± 2.1	10.231 ± 0.658	[42]
		dorsal roots		
L4	3302 ± 777	68.8 ± 2.0	22.119 ± 2.240	[42]
	2731	–		[53]
L5	3645 ± 363	65.0 ± 2.9	20.169 ± 1.159	[42]
L6	4425 ± 341	65.9 ± 3.4	19.178 ± 1.196	[42]
		nerves		
proximal sciatic	7599 ± 471	51.9 ± 3.5	13.081 ± 0.768	[42]
distal sciatic	8270 ± 1310	49.7 ± 2.6	16.861 ± 1.239	[42]
overall sciatic	7800 (efferent: 1600)	–		[45]
	7938	–		[54]
peroneal	1629 ± 53	46.2 ± 2.2	15.834 ± 1.527	[42]
	1900 (efferent: 588)	–		[45]
tibial	4262 ± 331	53.8 ± 2.4	12.991 ± 0.596	[42]
	4500; (efferent: 1014)	–		[45]
sural	920 ± 234	50.7 ± 3.4	21.434 ± 2.195	[42]
	1050	–		[45]
	956	–		[55]
cutaneous branch	439 ± 3	57.0 ± 0.8		[42]

Data are presented as means $\pm$ S.E.M. On average, the dorsal roots contain significantly more fibers than the ventral ones[42]. Moreover, the dorsal root fiber counts systematically varied with the root level ($N[f] = 145.2 + 693.8 \cdot level$, where the level varied from 4 to 6 for L4–L6, respectively), which was not the case for the ventral roots.

Another approach was introduced in [58]. The nerve diameter histograms were modeled as mixtures of 2 lognormal curves. The optimal parameter values were identified by means of least-squares minimization procedure. The authors identified 2 populations in the rat peroneal nerve: one with a peak at 3.53 μm (spread 0.46) and share of 59.8% and another with a peak at 8.54 μm (spread 0.23) and share of 40.2%. As can be seen from Fig. 9, a mixture of $A\gamma$ and $A\delta$ fibers match well the so-called "$A\beta$" population described in the study.

Both studies made prior assumptions about the number of components in the studied nerves and roots. A different goal was set in [42]. The authors tried to determine the optimal number of fiber populations, which could fit a given nerve histogram. It was found that the optimal models of the dorsal roots, the ventral roots, the sciatic, and the peroneal nerve contained three populations of fibers. The models are presented in Figures 3–9. It was found that the optimal models of the tibial and the sural nerves contained two populations of fibers (Figs. 10(a) and 11(a)). On the other hand, the use of only two-component models

Table 3. Classification of the A-fibers in the rat

	$d[f]_{border}$		inferred CV_{border}	
	low	high	low	high
$A\alpha^2$-motor	10.18	–	58.0	–
$A\alpha^1$-motor	6.76	10.18	$31.1 - 38.5$*	58.0
$A\alpha^2$-sensory	10.18	–	58.0	–
$A\alpha^1$-sensory	7.17	10.18	$33.0 - 40.8$*	58.0
$A\beta$	3.64	7.17	16.8	$33.0 - 40.8$*
$A\gamma$	1.00	6.76	4.6	$31.1 - 38.5$*
$A\delta$	1.00	3.64	4.6	16.8

Intercepts between components in the size distributions are considered as cut-off values for the classification of the nerve fibers. Intercepts were calculated according to the equation:

$$d[f]_{border} = \exp \frac{\left(\frac{\ln m_b}{w_b^2} - \frac{\ln m_a}{w_a^2}\right) \pm \sqrt{\left(\frac{\ln m_b}{w_b^2} - \frac{\ln m_a}{w_a^2}\right)^2 - \left(\frac{1}{w_b^2} - \frac{1}{w_a^2}\right)Q}}{\frac{1}{w_b^2} - \frac{1}{w_a^2}} \tag{2}$$

where

$$Q = \frac{\ln^2 m_b}{w_b^2} - \frac{\ln^2 m_a}{w_a^2} + 2\ln \frac{w_b \, m_b \, a_a}{w_a \, m_a \, a_b} + w_b^2 - w_a^2$$

m – peak parameter, w – spread parameter, a – share of the component; the indices a and b denote arbitrary sub-populations. The derivation of the equation is described in Appendix B.2.2.. The borders in terms of conduction velocities were calculated as:

$$CV_{border} = k_{pop} \, d[f]_{border} \tag{3}$$

where CV denotes conduction velocity and the index pop denotes different fiber populations and k is the coefficient of Arbuthnott, Boyd and Kalu. The cut-off borders between $A\beta$ and $A\gamma$ fibers are given in ranges of conduction velocities because values differ if for the same $d[f]$ is applied $k_{pop} = 4.6$ ($A\beta/A\gamma$-fibers) or $k_{pop} = 5.7$ ($A\alpha$-fibers) (asterisks).

can make interpretation of the obtained result difficult. As can be seen in Figs. 10(b) and 11(b), addition of a 3rd component could improve the anatomical classification.

Lognormal population models are described by the equation:

$$LNn\,(d[f]) = \sum_{i=1}^{n=2;\,3} a_i p\,(d[f]|m_i, w_i) \tag{4}$$

where a_i is the share of the component i and

$$p\,(d[f]|m, w) = \frac{e^{-\frac{w^2}{2}}}{\sqrt{2\pi}\,w\,m} \exp\left[-\frac{1}{2w^2}\left(\ln \frac{d[f]}{m}\right)^2\right]$$

is the lognormal probability density function (p.d.f) with parameters m and w (see Appendix A.). The averaged parameter values of the optimal models are presented as tables below Fig. 3 through 9. Functional identities of the statistically-discerned fiber populations are assigned according to Table 3 (see the discussion below).

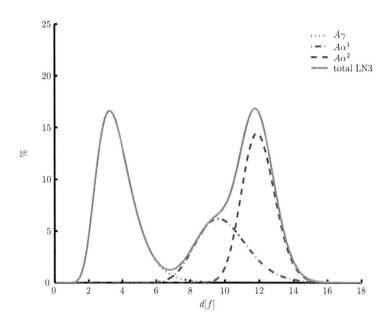

vetral L4	$A\gamma$	$A\alpha^1$	$A\alpha^2$
m[μm]	3.25 ± 0.19	9.62 ± 0.57	11.87 ± 0.58
w	0.30 ± 0.02	0.15 ± 0.02	0.07 ± 0.01
a[%]	42.90 ± 2.40	22.60 ± 4.77	34.50 ± 4.70

Notations: m – peak parameter; w – spread parameter; a – share; total – LN3($d[f]$). Data are presented as means ± SEM.

Figure 3. Average LN3 model of the ventral root L4.

The results presented in [42] suggest that the large myelinated $A\alpha$ fibers most-likely form 2 sub-populations in the ventral roots. This finding corresponds to previous findings reported in [59], who also showed 2 peaks in the histogram in the $A\alpha$ fiber range of cat L5 ventral roots. So-discerned fiber populations correspond with earlier measurements in the L5 dorsal and ventral roots and the proximal sciatic nerves[49]. In the tibial nerve, the peak position of the afferent fiber diameter histogram described by Schmalbruch[45] matched the peak of the $A\beta$ and the tail the $A\delta$ fibers. The peak positions of the reconstructed motor fiber histograms from the same study correspond with the $A\gamma$ and $A\alpha^1$ peaks, respectively [7].

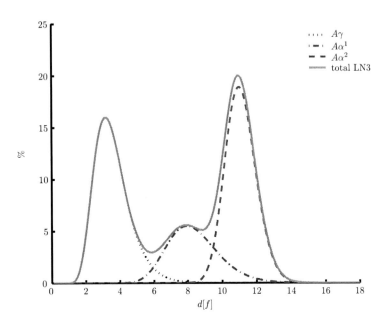

ventral L5	$A\gamma$	$A\alpha^1$	$A\alpha^2$
m[μm]	3.15 ± 0.16	7.94 ± 0.76	10.98 ± 0.47
w	0.29 ± 0.04	0.18 ± 0.04	0.08 ± 0.01
a[%]	38.20 ± 3.48	20.00 ± 4.65	41.80 ± 3.21

The peak positions of the $A\gamma$ and $A\alpha^2$ fibers matched the corresponding peaks described by [49] for the rat L5 ventral roots. Parameter notations are identical to Fig. 4. Data are presented as means ± S.E.M.

Figure 4. Average LN3 model of the ventral root L5.

3.3. Classification of the Fiber Populations

So-described fiber population models could be used for the purposes of nerve fiber classification. It is reasonable to assume that a fiber belongs to a certain fiber population if its size $d[f]$ falls within the interval where the population's p.d.f. $p(d[f]|m,w)$ is larger than the neighboring components (see Appendix B.). For example, a nerve fiber can be classified as $A\beta$ if

$$p(d[f]|A\beta) > p(d[f]|A\alpha)$$

The intercepts between components were, therefore, considered as cut-off borders between the different fiber populations. An anatomical classification of the nerve fibers based on the population models is proposed in Table 3. The left part of the table is based on the population mixture models described in Sec. 3.2.. The right part of the table is based on the inferred conduction velocities according to Eq. 3. The following ordering pattern about the fiber diameters can be discerned from Table 3:

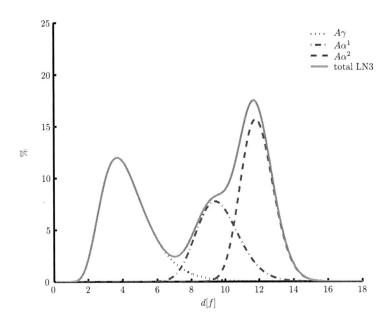

ventral L6	$A\gamma$	$A\alpha^1$	$A\alpha^2$
m[μm]	3.69 ± 0.20	9.41 ± 0.54	11.81 ± 0.56
w	0.33 ± 0.02	0.13 ± 0.02	0.08 ± 0.01
a[%]	38.70 ± 3.30	24.00 ± 15.50	37.30 ± 15.40

Parameter notations are identical to Fig. 3. Data are presented as means $\pm$ S.E.M.

Figure 5. Average LN3 model of the ventral root L6.

$$A\alpha^2 > A\alpha^1 > A\beta \geq A\gamma > A\delta$$

The cut-off border for the $A\alpha$-motor fibers is taken as the averaged value of the intercept between the $A\alpha$ and $A\gamma$ fiber populations in the ventral roots. In addition, the $A\alpha$-motor fibers are split into 2 populations with a cut-off border the intercept between $A\alpha^1$ and $A\alpha^2$ components. The cut-off border for the $A\alpha$-sensory fibers is taken as the averaged value of the intercept between the $A\alpha$ and $A\beta$ fiber populations in the dorsal roots. In addition, the $A\alpha$-motor fibers are split into 2 populations for reasons of symmetry similar to the motor fibers. The cut-off border for the $A\delta$ fibers is taken as the averaged intercept between the $A\beta$ and $A\delta$ populations in the dorsal roots and the sural nerve. The smallest fibers, which could be measured light-microscopically in our material were 1 μm in diameter that corresponded to conduction velocity of 4.6 m/s. Consequently, this value was taken as the low cut-off border for the $A\delta$ and $A\gamma$ fiber classes. By using so-estimated borders between the $A\alpha$, $A\beta$, $A\gamma$, and $A\delta$ fiber classes (Table 3) it was possible to identify the functional identity of a given fiber population.

It can be noticed that so-discerned $A\beta$ fiber populations overlap to a large extent with

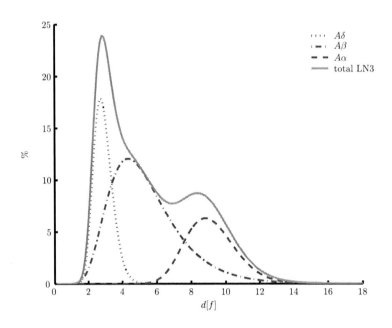

dorsal L4	$A\delta$	$A\beta$	$A\alpha^1$
m[μm]	2.73 ± 0.14	4.35 ± 0.36	8.81 ± 0.48
w	0.26 ± 0.05	0.21 ± 0.04	0.20 ± 0.06
a[%]	23.70 ± 6.81	53.70 ± 7.45	22.6 ± 13.68

Parameter notations are identical to Fig. 3. Data are presented as means $\pm$ S.E.M.

Figure 6. Average LN3 model of the dorsal root L4.

the neighboring populations. Therefore, relying only on one parameter, in this case $d[f]$, can be problematic, especially in the peripheral nerves (Fig. 9). Ideally, nerve fibers should be classified by larger morphological feature sets, for example including the g-ratio, circularity, etc.

3.4. Calculated Cut-off Borders Compared to Literature Data

There are no systematic experimental studies about the physiological nerve fiber classification in the rat. In most of the studies, the authors did not disclose how they arrived at the reported cut-off values or they made arbitrary choices. For example, Harper et al. [60] designated $A\alpha$ fibers in the range of 30–55 m/s; $A\beta$ fibers in the range of 14–30 m/s and $A\delta$ fibers in the range of 2.2–8 m/s. However, the authors admitted that the choice was arbitrary. Nevertheless, available literature allows for the following summary to be made:

Aα motor fibers: Bakels and Kernell[61] discerned 2 populations of motor fibers in the *Gastrocnemius*: "fast" with CV in the range of 41–85 m/s (7.2–15 μm)[5] and "slow"

---
[5] The numbers in brackets after the CVs denote inferred fiber diameters according to Arbuthnott, Boyd and

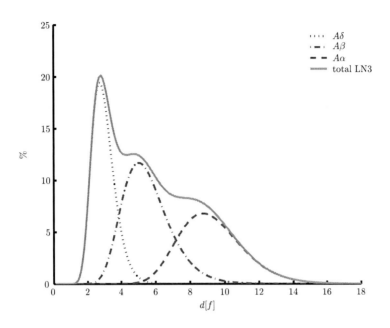

dorsal L5	$A\delta$	$A\beta$	$A\alpha^1$
m[μm]	2.67 ± 0.19	5.33 ± 0.80	8.74 ± 1.08
w	0.23 ± 0.05	0.25 ± 0.04	0.20 ± 0.04
a[%]	31.6 ± 4.85	38.0 ± 9.55	30.4 ± 9.55

The peak positions of the $A\delta$, $A\beta$ and $A\alpha^1$ populations match the peak positions of the histograms of the same root in [49]. Parameter notations are identical to Fig. 3. Data are presented as means ± S.E.M.

Figure 7. Average LN3 model of the dorsal root L5.

with CV in the range of 33–67 m/s (5.8–11.8 μm). Lewin and McMahon[62] found a peak for the $A\alpha$ motor fibers in the *Gastrocnemius* at 47.5 m/s (8.33 μm). Andrew and Part[63] measured CV for the $A\alpha$ fibers in in the range 33–59 m/s (95% confidence interval) in the *Soleus*. This corresponds to the range 5.8–10.4 μm.

$A\alpha$ sensory fibers: In the caudal muscles, Russell[64] measured sensory $A\alpha$ fibers having CV between 32 (5.6 μm) and 52 m/s (9.1 μm) with a peak at 38 m/s (6.7 μm). De-Doncker et al.[65] found a peak in the *Soleus* spindle afferent units $A\alpha$ at 43.3 m/s (7.6 μm). The corresponding border between the $A\alpha$ and $A\beta$ fibers could be estimated at 38 m/s (6.7–8.5 μm).

$A\beta$ sensory fibers: A review on the $A\beta$ fiber and sensory neuron properties can be found in [1]. De-Doncker et al.[65] found a peak in the *Soleus* $A\beta$ spindle afferent units at 33.9 m/s (7.37 μm). Russell[64] discerned sensory $A\beta$ fibers with CV between

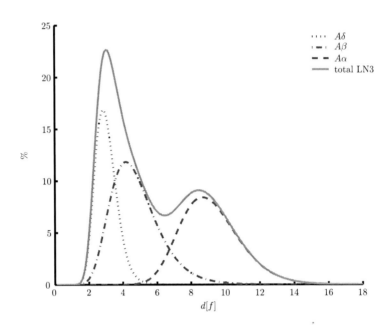

dorsal L6	$A\delta$	$A\beta$	$A\alpha^1$
m[μm]	3.03 ± 0.15	4.64 ± 1.01	9.44 ± 0.76
w	0.21 ± 0.05	0.30 ± 0.03	0.19 ± 0.03
a[%]	25.7 ± 6.53	38.9 ± 7.27	35.4 ± 8.29

Parameter notations are identical to Fig. 3. Data are presented as means $\pm$ S.E.M.

Figure 8. Average LN3 model of the dorsal root L6.

16.0 (3.5 μm) and 36.0 m/s (7.8 μm) with a peak at about 26.0 m/s (4.6 μm). In the rat sural and plantar nerves, Leem et al.[66] observed bimodal distribution of the CVs with a peak in the range of 32–44.5 m/s presumably in the range of the $A\beta$ fibers. This peak corresponds to the range 6.8–9.5 μm. Authors accepted a cut-off border between the $A\beta$ and $A\delta$ classes at 24.0 m/s (5.2 μm). Sanders and Zimmermann[67] accepted a border between the $A\beta$ and $A\delta$ classes at 25.0 m/s (5.4 μm) in measurements of the glabrous skin. Lewin and McMahon[68] found a peak at about 37.5 m/s (8.2 μm) for a mixed population of $A\alpha$ and $A\beta$ fibers innervating the skin.

Aγ motor fibers: Russell[64] measured CV for the $A\gamma$ fibers in the range between 4.0 (0.87 μm) and 24.0 m/s (5.2 μm). Andrew and Part[63] measured CV for the $A\gamma$ fibers in the range 14.9–25.5 m/s (95% confidence interval). This corrsponds to the range 3.2–5.5 μm. Lewin and McMahon[62] found a peak for the $A\gamma$ motor fibers in the *Gastrocnemius* at 17.5 m/s (3.8 μm). Reported value corresponds well with the peak of the $A\gamma$ fibers in Fig. 5.

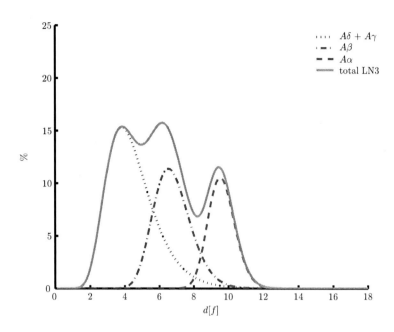

peroneal	$A\delta$ and $A\gamma$	$A\beta$	$A\alpha$
m[μm]	3.83 ± 0.19	6.53 ± 0.22	9.53 ± 0.30
w	0.33 ± 0.04	0.16 ± 0.03	0.08 ± 0.01
a[%]	49.6 ± 5.29	30.2 ± 5.90	20.2 ± 2.31

Parameter notations are identical to Fig. 3. Data are presented as means ± S.E.M.

Figure 9. Average LN3 model of the peroneal nerve.

$A\delta$ **sensory fibers:** In the rat sural nerve, Leem et al.[66] observed bimodal distribution with one of the peaks at 13.6 m/s (3.0 μm) in the range of the $A\delta$ fibers. Handwerker et al.[69] distinguished $A\delta$ fibers with conduction velocities in the range of 2.2 (0.5 μm) to 18.3 m/s (4.0 μm) in the skin. Gokin et al.[70] accepted a range of the $A\delta$ fibers between 2.2 m/s (0.5 μm) and 19.7 m/s (4.3 μm) after Handwerker et al. [69]. Lewin and McMahon[68] found a peak at about 25.0 m/s (5.4 μm) in the skin.

The literature data for the $A\alpha$-motor and sensory fibers correspond well with the cut-off borders proposed in Table 3. The data for the $A\alpha$-sensory fibers also correspond to Table 3, with the exception of ref. [64], where the CV appears underestimated. The data for $A\gamma$ and $A\delta$-fibers also correspond with the cut-off borders.

On the other hand, some discrepancies for the $A\beta$-fibers could be noticed. Presumed $A\beta$ peaks in the histograms of the measured CVs in the sural and plantar nerves [66] appear quite broad and on close inspection actually appear bimodal with a notch at about 40 μm, which could be expected from Table 3.

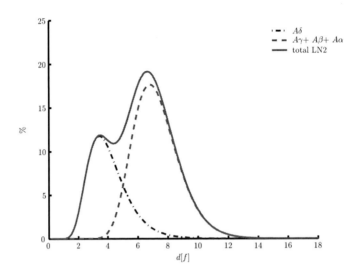

(a) LN2 model. Note that there is no clearcut distinction between $A\gamma$, $A\beta$ and $A\alpha$ fibers.

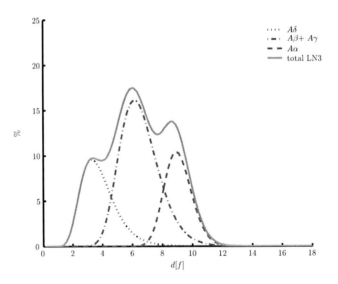

(b) LN3 model. Note that the $A\alpha$-population is now discernible

Model parameters are presented in Table 5.

Figure 10. Average population models of the tibial nerve.

Discrepancies could arise from the classification procedures (e.g., without the expectation for a possible presence of $A\alpha$-fibers in the sural nerve authors would classify all large fibers as $A\beta$) or from the experimental conditions. Many factors may influence CV

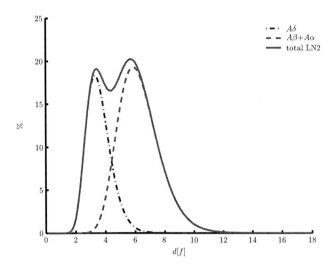

(a) LN2 model. Note that there is no clear cut distinction between the $A\alpha$ and the $A\beta$ fibers

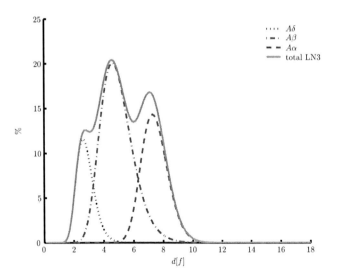

(b) LN3 model. Note that the $A\alpha$ population is now discernible

Model parameters are presented in Table 6.

Figure 11. Average population models of the sural nerve.

including the age or body weight of the animal, the recording site along the nerve[6], the

---

[6]Fibers of the same neurons conduct more slowly in the dorsal root than in the peripheral nerve [71].

temperature of the preparation[7], and whether or not utilization time[8] is included in the calculation (review in [1]).

In summary, proposed anatomical classification matches quantitatively available physiological data and could be used in future anatomical studies in the PNS. It is plausible to believe that the same cut-off values would be applicable in other closely-related rodent species—for example, in the mouse and guinea pig.

4. Functional Topography of the Nerves

The functional topography of nerve fibers can have an impact on the obtained spatial selectivity during peripheral nerve stimulation and recording. As outlined in several studies, variation of the site of insertion of microelectrodes results in different patterns of contraction of the peripheral nerves during stimulation[3]. Similar patterns are observed also in recording studies. It was found that recorded activity could vary reproducibly with the position of the recording site in the nerve. Using a microneurographical technique, Schady et al.[72] could discriminate some of the fascicles located in the upper arm, which projected to a single digital interspace. Modelling studies of the influence of various cuff electrode configurations outlined the importance of the fascicle geometry for the resulting selectivity [4].

Therefore, the type of nerve fibers' functional topography is an important design constraint for the development of neural prostheses for PNS. Notably, not all types of peripheral nerve electrodes could have equal performance, depending on the type of the motor functional topography.

Knowledge of the functional fiber topography also may be important for the interpretation of the studies of axonal regeneration and nerve repair. For example, it was shown that the path-finding choices of sensory axons depend on the motor axons [73]. Therefore, for successful functional regeneration, motor axons should be properly guided to restore their original functional topography and proper innervation targets.

4.1. Topography of Nerves and Dorsal Root Ganglia

The capability to demonstrate some topographical organization within PNS structures depends very much on the choice of methods of study. This statement can be supported by two examples.

- In the dorsal root ganglia, the set of enzyme-histochemical, immuno-histochemical and morphometric approaches (overview in [74]) failed to show a correlation between the site of the target muscle in the extremity and the position of the cell bodies in the individual ganglion (see also [75, 76, 77, 78]). Conversely, by means of retrograde

---

[7]It is empirically established that $CV[T] = CV[T_0] \cdot Q_{10}^{\frac{T-T_0}{10}}$, where T_0 is the measurement temperature. Q_{10} for mammalian myelinated nerve fibers is approximately 1.6 in the range of 27–37 °C [20].

[8]The utilization time is the time taken for an action potential to be generated after application of an electrical stimulus and unless excluded it causes a reduction in the calculated CV, creating a proportionately greater error when the latency is short. If utilization time is not excluded this causes an underestimate of CV, which is greater for faster conducting fibers especially in smaller animals with short conduction distances [71].

tracer studies, Wessels et al. [79, 80, 81] showed topographic mapping between some parts of a nerve and its corresponding dorsal root ganglia for all hind limb nerves (see also [82]).

- Historically, the literature has been indecisive about the kind of organization of the myelinated fibers in peripheral nerves. In the early XXth century, two contradicting views were promoted for the organization of nerves. While several investigators promoted "cable-like" fascicle organization [83, 84, 85, 86], others described some kind of "plexiform arrangement" of the fascicles within a nerve [87, 88, 89, 90]. By studying the clinical manifestations of the partial nerve injuries caused by nerve injuries from bullet wounds, Dejerine[91] was able to attribute motor or sensory groups of fibers to specific fascicles of the ulnar nerve at the elbow (review in [5]). Peripheral neuropathies associated with war injuries were also investigated using electrical stimulation in [92] and [93] who also concluded in favor of the cable organization. The results of intraneural stimulation experiments in the pioneering animal studies varied with the technique and the proximo-distal localization and were not conclusive. For example, stimulation of cat single peroneal fascicles at the knee level resulted in contraction of individual muscles [90], whereas stimulation at the level of the ischial tuberosity resulted in contraction of all muscles supplied by the sciatic nerve [94].

  In the 1940s, Sunderland[6] attempted to reconstruct the longitudinal course of fascicles by microdissection. His basic conclusion was that the complexity of fascicular rearrangements in the mid and proximal segments of nerves *"excluded the possibility of groups of nerve fibers being confined throughout their course to a particular funiculus (fascicle)"*. This became the commonly-accepted view about the internal structure of the nerves. While technically correct, Sunderlands's observations were very much limited by the employed gross dissection technique.

From the presented overview it is apparent that microdissection studies alone have very limited potential to reveal the presence of any particular functional topography. The so-outlined problems could be solved if neuronal tracing or electrophysiological techniques were applied instead. Microneurographic studies in men were able to demonstrate reproducibly intrafascicular concentration of the sensory axons[72, 95, 96, 97]. Clustering of the cutaneous afferent fibers was also demonstrated electrophysiologically in the cat saphenous nerve [98]. *Anatomic* evidence supporting a more-organized view on the topography of some nerves came primarily from *in vivo* retrograde tracing studies. Musculotopic organization of the motor axons was demonstrated in the *recurrent laryngeal nerve* in the cat [99]; the *oculomotor* [100] and *hypoglossal* nerves in the rat [101] and in the *segmental nerves* for the gluteal muscle fibers in the frog [102]. Cable-like fascicular anatomy was described also in the *median nerve* of the macaque [103] and the *musculocutaneous nerve* in the rat [104]. It was also suggested that the rat *sciatic nerve* fibers were grouped by their spinal level of origin[105].

Functional topography of nerve fibers can be revealed if the studied fiber population is specifically marked by some kind of a retrograde tracing substance deposited in the studied organ (for example the *Gastrocnemius* muscle). The resulting map of marked fibers would then represent the original population of fibers innervating the organ. Conclusions drawn from the distribution of this set of points will also be true for the topography of the original fiber population. Such an approach was elaborated in [7].

If the marked fiber is represented only by one point, then the set of all points, i.e., the spatial pattern representing all marked fibers, can be analyzed conveniently by the tools developed in spatial statistical analysis (see for example [106]). In the framework of hypothesis testing, observed patterns of nerve fibers can be compared against realizations of various types of stochastic spatial point processes, notably the completely spatially-random (CSR) Poisson process in the plane (see Sec. 5.2.). The non-Poisson, e.g. "non-random", arrangements then fall into two categories: (i) "clustering", where the objects tend to bundle closer than by a random arrangement; and (ii) "regularity", where the objects tend to be sparser than under a random arrangement. Some useful properties of the Poisson spatial processes (i.e., the CSR patterns) are summarized in Appendix C..

4.2. Spatial Analysis of the Ventral Root Topography

The analysis of the spatial arrangement of objects can be approached in several ways (see Sec. 5.2. for an overview and discussion). In this section we focus on 4 approaches: the Nearest-neighbor-analysis, the K-function analysis, the Voronoi analysis and the local clustering analysis.

Table 4. Summary of the presented cases, ventral root L6

case ID	$N[ax]_{total}$	$A_{prof}, \mu m^2$	$\lambda[ax]\cdot 10^{-3}, \mu m^{-2}$	A_f
N1570[a]	101	72545	1.93	0.0316
N1543[a]	138	85485	1.61	0.0305
N1547[b]	116	122621	0.946	0.0223
N1551[c]	102	139158	0.733	0.0163
N1549[d]	126	136838	0.921	0.0254
N1556[d]	119	137322	0.867	0.0221
Average	117	115663	1.08	0.0247
S.E.M.	6	11956	0.14	0.0023

Summary of the automatic measurements published in [8]. Gastrocnemius muscles of adult rats were injected with the retrograde tracer Fluoro-Gold and after 3 days survival time the spinal roots and the hind limb peripheral nerves of the animals were harvested and the tracer fluorescence was revealed. Measurements belong to the following experimental animals: a – A1120, b – A1119, c – A1121, d – A1134. A_f – area fraction of the axonal signal.

Measurements, which are analyzed further, are presented in Table 4. Morphometric data come from the tracing experiments described in [8]. Gastrocnemius muscles of adult rats were injected with the retrograde tracer Fluoro-Gold; following certain survival time the tracer fluorescence was revealed in cross-sections of the L6 spinal roots and the hind limb peripheral nerves. The Fluoro-Gold-positive axons were automatically detected at expected sensitivity level A_f=0.5 using custom-written image-processing software based on the program *ImageJ* (W. Raspband and contributors, National Institutes of Health, Bethesda, Maryland, USA).

4.2.1. Nearest-neighbor Analysis

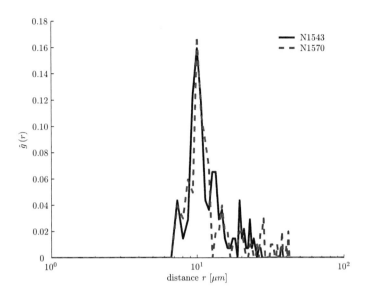

The peaks in the distributions are situated at about 10 μm. At small scales, the distribution showed marked differences compared to CSR, since there were no axons situated at less than 6 μm. This finding corresponded well with the size of the individual axons (not shown). On the other hand, the peaks positions approximately corresponded to the expected modes in CSR patterns (10.7 and 9.94 μm respectively; Eq. 54). Histograms are computed using 1000 classes of 0.67 μm each.

Figure 12. Nearest neighbor spatial analysis of two cases.

Pair-wise interactions of the *Gastrocnemius* motor fibers at the level of the L6 ventral root were studied by means of Nearest-neighbor (NN) analysis. The NN-analysis belongs to the group of distance-based methods. The method is described in Sec. 5.2.. This type of analysis is sensitive mostly to small-scale features of the spatial arrangement and specifically to deviations from CSR towards regularity [106]. The nearest-neighbor distance distribution of the Fluoro-Gold-positive axons is presented in Fig. 12. From the nearest-neighbor analysis only, the clustering of the axons, which is present at larger scales was not evident.

4.2.2. K-function Analysis

The arrangement of the *Gastrocnemius* motor fibers was also studied simultaneously at multiple scales using the Ripley's $K(r)$ function. K-function analysis belongs to the group of distance-based methods. The method is described in Sec. 5.2.. If the border effects are neglected, then for a CSR process it holds $K(r) = \pi r^2$ where r is the distance, e.g., the scale of observation. For regular patterns, $K(r) < \pi r^2$ while for clustered patterns $K(r) > \pi r^2$. Due to its quadratic form, plots of the K-function are often inconvenient for visual inspection. Therefore, the above-mentioned properties of $K(r)$ are used in the definition of a "derivative" function $L(r)$, which is more convenient to inspect visually:

$$L(r) = \sqrt{\frac{K(r)}{\pi}} - r$$

Positive deviations of $L(r)$ indicate clustering of the objects, while negative indicate regularity of the pattern.

$L(r)$ was estimated for the dataset described in Table 4. Results for 2 of the cases are presented in Fig. 13 and Fig. 14. As expected from its properties, $L(r)$ was more sensitive than $G(r)$ in the detection of departures toward clustering at large scales.

Results presented in Fig. 13 and Fig. 14 show two distinct trends. *At small scales,* below approx. 15 μm, Gastrocnemius axons were situated in more regular patterns corresponding to the average size of the complete fiber (i.e., axon + myelin sheath). This finding corresponded with the observed minimal spacing between the axons, as shown by their nearest-neighbor-distributions (Fig. 12). *At large scales,* the axons were situated in more clustered patterns. The clustering was most pronounced at scales between 100 and 150 μm.

The K-function analysis can be extended if other types of information about the nerve fibers become available. Such information can be provided, for example, by the axon size, which in turn could enable size-based classification to be performed [8]. Then one could use bivariate generalizations of the K-function to study the spatial co-variation of the $A\alpha$ and $A\gamma$ axons.

4.2.3. Tesselation Analysis

An entirely different approach follows the partition-based methods. These approaches divide the space between the objects into polygons according to some geometrical rule. The set of Voronoi polygons, called Voronoi tessellation[9], provides a natural polygonal partition of a point pattern (see, for example, [107]). The set of Voronoi polygons, which resembles a mosaic, gives a visual impression of the distribution of nerve fibers While providing an excellent pictorial impression, these methods are very difficult to handle analytically and hence it is difficult to test whether or not the objects under study follow some expected distribution. The tessellation approach to the study of the spinal root functional topography was introduced for the first time in [7]. The Voronoi tessellations of the cases N1543 and N1570 are demonstrated in Fig. 15.

4.2.4. Local Spatial Analysis

So-far demonstrated conventional spatial analytical methods do not provide the means to directly demonstrate the clustered objects. Instead, clustering of objects is only inferred. To overcome this serious limitation and in order to reveal the functional topography of nerve fibers in a cross section we devised an approach, which is able to test for the occurrence of clusters and to visualize them in the anatomical context of the studied nerve sample [7]. The approach is presented in detail in Sec. 5.4..

---

[9]The Voronoi polygon of a point is the region of space closest to that point than to any other point of the sample. The approach is also known as Dirichlet tessellation or Thiessen polygons.

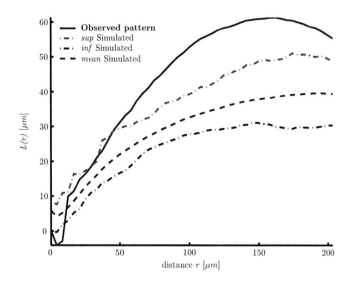

(a) L(r) plot. Simulated patterns show deviations from CSR due to the finite sizes of the nerve profiles.

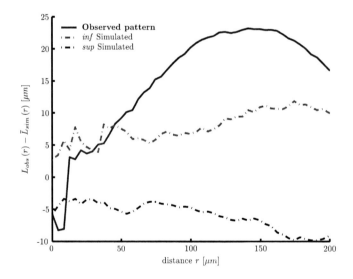

(b) De-trended plot of *L(r)*. The spatial distribution of fibers shows regularity at distances below 10 μm and clustering at distances above 45 μm. The maximal deviation from CSR can be observed at 150 μm.

Notations: $\bar{L}_{sim}(r)$ – average over simulated patterns; $L_{obs}(r)$ – L-function of the observed pattern of Fluoro-Gold-positive axons; *sup – supremum*; *inf – infumum*. 100 patterns were sampled from a pool of 2000 simulated points belonging to a realization of a homogeneous Poisson process.

Figure 13. K-function spatial analysis of case N1543.

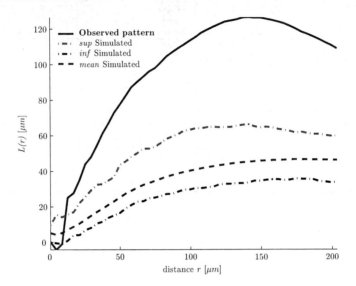

(a) L(r) plot, case N1570. Simulated patterns show deviations from CSR due to the finite sizes of the nerve profiles.

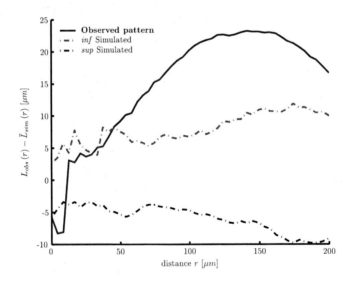

(b) De-trended plot of L(r). The spatial distribution of fibers shows regularity at scales below 10 μm and clustering at scales above 45 μm.

Notations and analysis are identical to Fig. 13. The maximal deviation from CSR can be observed at 140 μm.

Figure 14. K-function Spatial Analysis of Case N1570.

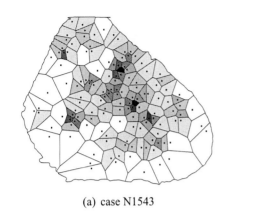 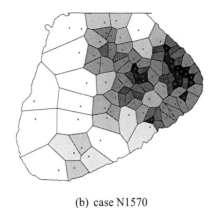

(a) case N1543   (b) case N1570

Voronoi tessellations were calculated for the simulated and the experimental data sets using the software program Voron [108]. The approach was introduced in [7]. The gray intensity corresponds to tile size (light - large, dark - small density). In both cases identical gray shading is used.

Figure 15. Tessellations of two experimental cases.

The spatial pattern of fibers P is considered to partition into a non-clustered, "CSR-like" part $C(r)$ and a clustered part $S(r)$. Partitioning is considered to be a function of the scale of observation r:

$$T(r) : P \longrightarrow C(r) \cup S(r) \qquad (5)$$

To perform this partitioning, we compute an indicator function $LC_p(r)$ measuring the local spatial fiber density around any given nerve fiber. Thresholds, measuring the "baseline" level of clustering in the pattern, are estimated by Monte-Carlo simulations of CSR patterns in the same area of study. In the particular examples (Figs. 16 through 19), the thresholds were computed from 200 simulations of CSR patterns. The "baseline" threshold level $T_\alpha(r)$ was conveniently set at the 95-th percentile of the simulations' distributions. All the points having $LC_p(r)$ values exceeding the "baseline" are considered to take part in the clustered pattern. Results presented here and in [7] indicate the presence of clustering of the motor fibers innervating the Gastrocnemius muscle at the level of the L6 ventral spinal root.

Cluster geometry could be further reconstructed by Gaussian kernel interpolation. The locations of the observed Fluoro-Gold-positive axons are "blurred" with the kernel $K_G(x, y \mid s)$ until some kind of probabilistic cluster density map is constructed. The approach is explained in more details in Sec. 5.4.3.. Results are presented in Figs. 16 through 19. The topography of the clusters inferred from $S(r)$ was reconstructed for several different scales of observation: 50, 100, 150, 200 μm. To relate detected clusters to ventral root microscopic anatomy the cluster density maps were superimposed on the tissue borders (Figs. 16 through 19). From the figure it is apparent that clusters of motor fibers were a robust feature of the ventral roots at all studied scales. Density maps were also similar in their dimensions and configuration (see for example Figs. 16 and 17).

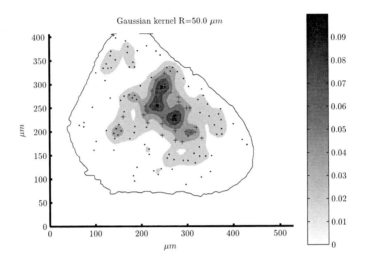

(a) Cluster density map $\Psi_G(x,y\,|r)$ at $r = 50\,\mu m$

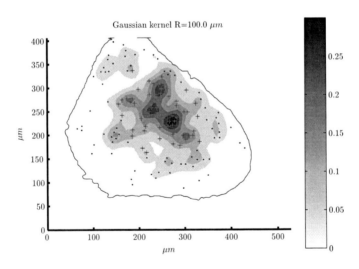

(b) Cluster density map $\Psi_G(x,y\,|r)$ at $r = 100\,\mu m$

Locations of the Fluoro-Gold-positive axons are represented by dots. Contours of the L6 ventral roots are drawn by solid lines. The axons for which $LC_p(r)$ exceeds the threshold of "randomness" are marked by crosses. Density maps are computed using the equation:

$$\Psi_G(x,y\,|r) = \frac{1}{N}\sum_{p=1}^{N} LC_p(r)\, K_G(x - x_p, y - y_p\,|s) \qquad (6)$$

where N is the number of Fluoro-Gold-positive axons and $K_G(x,y\,|s)$ is a Gaussian kernel parametrized by the scale parameter s (see also Sec. 5.4.3.). Map levels are coded by the gray tone intensities as indicated by the calibration bar.

Figure 16. Influence of the scale on the observed clustering, case N1543, I.

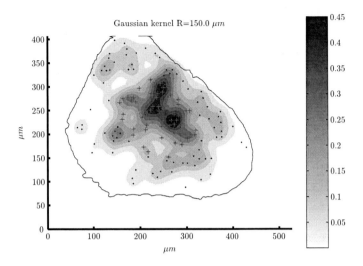

(a) Cluster density map $\Psi_G(x,y\,|r)$ at $r = 150\ \mu m$

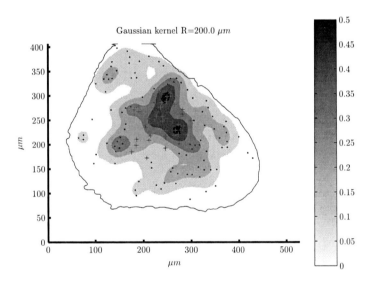

(b) Cluster density map $\Psi_G(x,y\,|r)$ at $r = 200\ \mu m$

Notations and analysis are identical to Fig. 16.

Figure 17. Influence of the scale on the observed clustering, case N1543, II.

4.2.5. Summary of the Spatial Analysis

Presented analysis and the findings already described in [7] and [8] could be summarized as follows:

1. It was shown that clustering was a robust feature of the observed tracing patterns at

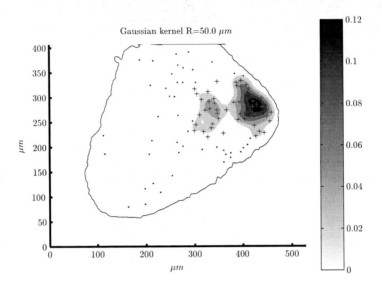

(a) Cluster density map $\Psi_G(x, y | r)$ at $r = 50\ \mu m$

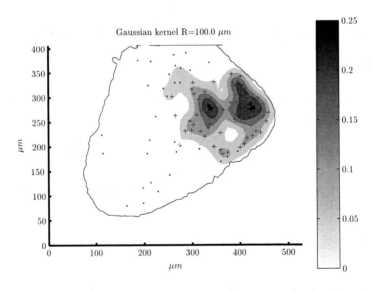

(b) Cluster density map $\Psi_G(x, y | r)$ at $r = 100\ \mu m$

Notations are identical to Fig. 16.

Figure 18. Influence of the scale on the observed clustering, case N1570, I.

scales above 50 μm.

2. At small scales, *Gastrocnemius* nerve fibers behaved like a regular pattern. This corresponds with the fact that the fibers have finite dimensions of the same scale.

3. The local spatial analysis showed that the cluster geometry varied only slightly with

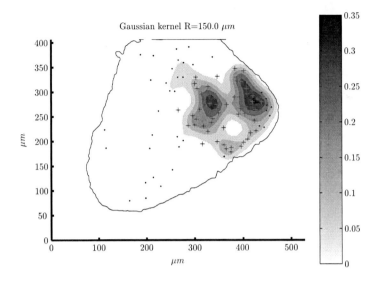

(a) Cluster density map $\Psi_G(x, y \,|\, r)$ at $r = 150\ \mu m$

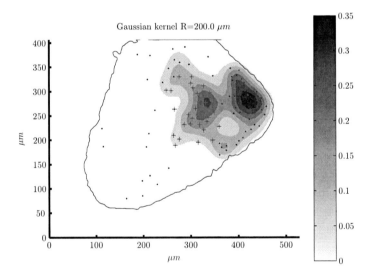

(b) Cluster density map $\Psi_G(x, y \,|\, r)$ at $r = 200\ \mu m$

The "clustered" points shift toward the center of the pattern probably due to border effects. Notations are identical to Fig. 16.

Figure 19. Influence of the scale on the observed clustering, case N1570, II.

the scale of observation.

4. Cluster density maps produced by the local spatial analysis correspond to the tessellation analysis as indicated by the density shadings of the tiles in Fig. 15. However,

the type of underlying process and the scale at which clustering occurred could not be inferred from the Voronoi partition.

Taken together these findings suggest that *Gastrocnemius* motor fibers were musculotopically organized in the studied examples of the L6 ventral root.

4.3. Functional Implications

The functional implications of the presented findings can be discussed in two directions. First, functional topography of nerve fibers could be used for further development of neural prostheses.

- From presented data it can be concluded that approaches for spatially-selective nerve stimulation should target the operational range of $10 - 200 \ \mu m$. The lower bond corresponds to the observed peak in the nearest-neighbor distance histograms, while the upper bond – to the maximal scale of clustering. It is interesting to note, that this upper bond corresponds to the size of individual fascicles in the sciatic nerve of man.

- Reported spatial data could be used to build more realistic models of selective fiber activation to test different types of implantable electrodes.

- Observed scale of clustering can help explaining the notorious performance of the sieve-electrodes [109, 110]. So far tested designs of sieve electrodes had relatively small openings of the sieve. It could be speculated that to allow a "cluster" of motor fibers to regenerate, the diameter of the sieve opening should be in the same range.

Secondly, it can be speculated that by analogy with the DRG organization [79] observed musculotopy is not isolated only to one particular spinal root. Such organization would correspond with the musculotopy observed in other parts of the motor system, notably the motor neuronal columns in the spinal cord [111, 112]. Observations in cats suggest that the flexor groups of motoneurons in the spinal cord are arranged in such a way that each main mass of cells tends to be concerned with the innervation of muscles, which move the same joint [111].

Although we have demonstrated musculotopical organization of the representation of one particular muscle, another question remains open: Do different muscles share the same topographical space or do they have different projections? In the rat spinal cord, the flexor muscle nuclei do not overlap much with the extensors' nuclei [113]. Therefore, if the arrangement of motor nuclei corresponds to the map in the ventral root then, by analogy with the separate location of the flexor and extensor motor columns, it can be hypothesized that the motor fibers innervating flexor and extensor muscles would have separate representations at the level of the ventral root.

4.4. Origin of the Observed Clustering

It is plausible to hypothesize that observed clustering of the motor fibers is caused by the action of a spatio-temporal gradient of positional cues within the spinal root, which guides the growth of motor axons to innervate appropriate target muscles in a topographical manner. Several arguments could support this view.

Firstly, other parts of the spinal motor system are organized approximately musculo-topically (see Sec. 4.3.). It was demonstrated that some motor nuclei form topographical projections onto their motor targets during the embryonic development that are refined after birth [114, 115, 116] and are disrupted if the nerve was severed and regenerated [117, 118]. In most cases, the rostro-caudal location of the axis of motoneuronal cell bodies is mapped onto either the rostro-caudal axis [119] or the antero-posterior axis of a muscle [120]. Therefore, during development the spinal cord motoneurons project to predictable locations within a particular muscle according to their position in the motor nucleus

Secondly, during development motor axons are able to grow to their correct muscle targets because the axons can respond to specific limb-associated cues [10, 121, 122, 75, 123]. Different positional cues and mechanical interactions inside the nerve are thought to play a role in the "routing" process (for overviews see [124] and [125]). Actions of positional gradients of substances, such as the cell-adhesion molecules (CAM), have been implied in development and regeneration of the amphibian [126] and in the development of the avian limbs [73]. In contrast, the process of segmentation is not essential for the precise innervation of muscle targets by motor neurons [127, 128].

In theory, further stochastic modeling could describe the most likely spatial model, which is able to produce the observed functional fiber topography. This model could help finding a biologically-meaningful dynamic mechanism able to produce observed topographical organization. Such models could further elucidate the spatial mechanisms of axonal path acting during normal development and the differences, which were described during regeneration [129].

5. Innovative Methodology

5.1. Population Mixture Modeling

Population mixture modeling can give a comparative framework for the studies of mechanisms and, consequently, treatments of some pathological conditions such as traumatic nerve injuries, neuropathies and nerve regeneration. Lognormal population mixture models were already used to study nerve regeneration [58, 130, 131, 132]. Fiber size distributions could be separated reproducibly in a number of components using a systematical statistical procedure [57, 58, 42]. Moreover, it was possible to assign a functional modality to these components.

Results presented here and in [8] and [42] demonstrate that in most of the cases the use of two-component models is not sufficient. In contrast, it may be important to use multicomponent analysis in the search of an optimal nerve fiber population model. The following process steps can be outlined in such a procedure:

1. morphometry and assembly of the histograms;

2. fitting of the histograms;

3. model selection.

The morphometric protocol and the initial processing of the data are beyond the scope of this section. These are described well in numerous publications (see, for example, [58]

5.1.1. Histogram Fitting

Normalized histograms of $d[f]$ (range 0-18 μm) are normally calculated using 180 classes of equal bin size of 0.1 μm.

Fiber size histograms were fitted in sequentially against several types of distributions: 1 component Gaussian distribution and 1 to 5 component lognormal mixture distributions: LN1 – LN5. The parameter selection was performed by least squares minimization criterion.

The corresponding functions are described by the following equations:

Gaussian function

$$N(x) = Fe^{-\frac{(x-m)^2}{2w^2}}$$

(7)

where m - mean; w - standard deviation; F - class frequency at the mode value (i.e. at m).

Lognormal functions

$$LNn(x) = \sum_{i=A,B,C,D,E}^{n} F_i e^{-\frac{(\ln x - \ln m_i)^2}{2w_i^2}}$$

(8)

where n denotes the number of components, m – peak position (i.e. mode value), w – spread parameter; F – class frequency at the mode value (i.e., population weight parameter).

The forms of these functions are selected in a way to avoid non-linear interactions between the parameters as much as possible. The actual share of each component from the lognormal models was estimated numerically.

5.1.2. Optimal Model Selection

The optimal models were selected according to a combination of three criteria:

1. The value of the Schwartz-Bayesian information criterion (SBIC) [133]:

$$SBIC_p = n \ln \frac{1}{n} \sum_{i}^{n} (F_i[d]_{obs} - F_i[d]_{fit})^2 + p \ln n$$

(9)

where n is the number of classes in the fitted histogram, p the number of free parameters (i.e., 3, 3, 6, 9, 12 and 15 for the Gaussian and LN1 - LN5 models, respectively), "obs" denotes the observed, "fit" the fitted frequency in the sample histogram and i is the class.

As could be seen from its formula, SBIC information criterion is a compromise between the minimization of the error and the numbers of the parameters employed to do so by inclusion of a penalizing term for the addition of new parameters. According to the general properties of SBIC, the optimal model minimizes the criterion value compared to all the other (non-optimal) models.

2. Occurrence of populations with less than 5% of share in the sample

Due to the choice of the class size, such models exhibited sharp spikes that were not comparable with the actual histograms and were considered over-fitted independently of the value of SBIC. In this case, the model with the second smallest SBIC value was selected as optimal.

3. Quality of histology

In case of unequivocal choice of model for a particular type of nerve or spinal root the histological sections were also inspected and the sample areas checked for tissue defects. In this case, the sections with some lower quality were excluded from the model selection scheme. However, they were retained for the calculation of the parameter means and SEMs.

5.2. Spatial Analysis

Spatial analysis could bring about better understanding of the microscopic anatomy of the central and peripheral nervous systems. The following examples from literature could support this statement.

- It was demonstrated that the regularity of the spatial arrangement, which retinal cells exhibit is beneficial for the uniform sampling of the visual field (recent overview in [134]).

- Spatial analysis revealed also the mechanistic rules by which the cellular pattern is formed in the retina during development [135] and regeneration [136]. Dynamic mathematical models developed further suggested that the regularity of the receptor mosaics was produced by two independent biological events: one embodying the exclusion zone around each receptor cell; and another, specifying the local density of a given receptor type [137]. Different modeling studies revealed also the importance of the interplay of mechanisms, such as cell death, cell motility and lateral inhibition for the generation of the final spatial pattern [138].

- Studies of variety of neurodegenerative disorders suggested that brain lesions often exhibit common spatial patterns that correlate with their pathogenesis [139]. Specific examples can be given by the Creutzfeldt-Jakob's disease [140], Alzheimer's disease [141, 142], and Lewy-bodies' dementia [143].

5.3. Conventional Analytical Tools

There are numerous spatial analytical methods currently used in different fields of science (for comprehensive descriptions see [106, 144, 145, 146, 147]). However, only very few of them were introduced in neurosciences. Most of these methods found their way from ecological or epidemiological applications [148]. In general, these methods can be divided into count-based and point-based.

Count-based methods usually divide the field of study into a number of quadrants and compare the observed numbers of objects against the counts that could be found if the objects were distributed randomly. The quadrant-count distribution of a CSR process approximates the χ^2_{n-1} distribution where n denotes the number of quadrants [106]. A useful visualization tool of the quadrant count method is the plot of the ratio of Variance to Mean (V/M ratio) against the size of the quadrants (i.e., scale). Due to the properties of the Poisson distribution, the V/M ratio of a CSR process is equal to 1. For aggregated processes it is higher than 1, while for processes with repulsion it is less than 1. An advantage of this approach is that it can be done even on a spreadsheet. A major disadvantage is, however, that large inhomogeneities in space (such as tissue defects or spaces between fascicles) violate the assumptions of the χ^2-test and thus invalidate test results. Moreover, complicated tissue borders introduce intractable border effects and thus also violate the assumptions of the χ^2-test. Other limitations of the count-based methods are that the partitioning and respectively the consequent aggregation procedures are not translation-invariant. Therefore, a random translation of the microscopic field and hence, the starting point of the grid could alter the outcome of the analysis. If the studied process is not stationary (i.e., there is a global intensity trend) this bias would be even larger.

Distance or point-based methods usually compute some characteristic of the data based on the distances between the objects: for example the distance to the nearest neighbor of an object or the average number of neighbors within a certain distance of an object. These characteristics are then compared to some theoretical distributions of objects [106].

Nearest-neighbor distance distribution, conventionally denoted as $G(r)$ is defined as the probability that the distance from an arbitrary point to its nearest neighbor point is at most r. At short distances $G(r)$ is a crude measure of the degree of clustering and its values at long distances indicates the fraction of points that are greatly distant from each other. Practically, $G(r)$ is estimated as:

$$\hat{G}(r) = \frac{1}{n} \sum_{i \leq n} N[\min_{i \neq j}(d_{i,j}|i) \leq r] \tag{10}$$

where N denotes the number of points having $d_{i,j} \leq h$ where $d_{i,j}$ is the distance between any points) and $\min_{i \neq j}(d_{i,j})$ denotes the distance to the nearest neighbor; n is the total number of points in the area of the study.

Ripley's K-function, conventionally denoted as $K(r)$ measures the expected number of points that are within a given distance to a randomly chosen point. $K(r)$ is defined as

$$K(r) = \lambda^{-1} \cdot E\,[\#\text{ extra events within distance r of a randomly chosen event}]$$

where λ is the density (number per unit area) of events. $K(r)$ describes characteristics of the point processes at many distance scales. Alternative summaries (e.g. nearest-neighbor distance distribution) do not have this property. The definition of the K-function assumes stationary of the point process. $K(r)$ does not uniquely define the point processes in the sense that two different processes can have the same $K(r)$ function [149]. Practically, $K(r)$ is estimated as:

$$\hat{K}(r) = \frac{A}{n(n-1)} \sum_i \sum_{j \neq i} \frac{N\,[d_{ij} \leq r]}{w_{ij}} \tag{11}$$

Quantitative Microscopic Analysis of Myelinated Nerve Fibers 243

where N denotes the number of points having $d_{i,j} \leq r$ where $d_{i,j}$ is the distance between any points); w_{ij} is an edge-effect correction factor [149]; n is the total number of points in the area of the study. Although $\hat{K}(r)$ can be estimated for any r, it is common practice to consider only $r < 1/2$ of the shortest dimension of the study area A.

In general, only few statistical tests are available for comparing different point patterns. The most general approach for comparison against a spatial pattern with known generation mechanism is by means of Monte-Carlo simulations. For example, if one aims to compare against CSR as the simplest alternative, series of CSR Monte-Carlo simulations are performed and for each of them some exploratory descriptor function is calculated.

Without diminishing generality we can give an example by $K(r)$. The lower simulation envelope $L(r) = \inf\{K_s(r)\}$ (where s denotes simulation) and the upper simulation envelope $U(r) = \sup\{K_s(r)\}$ are computed and the observed function is compared against them. For point patterns with repulsion between the points generally holds $K_{observed}(r) < L(r)$ while for point patterns that show clustering holds $K_{observed}(r) > U(r)$. Accordingly, CSR is rejected for the scales where either of the inequalities holds.

5.4. Local Spatial Analysis

In the context of spatial analysis, the main difficulties in front of a method applied to a nerve cross section are its finite geometry and its complex topology introduced by the tissue defects and borders. The finite geometry makes most of the analytical methods inapplicable, because they assume unbounded space and are greatly affected by border effects. The tissue defects violate another important assumption - the homogeneity of space. Altogether, these features of nerve cross sections make the use of global spatial descriptors very limited. To solve these problems, a four-step analytical approach was elaborated in [2, 7]. The following process steps can be outlined:

1. computation of the observed Local Clustering function $LC_p(r)$;

2. computation of $LC_p(r)$ for the simulated patterns;

3. thresholding;

4. cluster geometry reconstruction.

5.4.1. Local Clustering Function

The function $LC_p(r)$ measures the local point density, i.e., the local "amount" of clustering around each point p in the pattern. $LC_p(r)$ is formally defined as the number of neighboring points within the radius r from the original point p belonging to point pattern Q:

$$LC_p(r) = \mathbf{N}[(d_{p,j} \leq r) \mid (x_j, y_j) \in Q] \qquad (12)$$

where $\mathbf{N}$ is the counting operator and $d_{p,j}$ is the distance from an arbitrary point (x_j, y_j) to p.

5.4.2. Clustering Threshold Function

As $LC_p(r)$ measures local density, clustering can only be present if the function exceeds its expected value under a "non-clustered" distribution. Thus, in order to test locally whether the observed pattern of fiber locations is more clustered than a CSR pattern (an obvious null hypothesis) we introduced a parameterized clustering threshold function $T_\alpha(r)$ depending on the significance parameter α and the scale parameter r. The α-parameter expresses the probability that the local "amount" of clustering $LC_p(r)$ exceeds a certain threshold value in an associated CSR point process:

$$P\left[LC_p(r) > T_\alpha(r) | p \in CSR\right] = \alpha \tag{13}$$

Accordingly, if the "amount" of clustering of the observed pattern exceeds the "amount" present in CSR $LC_p(r) > T_\alpha(r)$ (e.g. the null hypothesis is locally rejected) one can infer the existence of clustering in the local neighborhood r around the particular point p. In infinite isotropic space, $T_\alpha(r)$ can be computed analytically. However, in the cross section the tissue borders and tissue defects introduce distortions that are intractable analytically. Therefore, $T_\alpha(r)$ was estimated from series of simulated CSR point patterns Q_{CSR} only inside the nerve tissue borders. Simulated patterns were sampled on the condition to have the same global intensity λ as the observed pattern. $T_\alpha(r)$ was numerically estimated as the inverse of the α-quantile of the empirical probability distribution function $\hat{P}_\alpha[LC_p(h)]$ averaged across all simulations:

$$\hat{T}_\alpha(r) = \frac{1}{N_{sim}} \sum_{j}^{N_{sim}} \hat{P}_{\alpha,j}^{-1}\left[LC_p(r) | p \in Q_{CSR}\right] \tag{14}$$

where α was conventionally set to 0.95. Consequently, only 5% of the points were expected to exceed the threshold $T_{0.95}$.

In this manner, $T_\alpha(r)$ can provide partition of the original pattern:

$$T_\alpha(r) : P \longrightarrow C(r) \cup S(r)$$

into a "clustered" part $S(r)$ and its complementary "non-clustered" part $C(r)$. The set of all local clustering functions exceeding the clustering threshold is defined as the Global clustering set $S(r)$:

$$S(r) = \{p \in Q \mid LC_p(r) > T_\alpha(r)\} \tag{15}$$

In this way all the local information concerning the pattern can be preserved.

5.4.3. Reconstruction of the Cluster Geometry

If one considers clustering to be a realization of an unknown spatial process, then kernel interpolation (e.g., krigging) could be used to estimate the process. A natural candidate for such a procedure is the Gaussian kernel interpolation, where the locations of the observed events (e.g., Fluoro-Gold-positive axons) are "blurred". In this way a kind of probabilistic cluster density map is constructed:

$$\Psi_s(r|s) = \frac{1}{2\pi s^2 N} \sum_{p\in P}^{N} LC_p(r) K_G(x - x_p, y - x_p |s) \tag{16}$$

$$K_G(x, y |s) = e^{-\frac{(x-x_p)^2+(y-y_p)^2}{2s^2}} \tag{17}$$

$$s = \sqrt{\frac{\pi r^2}{4\hat{\lambda}\hat{K}(r)}} \tag{18}$$

Cluster geometry can be outlined through a geometric thresholding condition:

$$\Psi_s(r) \geq T_G(r) \tag{19}$$

where $T_G(r)$ can be a spatially-varying thresholding surface.

5.4.4. Amount of Clustering

Since $S(r)$ is not corrected for edge effects, as an estimate for the amount of clustered fibers $\mathbf{N}[S(r)]$ could be rather conservative. A possible improvement of such estimation technique could be attained by multiplying the area occupied by clustered fibers, as determined by the thresholding condition, with the estimate of the overall intensity of the fibers. Then the equation:

$$N_{clustered} = \hat{\lambda} \cdot A[\Psi(r) \geq T_G(r)] \tag{20}$$

could be used to estimate the number of clustered fibers.

5.4.5. General Applications of the Local Spatial Analysis

The presented approach is not limited solely to investigations of normal functional topography of the nerves. So far, studies on pathological nervous mechanisms in the peripheral nervous system compare only estimates of the numbers, density and mean size of the fibers in various pathological conditions but not their spatial distribution [150]. The presented method allows going into detail while studying the spatial aspects of pathological mechanisms that act in the peripheral nerves. For example, in the peripheral neuropathies, in conditions occurring after exposure to certain drugs or induction of a pathological gene, the mechanism of progressing demyelination can be studied as it progresses in the space of the nerve. Clustering features of the demyelination that could be revealed by the method would allow one to better compare animal models of neuropathies to the diseases characteristics observed in humans.

The local spatial analysis is straightforward in its interpretation. Its major advantages are that individual clusters can be localized and correlated to other anatomical landmarks such as the tissue borders, the approach can deal with arbitrary patterns, and maps of the cluster density can be constructed for different scales of observation.

Appendices

A. Some Properties of the Lognormal Distribution

The lognormal distribution has a p.d.f. typically defined as:

$$p(x|\mu, w) = \frac{1}{\sqrt{2\pi}\, w\, x} e^{-\frac{1}{2w^2}\ln^2(\frac{x}{\mu})} \tag{21}$$

where w is the spread parameter and μ is the scale parameter. Statistical properties of the lognormal distributions can be found in [151]. The mode (i.e. the peak position) of the lognormal distribution is given by the expression:

$$m = \mu e^{-w^2} \tag{22}$$

The maximum is given then by:

$$p(\mu) = \frac{e^{\frac{w^2}{2}}}{\sqrt{2\pi}\,\mu\, w}$$

The lognormal distribution can be also re-parametrized about its mode as:

$$p(x|m, w) = \frac{e^{-\frac{w^2}{2}}}{\sqrt{2\pi}\, w\, m} e^{-\frac{1}{2w^2}\ln^2(\frac{x}{m})} \tag{23}$$

In this case, the maximum is reached at $x = m$. Following this formulation, it can be shown that the expectation of an arbitrary power p of the variable x (i.e., x^p) is:

$$E[x^p] = m^p\, e^{\frac{p(p+2)}{2} w^2} \tag{24}$$

Therefore, the mean and the variance of the lognormal distribution can be expressed by:

$$E[x] = m\, e^{\frac{3}{2} w^2} \tag{25}$$

$$Var[x] = E^2[x](e^{w^2} - 1) \tag{26}$$

B. Classification of Measurements into Mixture Models by Maximum Likelihood

In this section we will develop an optimal strategy for classification of objects based on their probability of observation. The argument is based in part on [152].

We will classify a given object represented by an instance measurement into one of n a priori defined classes.

B.1. The Maximum Likelihood Principle

Let us denote the classes by A_1 through A_n and assume that they are mutually exclusive and form a complete set of observations $\mathcal{O}$. In other words, $A_i \cap A_j = \emptyset$ and $\bigcup_i^n A_i = \mathcal{O}$. Let us assume that we must base our decision on the measurement of a scalar object variable $X \in \mathbf{R}$.

If we have observed a particular instance of $X \to x$ can we tell which class of object was most likely presented?

Let us build the following parametrized classifier:

$$C_\xi : x \longrightarrow \{A_1, \ldots, A_n\} \tag{27}$$

where $\xi = \{\xi_1 \leq \xi_2 \leq \ldots \leq \xi_n\}$ is an ordered threshold vector with components $\xi_i \in \mathbf{R}$. For simplicity let us further consider the case where the desired class is A_a. The classifier C_ξ divides the x-axis in $\mathbf{n}$ intervals so that

$$C_\xi (\xi_{a-1} < x \leq \xi_a) = A_a$$

and assuming that $\xi_0 = -\infty$ and $\xi_{n+1} = \infty$. Let us also assume that the instance measurement $x \in A_a$ is drawn from A_a with marginal probability $P(x|A_a)$ and p.d.f. $p(x|a)$.

The total probability of a correct classification then is

$$P_C = P(x \in A_a) \cdot P[C(x) = A_a | x \in A_a] + \\ + \sum_{i \neq a}^{n-1} P(x \in A_i) \cdot P[C(x) = A_i | x \in A_i] \tag{28}$$

Let us define the following abbreviated notations concerning A_a:

$$P(a) \equiv P(x \in A_a) \tag{29}$$
$$P(a|a) \equiv P[C(x) = A_a | x \in A_a] \tag{30}$$

From the definitions above and the properties of probability distributions it follows that

$$P(a|a) = \int_{\xi_{a-1}}^{\xi_a} p(u|a)\, du \tag{31}$$

Eq. 28 can be reformulated using the definitions and notations above in the following manner:

$$P_C = P(a) P(a|a) + \sum_{k \neq a}^{n-1} P(k) P(k|k) \tag{32}$$

Substituting eq. 31 into eq. 32 leads to:

$$P_C = P(a) \int_{\xi_{a-1}}^{\xi_a} p(x|a)\, dx + \sum_{k \neq a}^{n-1} P(k) \int_{\xi_{k-1}}^{\xi_k} p(x|k)\, dx \tag{33}$$

To find the threshold value ξ_a where the condition $P_c(\xi_a)$ is maximized, we need to solve the equation:

$$\frac{\partial}{\partial \xi_a} P_C(\xi_a) = 0 \tag{34}$$

This is equivalent to the equation:

$$\frac{\partial}{\partial \xi_a}\left[P(a) \int_{\xi_{a-1}}^{\xi_a} p(x|a)\,dx + \sum_{\substack{k \neq a}}^{n-1} P(k) \int_{\xi_{k-1}}^{\xi_k} p(x|k)\,dx \right] = 0 \tag{35}$$

From the ordering properties of ξ it follows that the derivatives of all but one of the terms in the sum vanish. Therefore,

$$P(a)\,p(\xi_a|a) - P(a+1)\,p(\xi_a|a+1) = 0 \tag{36}$$

and finally

$$P(a)\,p(\xi_a|a) = P(a+1)\,p(\xi_a|a+1) \tag{37}$$

These considerations are generalizable also to vector variables. In the latter case, the reasoning is applicable by induction to all individual components of the vector.

B.2. Applications in Mixture Models

Let us define a mixture model by:

$$p(x) = \sum_{i}^{n} P(A_i)\,p(x|A_i) \tag{38}$$

where $\sum_{i}^{n} P(A_i) = 1$ and $p(x|A_i)$ is the p.d.f. of the class A_i.

The probability that a measurement vector x belongs to class A_i is $p(A_i|x)$ and this posterior probability can be computed via the Bayes theorem as:

$$p(A_i|x) = \frac{p(x|A_i)\,P(A_i)}{p(x)} \tag{39}$$

where $P(A_i)$ is the prior probability of class A_i. According to the adopted notations eq. 39 can be reformulated as:

$$p(A_i|x) = \frac{P(i)\,p(x|i)}{p(x)} \tag{40}$$

Therefore, eq. 37 is equivalent to

$$p(A_i|x) = p(A_{i+1}|x) \tag{41}$$

In other words, thresholds between classes are defined by the intercepts of the posterior probabilities.

B.2.1. Gaussian Mixture Models

Gaussian mixture models are defined by

$$P\left(x\mid\theta\right)=\sum_{i}^{n}\frac{a_i}{\sqrt{2\pi}\,\sigma_i}\cdot e^{-\frac{(x-m_i)^2}{2\sigma_i^2}} \tag{42}$$

where $\theta=\{m,\sigma\}$ is the parameter vector.

Intercepts of any two arbitrary components in a Gaussian mixture distribution can be obtained by solving the equation:

$$\frac{a_a}{\sqrt{2\pi}\,\sigma_a}\cdot e^{-\frac{(x-m_a)^2}{2\sigma_a^2}}=\frac{a_b}{\sqrt{2\pi}\,\sigma_b}\cdot e^{-\frac{(x-m_b)^2}{2\sigma_b^2}} \tag{43}$$

After taking a logarithm:

$$\frac{(x-m_b)^2}{\sigma_b{}^2}-\frac{(x-m_a)^2}{\sigma_a{}^2}-2\log\frac{a_b\,s_a}{a_a\,s_b}=0 \tag{44}$$

This is equivalent to the elementary square equation:

$$\left(\frac{1}{\sigma_b^2}-\frac{1}{\sigma_a^2}\right)\cdot x^2-2\left(\frac{m_b}{\sigma_b^2}-\frac{m_a}{\sigma_a^2}\right)\cdot x+Q=0 \tag{45}$$

where

$$Q=\frac{m_b^2}{\sigma_b^2}-\frac{m_a^2}{\sigma_a^2}-2\log\frac{a_b\,\sigma_a}{a_a\,\sigma_b}$$

The roots of the equation are given by:

$$x_{1,2}=\frac{\frac{m_b}{\sigma_b}-\frac{m_a}{\sigma_a}\pm\sqrt{\left(\frac{m_b}{\sigma_b^2}-\frac{m_a}{\sigma_a^2}\right)^2-\left(\frac{1}{\sigma_b^2}-\frac{1}{\sigma_a^2}\right)Q}}{\frac{1}{\sigma_b^2}-\frac{1}{\sigma_a^2}} \tag{46}$$

B.2.2. Lognormal Mixture Models

Lognormal mixture models are defined as

$$P\left(x\mid\theta\right)=\sum_{i}^{n}\frac{a_i\,e^{-\frac{w_i^2}{2}}}{\sqrt{2\pi}\,w_i\,m_i}\cdot e^{-\frac{1}{2w_i^2}\ln^2\frac{x}{m_i}} \tag{47}$$

where $\theta=\{m,w\}$ is the parameter vector.

Intercepts of any two arbitrary components of a lognormal mixture distribution can be obtained by solving the equation:

$$\frac{a_a\,e^{-\frac{w_a^2}{2}}}{\sqrt{2\pi}\,w_a\,m_a}\cdot e^{-\frac{1}{2w_a^2}\ln^2\frac{x}{m_a}}=\frac{a_b\,e^{-\frac{w_b^2}{2}}}{\sqrt{2\pi}\,w_b\,m_b}\cdot e^{-\frac{1}{2w_b^2}\ln^2\frac{x}{m_b}} \tag{48}$$

where and a and b denote any 2 components of the mixture. After logarithmic transformation and grouping, it can be shown that eq. 48 is equivalent to the elementary square equation

$$\left(\frac{1}{w_b^2} - \frac{1}{w_a^2}\right) \cdot z^2 - 2\left(\frac{\ln m_b}{w_b^2} - \frac{\ln m_a}{w_a^2}\right) \cdot z + Q = 0 \tag{49}$$

where

$$Q = \frac{\ln^2 m_b}{w_b^2} - \frac{\ln^2 m_a}{w_a^2} + 2\ln\frac{w_b\, m_b\, a_a}{w_a\, m_a\, a_b} + w_b^2 - w_a^2$$

and $z = \ln x$. Therefore, the solution is given by:

$$\ln x_{1,2} = \frac{\left(\frac{\ln m_b}{w_b^2} - \frac{\ln m_a}{w_a^2}\right) \pm \sqrt{\left(\frac{\ln m_b}{w_b^2} - \frac{\ln m_a}{w_a^2}\right)^2 - \left(\frac{1}{w_b^2} - \frac{1}{w_a^2}\right)Q}}{\frac{1}{w_b^2} - \frac{1}{w_a^2}} \tag{50}$$

C. Properties of CSR Spatial Point Patterns

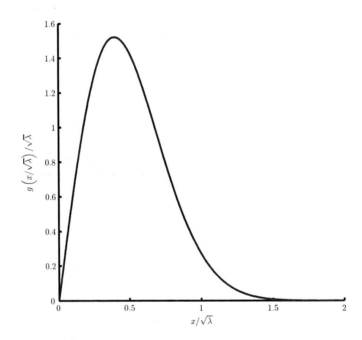

Figure 20. Plot of the nearest-neighbor probability density function.

In the framework of hypothesis testing, observed patterns of nerve fibers can be compared against realizations of various types of stochastic spatial point processes. A benchmark for such comparisons is the homogeneous Poisson process in the plane because it is the simplest and the best-studied spatial process. It is characterized by two important properties, integrated in the concept of Complete Spatial Randomness (CSR):

1. homogeneity - the intensity of the process is constant over the region of study;

2. spatial independence in the occurrence of the events - numbers of the observed points in neighboring regions do not correlate.

The CSR patterns obey the Poisson distribution [106]. The probability distribution to observe k objects in the cicrle with radius r is as follows:

$$P\left(r|x = k\right) = \frac{\left(\lambda\pi r^2\right)^k}{k!}\, e^{-\lambda\pi r^2} \tag{51}$$

Therefore, the nearest-neighbor-probability distribution of a CSR pattern is given by:

$$G\left(r\right) = 1 - P\left(r|x = 0\right) = 1 - e^{-\lambda\pi r^2} \tag{52}$$

The density of the nearest-neighbor probability distribution is as follows:

$$g\left(r\right) = 2\,\pi\,\lambda\,r\,e^{-\lambda\pi r^2} \tag{53}$$

where λ is the spatial density. The function is plotted in Fig. 20.
The mode of the distribution is given by

$$m = \frac{1}{\sqrt{2\,\pi\,\lambda}} \approx \frac{0.3989}{\sqrt{\lambda}} \tag{54}$$

and the corresponding maximum by

$$g\left(m\right) = \sqrt{\frac{2\,\pi}{e}}\,\lambda \approx 1.5203\,\sqrt{\lambda}$$

The expectation of the nearest-neighbor distance is given by:

$$x = \frac{1}{2\,\sqrt{\lambda}} = \frac{0.5}{\sqrt{\lambda}} \tag{55}$$

and the corresponding p.d.f value by:

$$g\left(x\right) = \pi\,e^{-\frac{\pi}{4}}\,\sqrt{\lambda} \approx 1.4324\,\sqrt{\lambda}$$

The $K\left(r\right)$-function of a CSR pattern is simply:

$$K\left(r\right) = \pi\,r^2 \tag{56}$$

D. Parameters of the Lognormal Population Models of the Tibial and Sural Nerves

Table 5. Tibial nerve population models

LN2	$A\delta$	$A\gamma + A\beta + A\alpha$
m[μm]	3.43 ± 0.12	6.80 ± 0.42
w	0.33 ± 0.02	0.21 ± 0.01
a[%]	35.3 ± 7.81	64.7 ± 7.82

LN3	$A\delta$	$A\gamma + A\beta$	$A\alpha$
m[μm]	3.30 ± 0.19	6.16 ± 0.54	8.93 ± 0.62
w	0.35 ± 0.04	0.21 ± 0.02	0.09 ± 0.02
a[%]	25.8 ± 3.9	50.8 ± 9.7	23.4 ± 10.5

Parameter notations are identical to Fig. 4. Data are presented as means $\pm$ S.E.M.

Table 6. Sural nerve population models

LN2	$A\delta$	$A\beta + A\alpha$
m[μm]	3.30 ± 0.21	5.87 ± 0.48
w	0.23 ± 0.03	0.22 ± 0.02
a[%]	35.9 ± 7.39	64.1 ± 7.39

LN3	$A\delta$	$A\beta$	$A\alpha$
m[μm]	2.46 ± 0.30	4.36 ± 0.61	7.17 ± 0.71
w	0.21 ± 0.04	0.22 ± 0.02	0.12 ± 0.03
a[%]	16.3 ± 6.16	52.1 ± 7.92	31.6 ± 12.25

Parameter notations are identical to Fig. 4. Data are presented as means $\pm$ S.E.M.

E. Glossary

A_f Area fraction [%].

$A[f]$ Area of the fiber profile [μm^2].

$A[f]_{rel}$ Relative area of the fibers, estimated by $\Sigma A[f]/A[s] \cdot 100$.

A_{prof} Area of the nerve profile [μm^2].

$A[s]$ Area of the sample [μm^2].

Bivariate K and L-functions are generalization of $K(r)$ and $L(r)$ to more than one type of event (e.g. in a multivariate spatial point process).

CNS Central Nervous System.

CSR Complete Spatial Randomness. It a special type of spatial process with the following properties: (i) homogeneity and (ii) spatial independence in the occurrence of the events Sec. 5.2.

DRG Dorsal root ganglion(a).

$d[f]$ Equivalent fiber diameter, estimated by $2\sqrt{A[f]/\pi}$ [μm].

Functional (fiber) topography is the spatial organization of nerve fibers with regard to their targets of innervation.

g-ratio is the ratio between the axonal diameter and the total fiber diameter (i.e. axonal diameter plus the thickness of the myelin sheath).

Homogeneous Poisson process is a synonym of CSR.

$K_G(x,y \mid s)$ Gaussian kernel with a scale parameter s.

K(r) is the Ripley's K-function (see *Sec.* 5.2).

λ[ax], λ[f] Spatial density of the nerve fibers, or respectively axons, $[\mu m^{-2}]$. It is estimated by

$$\lambda = \frac{N[f]_{sample}}{A[s]}$$

L(r) is the L-function. It is defined relative to $K(r)$:

$$L(r) = \sqrt{\frac{K(r)}{\pi}} - r$$

G(r) is the nearest-neighbor distance distribution (see *Sec.* 5.2).

N[f]$_{sample}$ Number of fibers in a sample.

PNS Peripheral Nervous System.

Ψ_C (x, y |r) Cluster density map with a scale parameter r.

p.d.f. Probability distribution function.

S.E.M. Standard Error of the Mean.

Spatial point process is a finite random subset of a given bounded region S. A realization of such a process is a spatial point pattern $x = \{x_1, \ldots, x_n; x_i \in S\}$ of a number of points contained in S.

SPP Spatial Point Pattern. It consists of the locations of the so-called events in a predefined study area.

CV Conduction velocity.

References

[1] Djouhri, L and Lawson, SN. $A\beta$-fiber nociceptive primary afferent neurons: a review of incidence and properties in relation to other afferent A-fiber neurons in mammals. *Brain Res / Brain Res Rev*, 2004. 46 2, 131–145.

[2] Prodanov, D. *Morphometric analysis of the rat lower limb nerves. Anatomical data for neural prosthesis design*. Ph.D. thesis, Twente University, Enschede, The Netherlands, 2006.

[3] Branner, A and Normann, RA. A multielectrode array for intrafascicular recording and stimulation in sciatic nerve of cats. *Brain Res Bull*, 2000. 51 4, 293–306.

[4] Deurloo, K and Holsheimer, J. Fascicular selectivity in transverse stimulation with a nerve cuff electrode: A theoretical approach. *Neuromodulation*, 2003. 6 4, 258–269.

[5] Stewart, JD. Peripheral nerve fascicles: anatomy and clinical relevance. *Muscle Nerve*, 2003. 28 5, 525–541. Available from http://dx.doi.org/10.1002/mus.10454.

[6] Sunderland, S. The intraneural topography of the radial, median and ulnar nerves. *Brain*, 1945. 68 4, 243–299.

[7] Prodanov, D; Nagelkerke, N; and Marani, E. Spatial clustering analysis in neuroanatomy: applications of different approaches to motor nerve fiber distribution. *J Neurosci Methods*, 2007. 160 1, 93–108. Available from http://dx.doi.org/10.1016/j.jneumeth.2006.08.017.

[8] Prodanov, D and Feirabend, HKP. Automated characterization of nerve fibers labeled fluorescently: Determination of size, class and spatial distribution. *Brain Res*, 2008. 1233, 35–50. Available from http://dx.doi.org/10.1016/j.brainres.2008.07.049.

[9] Prochaska, G. *De structura nervorum*. R. Graeffer, Vienna, 1779.

[10] Landmesser, L. The development of motor projection patterns in the chick hind limb. *J Physiol (Lond)*, 1978. 284, 391–414.

[11] Key, A and Retzius, G. *Studien in der Anatomie des Nervensystems und des Bindegewebes*, vol. 2. Samson & Wallin, Stockholm, 1876.

[12] Sunderland, S. *Nerves and nerve injuries*. Churchill Livingstone, Edinburgh and London, 1972.

[13] Thomas, P. *Peripheral neuropathy*. WB Saunders Co., Philadelphia, 1984.

[14] Ushiki, T and Ide, C. Three-dimensional organization of the collagen fibrils in the rat sciatic nerve as revealed by transmission- and scanning electron microscopy. *Cell Tissue Res*, 1990. 260 1, 175–184.

[15] Ushiki, T and Ide, C. Three-dimensional architecture of the endoneurium with special reference to the collagen fibril arrangement in relation to nerve fibers. *Arch Histol Jpn*, 1986. 49 5, 553–563.

[16] Thil, MA. *Nerve reactions to self-sizing cuff electrode implantation and electrical stimulation: Physiological and histological studies* . Ph.D. thesis, Université Catholic de Louvain, 2006.

[17] Erlanger, J and Gasser, H. *Electrical Signs of Nervous Activity.* University of Pennslyvania Press, Philadelphia, 1937.

[18] Guyton, A and Hall, J, (editors) *Textbook of Medical Physiology.* Saunders, 10th ed., 2000.

[19] Morgan, G; Mikhail, M; and Murray, M, (editors) *Clinical Anesthesiology.* McGaw-Hill Medical, 4th ed., 2005.

[20] Waxman, SG. Determinants of conduction velocity in myelinated nerve fibers. *Muscle Nerve*, 1980. 3 2, 141–150. Available from http://dx.doi.org/10.1002/mus. 880030207.

[21] Matsumoto, G and Tasaki, I. A study of conduction velocity in nonmyelinated nerve fibers. *Biophys J*, 1977. 20 1, 1–13.

[22] Tasaki, I and Matsumoto, G. On the cable theory of nerve conduction. *Bull Math Biol*, 2002. 64 6, 1069–1082. Available from http://dx.doi.org/10.1006/bulm.2002. 0310.

[23] Hursh, JB. Conduction velocity and diameter of nerve fibers. *Am J Physiol*, 1939. 127, 131–139.

[24] Gasser, HS and Erlanger, J. The role played by the sizes of the constituent fibers of a nerve trunk in determining the form of its action potential wave. *Am J Physiol*, 1927. 80, 527–547.

[25] Blair, EA and Erlanger, J. A comparison of the characteristics of axons through their individual electrical responces. *Am J Physiol*, 1933. 106, 524–564.

[26] Gasser, HS and Grundfest, H. Axon diameters in relation to the spike dimensions and the conduction velocity in mammalian nerves. *Am J Physiol*, 1939. 127, 393–414.

[27] Tasaki, I; Ishii, K; and Ito, H. On the relation between the conduction rate, the fibre diameter and the internodal distance of the medullated nerve fibre. *Jap J med Sci Biophys*, 1943. 9, 189 – 199.

[28] Hutchinson, NA; Koles, ZJ; and Smith, RS. Conduction velocity in myelinated nerve fibres of Xenopus laevis. *J Physiol*, 1970. 208 2, 279–289.

[29] Arbuthnott, ER; Boyd, IA; and Kalu, KU. Ultrastructural dimensions of myelinated peripheral nerve fibres in the cat and their relation to conduction velocity. *J Physiol (Lond)*, 1980. 308, 125–157.

[30] Arbuthnott, ER; Boyd, IA; and Kalu, KU. The relation between axon area, axon circumference, total fibre circumference and number of myelin lamellae for different groups of fibres in cat hind-limb nerves. *J Physiol (Lond)*, 1977. 273 2, 88P–89P.

[31] Boyd, IA and Kalu, KU. Scaling factor relating conduction velocity and diameter for myelinated afferent nerve fibres in the cat hind limb. *J Physiol (Lond)*, 1979. 289, 277–297.

[32] Sakaguchi, T; Okada, M; Kitamura, T; and Kawasaki, K. Reduced diameter and conduction velocity of myelinated fibers in the sciatic tnerve of a neurofilament-deficient mutant quail. *Neurosci Lett*, 1993. 153 1, 65–68.

[33] Necker, R and Meinecke, C. Conduction velocities and fiber diameters in a cutaneous nerve of the pigeon. *J Comp Physiol A*, 1984. 154, 817–824.

[34] Tackmann, W; Spalke, G; and Oginszus, HJ. Quantitative histometric studies and relation of number and diameter of myelinated fibres to electrophysiological parameters in normal sensory nerves of man. *J Neurol*, 1976. 212 1, 71–84.

[35] Rushton, WA. A theory of the effects of fibre size in medullated nerve. *J Physiol (Lond)*, 1951. 115 1, 101–122.

[36] Goldman, L and Albus, JS. Computation of impulse conduction in myelinated fibers; theoretical basis of the velocity-diameter relation. *Biophys J*, 1968. 8 5, 596–607. Available from http://dx.doi.org/10.1016/S0006-3495(68)86510-5.

[37] McIntyre, CC; Richardson, AG; and Grill, WM. Modeling the excitability of mammalian nerve fibers: influence of afterpotentials on the recovery cycle. *J Neurophysiol*, 2002. 87 2, 995–1006.

[38] Lloyd, D. Neuron patterns controlling transmission of ipsilateral hind limb reflexes in cat. *J Neurophysiol*, 1943. 6, 293 – 315.

[39] Boyd, I and Davey, M. *Composition of Peripheral Nerves*. E. & S. Livingstone Ltd., Edinburgh and London, 1968.

[40] Abruthnott, E; Boyd, I; and Kalu, K. Ultrastructure and conduction velocity of small myelinated peripheral nerve fibres. In: Kornhuber, M, (editor) *The Somatosensory System*, George Thieme, Stuttgart, pp. 168 – 175. 1975.

[41] Manzano, GM; Giuliano, LMP; and Nobrega, JAM. A brief historical note on the classification of nerve fibers. *Arq Neuropsiquiatr*, 2008. 66 1, 117–119.

[42] Prodanov, D and Feirabend, HKP. Morphometric analysis of the fiber populations of the rat sciatic nerve, its spinal roots, and its major branches. *J Comp Neurol*, 2007. 503 1, 85–100. Available from http://dx.doi.org/10.1002/cne.21375.

[43] Brunner, R; Zimmermann, P; and Klussmann, FW. Localization and neurophysiological properties of motoneurones of the M. triceps surae of the rat after retrograde labelling with Evans blue. *Cell Tissue Res*, 1980. 212 1, 73–81.

[44] Swett, JE; Wikholm, RP; Blanks, RH; Swett, AL; and Conley, L. Motoneurons of the rat sciatic nerve. *Exp Neurol*, 1986. 93 1, 227–252.

[45] Schmalbruch, H. Fiber composition of the rat sciatic nerve. *Anat Rec*, 1986. 215 1, 71–81.

[46] Hebel, R and Stromberg, MW. *Anatomy and Embryology of the Laboratory Rat*. BioMed Verlag, Worthsee, 1986.

[47] Rigaud, M; Gemes, G; Barabas, ME; Chernoff, DI; Abram, SE; Stucky, CL; and Hogan, QH. Species and strain differences in rodent sciatic nerve anatomy: implications for studies of neuropathic pain. *Pain*, 2008. 136 1-2, 188–201. Available from http://dx.doi.org/10.1016/j.pain.2008.01.016.

[48] Vleggeert-Lankamp, C. The role of evaluation methods in the assessment of peripheral nerve regeneration through synthetic conduits: a systematic review. Laboratory investigation. *J Neurosurg*, 2007. 107 6, 1168–1189. Available from http://dx.doi.org/10.3171/JNS-07/12/1168.

[49] Sima, A. Studies on fibre size in developing sciatic nerve and spinal roots in normal,undernourished, and rehabilitated rats. *Acta Physiol Scand Suppl*, 1974. 406, 1–55.

[50] LoPachin, RM; Ross, JF; Reid, ML; Das, S; Mansukhani, S; and Lehning, EJ. Neurological evaluation of toxic axonopathies in rats: acrylamide and 2,5-hexanedione. *Neurotoxicology*, 2002. 23 1, 95–110.

[51] LoPachin, RM. Acrylamide neurotoxicity: neurological, morhological and molecular endpoints in animal models. *Adv Exp Med Biol*, 2005. 561, 21–37.

[52] Langford, LA and Coggeshall, RE. Branching of sensory axons in the peripheral nerve of the rat. *J Comp Neurol*, 1981. 203 4, 745–750.

[53] Rao, RS and Krinke, G. Changes with age in the number and size of myelinated axons in the rat L4 dorsal spinal root. *Acta Anat (Basel)*, 1983. 117 3, 187–192.

[54] Jenq, CB; Chung, K; and Coggeshall, RE. Postnatal loss of axons in normal rat sciatic nerve. *J Comp Neurol*, 1986. 244 4, 445–450.

[55] Jeronimo, A; Jeronimo, CA; Filho, OAR; and Fazan, LSSVP. Microscopic anatomy of the sural nerve in the postnatal developing rat: A longitudinal and lateral symmetry study. *J Anat*, 2005. 206 1, 93–99.

[56] Varejao, AS; Melo-Pinto, P; Meek, MF; Filipe, VM; and Bulas-Cruz, J. Methods for the experimental functional assessment of rat sciatic nerve regeneration. *Neurol Res*, 2004. 26, 186 –194.

[57] Kaar, GF and Fraher, JP. The development of α and γ motoneuron fibres in the rat. I. A comparative ultrastructural study of their central and peripheral axon growth. *J Anat*, 1985. 141, 77–88.

[58] Vleggeert-Lankamp, CL; van den Berg, RJ; Feirabend, HK; Lakke, EA; Malessy, MJ; and Thomeer, RT. Electrophysiology and morphometry of the $A\alpha$- and $A\beta$-fiber populations in the normal and regenerating rat sciatic nerve. *Exp Neurol*, 2004. 187 2, 337–349.

[59] Dyck, PJ; Karnes, J; Sparks, M; and Low, PA. The morphometric composition of myelinated fibres by nerve, level and species related to nerve microenvironment and ischaemia. *Electroencephalogr Clin Neurophysiol Suppl*, 1982. 36, 39–55.

[60] Harper, AA and Lawson, SN. Electrical properties of rat dorsal root ganglion neurones with different peripheral nerve conduction velocities. *J Physiol*, 1985. 359, 47–63.

[61] Bakels, R and Kernell, D. Matching between motoneurone and muscle unit properties in rat medial gastrocnemius. *J Physiol*, 1993. 463, 307–324.

[62] Lewin, GR and McMahon, SB. Physiological properties of primary sensory neurons appropriately and inappropriately innervating skeletal muscle in adult rats. *J Neurophysiol*, 1991. 66 4, 1218–1231.

[63] Andrew, BL and Part, NJ. Properties of fast and slow motor units in hind limb and tail muscles of the rat. *Q J Exp Physiol Cogn Med Sci*, 1972. 57 2, 213–225.

[64] Russell, NJ. Axonal conduction velocity changes following muscle tenotomy or deafferentation during development in the rat. *J Physiol*, 1980. 298, 347–360.

[65] De-Doncker, L; Picquet, F; Petit, J; and Falempin, M. Characterization of spindle afferents in rat soleus muscle using ramp-and-hold and sinusoidal stretches. *J Neurophysiol*, 2003. 89 1, 442–449. Available from http://dx.doi.org/10.1152/jn.00153. 2002.

[66] Leem, JW; Willis, WD; and Chung, JM. Cutaneous sensory receptors in the rat foot. *J Neurophysiol*, 1993. 69 5, 1684–1699.

[67] Sanders, KH and Zimmermann, M. Mechanoreceptors in rat glabrous skin: redevelopment of function after nerve crush. *J Neurophysiol*, 1986. 55 4, 644–659.

[68] Lewin, GR and McMahon, SB. Physiological properties of primary sensory neurons appropriately and inappropriately innervating skin in the adult rat. *J Neurophysiol*, 1991. 66 4, 1205–1217.

[69] Handwerker, HO; Kilo, S; and Reeh, PW. Unresponsive afferent nerve fibres in the sural nerve of the rat. *J Physiol*, 1991. 435, 229–242.

[70] Gokin, AP; Philip, B; and Strichartz, GR. Preferential block of small myelinated sensory and motor fibers by lidocaine: In vivo electrophysiology in the rat sciatic nerve. *Anesthesiology*, 2001. 95 6, 1441–1454.

[71] Waddell, PJ; Lawson, SN; and McCarthy, PW. Conduction velocity changes along the processes of rat primary sensory neurons. *Neuroscience*, 1989. 30 3, 577–584.

[72] Schady, W; Ochoa, JL; Torebjork, HE; and Chen, LS. Peripheral projections of fascicles in the human median nerve. *Brain*, 1983. 106 (Pt 3), 745–760.

[73] Honig, MG; Frase, PA; and Camilli, SJ. The spatial relationships among cutaneous, muscle sensory and motoneuron axons during development of the chick hind limb. *Development*, 1998. 125 6, 995–1004.

[74] Feirabend, H and Marani, E. The dorsal root ganglion. In: Aminoff, M and Daroff, R, (editors) *Encyclopedia of the Neurological Sciences*, Elsevier, Amsterdam, vol. 4, pp. 33 – 34. 2003.

[75] Honig, MG. The development of sensory projection patterns in embryonic chick hind limb. *J Physiol (Lond)*, 1982. 330, 175–202.

[76] Molander, C and Grant, G. Cutaneous projections from the rat hindlimb foot to the substantia gelatinosa of the spinal cord studied by transganglionic transport of WGA-HRP conjugate. *J Comp Neurol*, 1985. 237 4, 476–484. Available from http://dx.doi.org/10.1002/cne.902370405.

[77] Molander, C and Grant, G. Laminar distribution and somatotopic organization of primary afferent fibers from hindlimb nerves in the dorsal horn. A study by trans-ganglionic transport of horseradish peroxidase in the rat. *Neuroscience*, 1986. 19 1, 297–312.

[78] Peyronnard, JM; Charron, LF; Lavoie, J; and Messier, JP. Motor, sympathetic and sensory innervation of rat skeletal muscles. *Brain Res*, 1986. 373 1-2, 288–302.

[79] Wessels, WJ; Feirabend, HK; and Marani, E. Evidence for a rostrocaudal organi-zation in dorsal root ganglia during development as demonstrated by intra-uterine WGA-HRP injections into the hindlimb of rat fetuses. *Brain Res / Dev Brain Res*, 1990. 54 2, 273–281.

[80] Wessels, WJ; Feirabend, HK; and Marani, E. Somatotopic organization in the sen-sory innervation of the rat hindlimb during development, using half dorsal root gan-glia as subsegmental units. *Eur J Morphol*, 1990. 28 2-4, 394–403.

[81] Wessels, WJ; Feirabend, HK; and Marani, E. Development of projections of primary afferent fibers from the hindlimb to the gracile nucleus: a WGA-HRP study in the rat. *Brain Res / Dev Brain Res*, 1991. 63 1-2, 265–279.

[82] Werner, G and Whitsel, BL. The topology of dermatomal projection in the medial lemniscal system. *J Physiol*, 1967. 192 1, 123–144.

[83] Stoffel, A. Ueber die Behandlung verletzter Nerven im Kriege. *München Med Wehn-schr*, 1915. 62, 201–203.

[84] Stoffel, A. Beitrage zu einer rationellen Nervenchirurgie. *München Med Wehnschr*, 1913. 60, 175–179.

[85] Putti, V. Sulla topografia fascicolare dei nervi periferici e piu specialmente dello sciatic popliteo externo. *Clinica Chir*, 1916. 24, 1021–1035.

[86] Barile, C. Sul reale valoro practico della topografia fascicolare dei nervi periferici (secondo Stoffel) per l'esecuzione dell anastomosi dei nervi degli arti. *Policlinico*, 1917. 24, 1177–1180.

[87] Heinemann, O. Ueber Schutzverletzungen der peripheren Nerven. Nebst anatomischen Untersuchungen über den inneren Bau der grossen Nervenstamme. *Arch klin Chir*, 1916. 108, 107–150.

[88] Dustin, AP. La fasciculation des nerfs. *Ambul Ocean*, 1918. 2, 135–154.

[89] Compton, AT. The intrinsic anatomy of the large nerve truncs of limbs. *J Anat*, 1917. 51, 103–117.

[90] Langley, JN and Hashimoto, M. On the structure of separate nerve bundles in a nerve trunc and on internal nerve plexuses. *J Physiol (Lond)*, 1917. 51, 318–345.

[91] Dejerine, J; Dejerine, A; and Mouzon, J. Les lésions de gros troncs nerveux des membres par projectiles de guerre. *Presse Med*, 1915. 40, 321–328.

[92] Marie, P; Meige, H; and Gosset, A. Les localisations motrices dans les nerfs périphériques. *Bull Acad Méd (Paris)*, 1915. 74, 789–810.

[93] Kraus, WM and Ingham, SD. Peripheral nerve topography. *Arch Neurol Psychiatry*, 1920. 4, 259–296.

[94] McKinley, JC. The intraneural plexus of fasciculi and fibers in the sciatic nerve. *Arch Neurol Psychiatry*, 1921. 6, 377–399.

[95] Hallin, RG. Microneurography in relation to intraneural topography: Somatotopic organisation of median nerve fascicles in humans. *J Neurol Neurosurg Psychiatry*, 1990. 53 9, 736–744.

[96] Marchettini, P; Cline, M; and Ochoa, JL. Innervation territories for touch and pain afferents of single fascicles of the human ulnar nerve. Mapping through intraneural microrecording and microstimulation. *Brain*, 1990. 113 (Pt 5), 1491–1500.

[97] Wu, G; Ekedahl, R; and Hallin, RG. Clustering of slowly adapting type II mechanoreceptors in human peripheral nerve and skin. *Brain*, 1998. 121 (Pt 2), 265–279.

[98] Roberts, WJ and Elardo, SM. Clustering of primary afferent fibers in peripheral nerve fascicles by sensory modality. *Brain Res*, 1986. 370 1, 149–152.

[99] Malmgren, LT; Lyon, MJ; and Gacek, RR. Localization of abductor and adductor fibers in the kitten recurrent laryngeal nerve: use of a variation of the Horseradish peroxidase tracer technique. *Exp Neurol*, 1977. 55 1, 187–198.

[100] Atasever, A; Durgun, B; Celik, HH; and Yilmaz, E. Somatotopic organization of the axons innervating the superior rectus muscle in the oculomotor nerve of the rat. *Acta Anat (Basel)*, 1993. 146 4, 251–254.

[101] Lee, S; Eisele, DW; Schwartz, AR; and Ryugo, DK. Peripheral course of genioglossal motor axons within the hypoglossal nerveof the rat. *Laryngoscope*, 1996. 106 10, 1274–1279.

[102] Brown, DR; Everett, AW; and Bennett, MR. Compartmental and topographical distributions of axons in nerves to the amphibian (Bufo marinus) glutaeus muscle. *J Comp Neurol*, 1989. 284 2, 231–241.

[103] Brushart, TM. Central course of digital axons within the median nerve of Macaca mulatta. *J Comp Neurol*, 1991. 311 2, 197–209.

[104] Bertelli, JA; Taleb, M; Saadi, A; Mira, JC; and Pecot-Dechavassine, M. The rat brachial plexus and its terminal branches: an experimental model for the study of peripheral nerve regeneration. *Microsurgery*, 1995. 16 2, 77–85.

[105] Montoya, GJ; Ariza, J; Sutachan, JJ; and Hurtado, H. Relationship between functional deficiencies and the contribution of myelinated nerve fibers derived from L-4, L-5, and L-6 spinolumbar branches in adultrat sciatic nerve. *Exp Neurol*, 2002. 173 2, 266–274.

[106] Diggle, PJ. *Statistical Analysis of Spatial Point Patterns* . Academic Press, London, 1983.

[107] Okabe, A; Sugihara, K; Boots, B; and Chiu, SN. *Spatial Tessellations: Concepts and applications of Voronoi diagrams* . Wiley, New Jersey, 2000.

[108] Duyckaerts, C; Godefroy, G; and Hauw, JJ. Evaluation of neuronal numerical density by Dirichlet tessellation. *J Neurosci Methods*, 1994. 51 1, 47–69.

[109] Negredo, P; Castro, J; Lago, N; Navarro, X; and Avendano, C. Differential growth of axons from sensory and motor neurons through a regenerativeelectrode: a stereological, retrograde tracer, and functional study in the rat. *Neuroscience*, 2004. 128 3, 605–615.

[110] Castro, J; Negredo, P; and Avendano, C. Fiber composition of the rat sciatic nerve and its modification during regeneration through a sieve electrode. *Brain Res*, 2008. 1190, 65–77. Available from http://dx.doi.org/10.1016/j.brainres.2007.11.028.

[111] Romanes, GJ. The motor pools of the spinal cord. In: *Organization of the spinal cord*, Progress in brain research, Elsevier, chap. 11, pp. 93–119. 1964.

[112] Jacobson, M. Development of nerve connections with muscle and peripheral sense organs. In: *Developmental Neurobiology*, Plenum press, book chapter 9, pp. 359–400. 3rd ed., 1991.

[113] Nicolopoulos-Stournaras, S and Iles, JF. Motor neuron columns in the lumbar spinal cord of the rat. *J Comp Neurol*, 1983. 217 1, 75–85.

[114] Bennett, MR and Lavidis, NA. Development of the topographical projection of motor neurons to amphibian muscle accompanies motor neuron death. *Brain Res*, 1981. 254 3, 448–452.

[115] Bennett, MR; Davies, AM; and Everett, AW. The development of topographical maps and fibre types in toad (Bufo marinus) glutaeus muscle during synapse elimination. *J Physiol (Lond)*, 1989. 409, 43–61.

[116] Brown, MC and Booth, CM. Postnatal development of the adult pattern of motor axon distribution in rat muscle. *Nature*, 1983. 304 5928, 741–742.

[117] Everett, AW and Brown, DR. Loss of the position-dependent reinnervation of regenerated toad (Bufo marinus)glutaeus muscle. *J Comp Neurol*, 1996. 366 2, 293–302.

[118] Brown, DR and Everett, AW. Compartmental and topographical specificity of reinnervation of the glutaeus muscle in the adult toad (Bufo marinus). *J Comp Neurol*, 1990. 292 3, 363–372.

[119] Laskowski, MB and Sanes, JR. Topographic mapping of motor pools onto skeletal muscles. *J Neurosci*, 1987. 7 1, 252–260.

[120] Hardman, VJ and Brown, MC. Spatial organization within rat motoneuron pools. *Neurosci Lett*, 1985. 60 3, 325–329.

[121] Lance-Jones, C and Landmesser, L. Motoneurone projection patterns in the chick hind limb following early partialreversals of the spinal cord. *J Physiol (Lond)*, 1980. 302, 581–602.

[122] Lance-Jones, C and Landmesser, L. Pathway selection by embryonic chick motoneurons in an experimentally altered environment. *Proc R Soc Lond B Biol Sci*, 1981. 214 1194, 19–52.

[123] Lance-Jones, C and Dias, M. The influence of presumptive limb connective tissue on motoneuron axon guidance. *Dev Biol*, 1991. 143 1, 93–110.

[124] Landmesser, L. Growth cone guidance in the avian limb: a search for cellular and molecular mechanisms. In: Letourneau, PC; Kater, SB; and Macagano, ER, (editors) *The nerve growth cone*, Raven, pp. 373–385. 1992.

[125] Goodman, CS. Mechanisms and molecules that control growth cone guidance. *Ann Rev Neurosci*, 1996. 19, 341–377.

[126] Maden, M. Positional information: knowing where you are in a limb. *Curr Biol*, 2002. 12 22, R773–R775.

[127] Tosney, KW. Proximal tissues and patterned neurite outgrowth at the lumbosacral level of the chick embryo: partial and complete deletion of the somite. *Dev Biol*, 1988. 127 2, 266–286.

[128] Tosney, KW. Somites and axon guidance. *Scanning Microsc*, 1988. 2 1, 427–442.

[129] Witzel, C; Rohde, C; and Brushart, T. Pathway sampling by regenerating peripheral axons. *J Comp Neurol*, 2005. 485 3, 183–190.

[130] Vleggeert-Lankamp, CLAM; de Ruiter, GCW; Wolfs, JFC; Pego, AP; Feirabend, HKP; Lakke, EAJF; and Malessy, MJA. Type grouping in skeletal muscles after experimental reinnervation: another explanation. *Eur J Neurosci*, 2005. 21 5, 1249–1256. Available from http://dx.doi.org/10.1111/j.1460-9568.2005.03954.x.

[131] Vleggeert-Lankamp, CLAM; de Ruiter, GCW; Wolfs, JFC; Pego, AP; van den Berg, RJ; Feirabend, HKP; Malessy, MJA; and Lakke, EAJF. Pores in synthetic nerve conduits are beneficial to regeneration. *J Biomed Mater Res A*, 2007. 80 4, 965–982. Available from http://dx.doi.org/10.1002/jbm.a.30941.

[132] Vleggeert-Lankamp, CLAM; Wolfs, J; Pego, AP; van den Berg, R; Feirabend, HKP; and Lakke, EAJF. Effect of nerve graft porosity on the refractory period of regenerating nerve fibers. *J Neurosurg*, 2008. 109 2, 294–305. Available from http://dx.doi.org/NS/2008/109/8/0294.

[133] Schwartz, G. Estimating the dimensions of a model. *Annals Stat*, 1987. 6, 461–464.

[134] Cook, JE. Spatial regularity among retinal neurons. In: Chalupa, LM and Werner, JS, (editors) *The Visual Neurosciences*, MIT Press, chap. 29, pp. 463–477. 2003.

[135] Cameron, DA and Carney, LH. Cellular patterns in the inner retina of adult zebrafish: quantitative analyses and a computational model of their formation. *J Comp Neurol*, 2004. 471 1, 11–25.

[136] Stenkamp, DL; Powers, MK; Carney, LH; and Cameron, DA. Evidence for two distinct mechanisms of neurogenesis and cellular pattern formation in regenerated goldfish retinas. *J Comp Neurol*, 2001. 431 4, 363–381.

[137] Galli-Resta, L; Novelli, E; Kryger, Z; Jacobs, GH; and Reese, BE. Modelling the mosaic organization of rod and cone photoreceptors with a minimal-spacing rule. *Eur J Neurosci*, 1999. 11 4, 1461–1469.

[138] Eglen, SJ and Willshaw, DJ. Influence of cell fate mechanisms upon retinal mosaic formation: a modelling study. *Development*, 2002. 129 23, 5399–5408.

[139] Armstrong, RA; Cairns, NJ; and Lantos, PL. What does the study of the spatial patterns of pathological lesions tell us about the pathogenesis of neurodegenerative disorders? *Neuropathology*, 2001. 21 1, 1–12.

[140] Armstrong, RA and Cairns, NJ. Spatial patterns of the pathological changes in the cerebellar cortex in sporadic Creutzfeldt-Jakob disease (sCJD). *Folia Neuropathol*, 2003. 41 4, 183–189.

[141] Pearson, RC; Esiri, MM; Hiorns, RW; Wilcock, GK; and Powell, TP. Anatomical correlates of the distribution of the pathological changes in the neocortex in Alzheimer disease. *Proc Natl Acad Sci USA*, 1985. 82 13, 4531–4534.

[142] Armstrong, RA. Is the clustering of neurofibrillary tangles in Alzheimer's patients related to the cells of origin of specific cortico-cortical projections? *Neurosci Lett*, 1993. 160 1, 57–60.

[143] Armstrong, RA. Analysis of spatial patterns in histological sections of brain tissue. *J Neurosci Methods*, 1997. 73 2, 141–147.

[144] Ripley, BD. *Statistical inference for spatial processes*. Cambridge University Press, Cambridge, 1st ed., 1991.

[145] Cressie, N. *Statistics for Spatial Data. Revised edition*. Wiley Series in Probability and Statistics, John Wiley & Sons, New York, 1993.

[146] Stoyan, D; Kendall, W; and Mecke, J. *Stochastic geometry and its applications*. John Wiley & Sons, 2nd ed., 1996.

[147] Haining, R. *Spatial Data Analysis: Theory and Practice*. Cambridge University Press, Cambridge, 2003.

[148] Armstrong, RA. Methods of studying the planar distribution of objects in histological sections of brain tissue. *J Microsc*, 2006. 221 Pt 3, 153–158.

[149] Dixon, P. Ripley's K-function. In: El-Shaarawi, A and Piegorsch, W, (editors) *Encyclopedia of Environmetrics*, John Wiley & Sons, Chichester, vol. 3, pp. 1796 – 1803. 2002.

[150] Dyck, PJ; Karnes, J; O'Brien, P; Nukada, H; Lais, A; and Low, P. Spatial pattern of nerve fiber abnormality indicative of pathologic mechanism. *Am J Pathol*, 1984. 117 2, 225–238.

[151] Weisstein, EW. Log Normal Distribution. In: *A Wolfram Web Resource*, CRC Press. 1999. Available from http://mathworld.wolfram.com/LogNormalDistribution.html.

[152] Rieke, F; Warland, D; de Ruyter van Steveninck, R; and Bialek, W. *Spikes: Exploring the Neural Code*. The MIT Press, Cambridge, MA, USA, 1999.

Index

A

acetylcholine, 13, 44, 47, 198
acetylcholinesterase, 50, 58
acid, 43, 56, 116, 122, 180
action potential, 11, 226, 256
acupuncture, 23
acute stress, 16
adaptation, 61, 184, 194, 208
adaptations, 135
adductor, 261
adenosine, 10, 12
adenosine triphosphate, 12
adhesion, 239
adolescent female, 204
adolescents, 200
adrenoceptors, 44, 91
adverse event, 25
affective dimension, 15, 21, 52
affective disorder, 205
afferent nerve, 257, 259
African Americans, 206
age, 80, 95, 109, 114, 118, 132, 169, 200, 201, 225, 258
ageing, 180
aggregation, 242
aggressive behavior, 18
agonist, 30, 47
albumin, 29, 97
alcohol, 27, 69, 70, 124, 206
allometry, xi, 183
alters, 108
ambiguity, 153
amino acids, 8, 97, 122, 123
amphibia, 134, 195, 239, 262, 263

amphibians, 122, 130, 133, 134, 142, 189
amplitude, 200, 201
amygdala, 2, 14, 16, 20, 33, 56, 198
analgesic, 11, 23, 37, 58, 136
anatomy, viii, 37, 59, 68, 69, 82, 87, 91, 146, 162, 164, 188, 203, 210, 213, 214, 227, 233, 241, 255, 258, 261
angiography, 49
angiotensin converting enzyme, 9
aniline, 70
anterior cingulate cortex, 24, 33, 198
antibody, 75, 76, 77, 88, 89, 97, 106, 107, 125, 131
antigen, 75, 76, 88
anti-inflammatory medications, 23
anxiety, 21, 200, 204
apoptosis, ix, 94, 109, 110, 112, 114, 117, 193
arbitration, xi, 184
arginine, 137, 141
arousal, 14, 33, 122, 129, 130, 131, 134, 197, 202, 204
arteries, vii, 1, 5, 12, 13, 30, 41, 44, 50, 51, 56
arterioles, 8, 12
artery, 7, 25, 28, 33, 41, 44, 45, 47, 48
aspartate, 8, 31, 35
assessment, 52, 258
assumptions, 148, 212, 213, 215, 242
astrocytes, 114
asymmetry, 204
ataxia, 51
ATP, 12
attacks, 8, 9, 12, 18, 22, 23, 25, 27, 28, 31, 35, 40, 43, 46, 47, 49, 51, 54, 55, 57
auditory cortex, 86, 87
authors, ix, x, xii, 107, 108, 109, 110, 111, 112, 113, 130, 135, 174, 179, 208, 212, 214, 215, 220, 224
autonomic activity, 203, 204, 205

autonomic nervous system, 33, 202
availability, viii, 59, 85, 130, 135, 201, 207
axon terminals, 143
axons, 4, 6, 13, 14, 19, 22, 30, 41, 50, 85, 108, 114, 161, 174, 176, 209, 226, 227, 228, 229, 230, 231, 233, 234, 238, 239, 244, 256, 258, 260, 262, 264

B

baroreceptor, 129, 139
basal forebrain, 98, 136, 180, 181
basal ganglia, 24, 142
basilar artery, 12
behavior, x, 14, 18, 38, 42, 50, 60, 122, 129, 131, 134, 138, 141, 143, 165, 203
benign, 56
bias, 73, 87, 199, 242
bicarbonate, 25
binding, viii, 29, 44, 59, 74, 75, 78, 79, 87, 88
bioavailability, 9
biochemistry, 208
biogeography, 195
biological activity, 98
biological rhythms, 133
biomarkers, 40
biotin, 98
birds, 122, 124, 126, 130, 131, 132, 133, 134, 135, 136, 140, 143
birth, 202, 204, 206, 239
birth weight, 202, 204, 206
blood, vii, viii, 1, 2, 5, 8, 9, 10, 11, 13, 24, 26, 28, 29, 30, 31, 32, 35, 38, 41, 45, 46, 48, 49, 50, 51, 55, 136, 198, 209, 210
blood flow, 9, 10, 11, 13, 30, 32, 35, 38, 41, 45, 48, 50, 55
blood supply, 1
blood vessels, viii, 2, 5, 8, 9, 11, 13, 26, 29, 30, 32, 41, 49, 50, 209, 210
blood-brain barrier, 46
body weight, 225
bone, 7, 173
boutons, 86, 89
brachial plexus, 262
bradykinin, 29
brain activity, 24
brain size, xi, 183, 192
brain stem, 4, 34, 57, 61
brain structure, 14, 24, 33
brain tumor, vii, 1

brainstem, viii, 2, 3, 4, 5, 7, 10, 11, 14, 16, 18, 20, 22, 24, 26, 29, 31, 33, 34, 36, 37, 39, 49, 52, 141, 198, 200
buffer, 21, 96, 97, 99, 124
bun, 228
burn, 39
burning, 4, 9

C

Ca^{2+}, 28, 51
calcitonin, viii, 2, 8, 24, 35, 36, 37, 38, 41, 42, 43, 44, 45, 46, 47, 51, 53, 55, 57, 58
calcium, vii, 2, 9, 10, 25, 27, 35, 38, 46, 75
calcium channel blocker, 25
calibration, 87, 234
cardiovascular disease, 32
cardiovascular function, 20
cardiovascular system, vii, xi, 18, 197
caregiving, 202
cataplexy, 142
cation, 9
causal relationship, 28
cDNA, 137, 140
cell body, 32, 70, 132
cell culture, ix, 93, 95, 98, 107, 109
cell death, vii, viii, 87, 93, 94, 95, 96, 99, 107, 108, 112, 114, 115, 116, 118, 119, 241
cell fate, 264
cell line, 112
cell surface, 94
central nervous system, vii, xii, 1, 8, 9, 23, 32, 33, 91, 107, 138, 140, 142, 207, 209
cephalgia, 54
cerebellum, 32, 118, 132, 133, 173
cerebral arteries, 8, 13, 25, 40, 41, 44, 51
cerebral blood flow, 12, 13, 25, 26, 27, 33, 34, 47, 50, 51, 56, 204
cerebral cortex, x, 5, 14, 19, 27, 33, 60, 69, 70, 72, 79, 80, 83, 87, 88, 89, 91, 162, 164, 165, 167, 198
cerebral hemisphere, 76, 184, 186
cerebrospinal fluid, 11, 23, 37, 47
channels, 10, 27
chemiluminescence, 97
chicken, 110, 115, 116, 117, 122, 131, 140
child maltreatment, 201
children, 25, 199, 200, 201, 203, 204, 205
cholinesterase, 90
chromosome, 27
cilia, 173

circadian rhythm, 24

circadian rhythmicity, 24

circulation, 15, 23, 24, 29, 41, 42, 43, 44, 45, 47, 49, 55

class size, 241

classes, xii, 4, 75, 194, 207, 211, 212, 213, 214, 219, 222, 229, 240, 246, 247, 248

classification, xi, xii, 24, 54, 85, 162, 171, 207, 208, 210, 211, 212, 213, 216, 218, 224, 226, 230, 246, 247, 257

clinical symptoms, 26

cloning, 9, 140

closure, 28, 37, 45, 55, 57

cluster headache, viii, 2, 3, 9, 12, 18, 22, 24, 25, 32, 33, 34, 41, 43, 48, 49, 51, 54, 56

clustering, 130, 151, 228, 229, 230, 231, 232, 233, 234, 235, 236, 237, 238, 242, 243, 244, 255, 265

clusters, 176, 230, 233, 245

CNS, 9, 11, 12, 31, 33, 52, 111, 114, 115, 117, 204, 208, 209

CO2, 98, 150

cocaine, 41

coding, 164

cognition, 160

cognitive abilities, 60

cognitive function, 90

cognitive impairment, 181

cognitive processing, 198

coherence, 204

collagen, 209, 210, 255

collateral, 156

colon, 198

commissure, 178

communication, vii, xi, 44, 154, 167, 197, 202, 204

complex behaviors, 61

complexity, 35, 135, 193, 194, 227

components, 115, 118, 167, 200, 209, 214, 215, 216, 218, 219, 239, 240, 247, 248, 249, 250

composition, vii, xii, 207, 208, 214, 258, 259, 262

comprehension, 69

compression, 209

computation, 208, 243

computational capacity, 67

concentration, 22, 28, 32, 102, 103, 105, 106, 108, 110, 227

conductance, 11, 32

conduction, 4, 28, 29, 198, 210, 211, 212, 213, 216, 218, 219, 223, 226, 256, 257, 259

confidence, 221, 222

confidence interval, 221, 222

confinement, 109

confusion, 72

connective tissue, 30, 96, 209, 210, 263

connectivity, 67, 84, 85, 87, 129, 178, 199, 213

consensus, 131

conservation, ix, 121, 122, 129, 133, 134, 192

contamination, 96

control, viii, 2, 10, 12, 13, 14, 16, 17, 20, 21, 33, 34, 37, 40, 48, 50, 93, 108, 111, 113, 114, 115, 134, 137, 141, 192, 198, 199, 203, 206, 263

cornea, 8

coronary arteries, 32

correlation, 101, 103, 108, 111, 112, 151, 152, 209, 214, 226

cortex, x, xi, 8, 13, 14, 15, 27, 32, 33, 34, 39, 60, 61, 63, 64, 65, 66, 67, 68, 69, 70, 71, 72, 73, 74, 75, 76, 77, 78, 80, 81, 82, 83, 85, 86, 87, 88, 89, 90, 118, 126, 127, 132, 133, 139, 145, 146, 147, 149, 150, 154, 155, 156, 161, 162, 163, 164, 171, 173, 174, 176, 177, 178, 181, 264

cortical localization, 69

cortical neurons, 60, 75

corticotropin, 137

coupling, 48

cranial nerve, vii, 1, 2, 5, 6, 7, 19, 33, 198

cranium, 173

creatine, 24

cross-sectional study, 53

CSF, 11, 23, 133

cues, 118, 238, 239

culture, ix, 94, 95, 109, 110, 111, 113, 117

cycles, 96, 130

cytoarchitecture, 60, 67, 82, 85, 87, 88, 179

cytochrome, x, 74, 91, 145, 148, 151, 152, 153, 154, 163, 164

cytokines, 95, 112, 117

cytometry, 116

D

data set, 233

dating, x, 165

death, 95, 108, 109, 111, 112, 114, 115, 117, 118, 119, 204, 263

decompression illness, 57

deep brain stimulation, 18, 25, 35

defects, 241, 242, 243, 244

definition, 136, 229, 242

degradation, 31, 44

dementia, 241

demyelination, 245

dendrites, 61, 70, 125, 174

density, 51, 67, 78, 80, 81, 94, 97, 126, 127, 133, 134, 185, 214, 233, 234, 235, 236, 237, 241, 242, 243, 244, 245, 251, 262

depolarization, 28, 29, 32, 35, 199

deposition, 172, 179, 180

deposits, 174, 176

depression, viii, 2, 23, 27, 28, 31, 43, 47, 56

deprivation, 95, 131, 135, 139

derivatives, 94, 248

detection, 54, 82, 97, 230

determinism, 203

developmental change, 108

developmental process, viii, 93, 94

deviation, 231, 232

diagnostic criteria, 25

dialysis, 36

differentiation, 32, 64, 94, 111, 112, 113, 117

diffusion, 84, 88, 91, 182, 209

digestion, 96

dilation, 10, 35

direct action, 109

disability, 3, 25, 48

discharges, 28

discipline, vii, 196

discourse, 208

discrimination, 149

disorder, 23, 24, 25, 139, 180, 182

displacement, 5

distortions, 244

distress, 200

divergence, 113

diversification, 62, 67

diversity, viii, 59, 60, 62, 63

division, 129

DNA, 73, 96

dogs, 69, 138

dominance, 19, 67, 88, 199

donations, 179

donors, 10

dopamine, 180, 182

dopaminergic, 114, 174, 178

dorsal horn, 2, 3, 4, 7, 8, 11, 13, 14, 16, 17, 18, 19, 20, 21, 33, 34, 35, 42, 45, 48, 51, 55, 57, 58, 260

drawing, 185

drugs, 12, 31, 32, 33, 43, 58, 135, 245

dry ice, 96, 124

dura mater, vii, 1, 6, 7, 8, 12, 30, 46, 47, 49

duration, 11, 23, 25, 31, 61, 113

DWI, 174

E

economic problem, 3

EEG, 204

elaboration, 206

electrocardiogram, 200

electrodes, 226, 238

electroencephalogram, 204

electron, 36, 41, 42, 164

electron microscopy, 41

ELISA, 97, 100, 103, 108

embolism, 36

embryo, 87, 116, 263

embryology, 181

emission, 26, 34, 35, 42

emotion, xii, 22, 160, 166, 197, 198, 199, 200, 201, 202, 203, 205

emotion regulation, xii, 197, 198, 199, 200, 201, 202, 203, 205

emotional experience, 3

emotional valence, 15

emotions, 13, 15, 203, 205

empathy, 203

encoding, 13, 40, 42

endocrine, 133

endorphins, 9

endothelium, 29

energy, vii, 2, 26, 38, 130

engagement, 199

enkephalins, 54

enlargement, 29

entorhinal cortex, 173, 180

environment, vii, xi, 123, 146, 197, 202, 263

environmental factors, viii, 2, 62, 66

epithelium, 96, 98, 181

equilibrium, 46

estrogen, 27, 56

ethology, 188

European Community, 149

event-related potential, 205

evolution, x, xi, 74, 83, 86, 88, 90, 121, 122, 129, 130, 139, 141, 183, 185, 192, 194, 195, 199

excitability, 35, 257

excitation, 45, 197

exclusion, 241

experimental condition, 224

exposure, 32, 108, 113, 206, 245

extensor, 238

Index

271

extraction, 87

extravasation, 12, 29

F

facial muscles, 199

facial nerve, 25

factor analysis, 191, 193

family, 9, 12, 18, 32, 94, 99, 112, 136, 141, 166, 189, 193, 195

fasciculation, 209, 261

fasting, 131

fauna, 166

fear, 21, 25, 200, 206

feelings, 15

females, 123, 201

ferret, 154, 155, 163

fiber bundles, 84

fibroblasts, 209

fidelity, 96

filters, 200

fingerprints, 78, 85, 91

fish, 122, 130, 134

fixation, 69, 79, 81, 82, 89, 90

flexibility, 64, 204

flexor, 57, 238

flight, 199

floating, 123, 124

fluid, 129, 130, 135

fluid balance, 130

fluorescence, 100, 103, 104, 228

focusing, 22

food, 18, 123, 130, 131, 134, 135, 138, 140, 141, 143, 146

food intake, 18, 138, 140, 141

foramen, 28, 44, 45, 49, 53, 54, 55, 186

foramen ovale, 28, 44, 45, 49, 53, 54, 55

Ford, 138, 141

forebrain, 14, 15, 22, 48, 75, 94, 127, 141, 189, 196, 198

formaldehyde, 69

Fourier transform technique, 200

fovea, 155

fractality, xi, 183

freezing, 90

frontal cortex, 22, 71, 163

frontal lobe, x, 24, 162, 163, 165, 166, 167, 173, 174

frustration, 200

functional changes, 49

functional imaging, viii, 18, 35, 54, 59

functional MRI, 24, 34, 85, 146

G

Gabon, 194

ganglion, ix, x, 4, 6, 7, 8, 10, 12, 31, 36, 39, 40, 41, 45, 46, 47, 53, 58, 93, 94, 95, 98, 99, 100, 101, 103, 104, 106, 107, 113, 114, 115, 116, 117, 118, 119, 145, 147, 148, 159, 226, 259, 260

gastrin, 9

gastrocnemius, 259

gastrointestinal tract, 11, 12

gate-control theory, 16

gel, 96, 98

gender, 135

gene, vii, viii, 2, 8, 24, 27, 30, 31, 35, 36, 37, 38, 39, 41, 42, 43, 44, 45, 46, 47, 50, 51, 53, 54, 55, 56, 57, 58, 73, 83, 85, 88, 91, 107, 110, 114, 115, 116, 117, 136, 138, 139, 204, 230, 245

gene expression, 38, 73, 83, 85, 91, 115, 136

gene therapy, 28, 55

gene transfer, 114

generalized anxiety disorder, 206

generation, 10, 29, 116, 195, 241, 243

genes, 28, 51, 73, 74, 83, 201

genetic mutations, 67

genetics, 47, 53, 57, 136

genotype, 206

genre, 194

glia, 117, 260

glucose, 136

glutamate, 8, 10, 27, 31, 32, 38, 44, 52, 73, 130, 141, 143

glycine, 56, 97, 98

gonads, 140

government, iv

gracilis, 7

grants, 202

granules, 70

graph, x, 145, 149, 150, 159, 160, 161

gray matter, viii, 2, 13, 21, 24, 48, 57, 184

grief, 205

grouping, 87, 250, 264

groups, x, 7, 61, 67, 73, 102, 105, 106, 133, 146, 176, 210, 212, 227, 238, 256

growth, 85, 89, 95, 111, 114, 115, 116, 117, 119, 184, 209, 238, 258, 262, 263

growth factor, 95, 114, 115, 116, 117, 119

growth rate, 184

guidance, 263, 264

H

harmony, 60
headache, vii, viii, 1, 2, 3, 5, 8, 9, 10, 13, 18, 19, 22, 23, 24, 25, 26, 27, 28, 29, 30, 31, 32, 33, 34, 36, 37, 38, 39, 40, 42, 45, 47, 48, 49, 51, 54, 55
health, 25, 203
heart rate, 198, 199, 200, 202, 204, 205, 206
heat, 39
heavy metals, 86
hemisphere, 68, 77
hemorrhage, vii, 1
heterogeneity, 91
hippocampus, 15, 75, 118, 132, 133, 180
histamine, 29, 49
histidine, 9, 40
histochemistry, 49, 91, 149
histogram, 212, 215, 217, 221, 223, 238, 239, 240, 241
histology, iv, 181, 241
holism, 155
homeostasis, ix, 121, 129, 131
homogeneity, 243, 251
Honda, 122, 136
hormone, 129, 136, 137, 138
HPA axis, 139
human animal, 201
human brain, 66, 69, 83, 88, 89, 91, 146, 173, 174, 175, 176, 177, 178, 180
human cerebral cortex, 72, 85, 90, 91, 167
human subjects, 8, 83
hybridization, 73
hybridoma, 75
hydrogen, 124
hydrogen peroxide, 124
hypersensitivity, 26
hypertension, vii, 1, 95, 116
hypoglossal nerve, 227, 262
hypothalamus, viii, ix, 2, 3, 13, 14, 16, 17, 19, 22, 24, 27, 33, 34, 35, 37, 44, 57, 121, 125, 126, 127, 129, 130, 131, 132, 133, 134, 136, 137, 138, 139, 140, 142, 198
hypothermia, 46
hypothesis, x, 51, 109, 113, 145, 147, 148, 149, 152, 153, 154, 159, 160, 250
hypothesis test, 250

I

identification, 14, 83, 85, 87, 124, 137, 139, 174, 193
identity, 219
idiopathic, 4, 49, 180, 182
illusion, 39
imagery, 67
images, 70, 81
immunoglobulin, 124
immunohistochemistry, 40, 76, 132
immunomodulator, 43
immunoreactivity, 7, 8, 18, 29, 31, 39, 40, 45, 46, 47, 51, 52, 53, 76, 80, 100, 106, 108, 111, 136, 137, 139, 140, 142, 143, 181, 182
impairments, 69
in vitro, ix, 29, 41, 45, 52, 94, 107, 109, 111, 113, 114, 116, 117, 134
in vivo, 9, 38, 39, 43, 58, 84, 86, 94, 95, 107, 109, 113, 116, 117, 118, 211, 227
incidence, 28, 252, 255
indices, xi, 183, 184, 188, 189, 203, 216
individual differences, 206
induction, 50, 95, 98, 116, 245, 248
inertia, 193, 194
infants, 199, 201, 205
inflammation, 4, 5, 9, 12, 20, 29, 32, 52, 57
inflation, 51
information processing, x, 53, 145, 147, 153, 154, 155, 178
inhibition, 3, 16, 17, 20, 21, 27, 34, 48, 55, 56, 61, 131, 200, 203, 241
inhibitor, 42, 44, 113
initiation, viii, 2, 22
injections, 86, 95, 117, 131, 132, 142, 152, 156, 158, 159, 260
injuries, 227, 239, 255
injury, 4, 15, 20, 29, 40, 116
insertion, 206, 226
insomnia, 141, 143
insulin, ix, 94, 95, 96, 97, 98, 103, 105, 106, 107, 111, 112, 114, 115, 116, 118, 119
integration, 18, 61, 63, 67, 83, 172, 206
integrity, ix, 94, 107
interaction, 14, 16, 28, 33, 46, 55, 76
interactions, 15, 16, 38, 107, 117, 229, 239, 240
interneurons, 5, 10, 11, 16, 21, 48, 76, 95, 174
interparental conflict, 203
interval, 198, 218
intramuscular injection, 124, 137

Index 273

intraocular, 109
ion channels, 9, 32
ion transport, 28, 51
ions, vii, 1, 26, 75, 86
ipsilateral, 4, 7, 11, 14, 19, 24, 30, 31, 34, 53, 198, 257
iron, 22
ischemia, 119
isolation, 75
isoleucine, 9, 40

K

K⁺, vii, 2, 11, 27, 40, 56

L

labeling, 48, 52, 78, 98, 100, 125, 159, 180, 198, 206
labor, xii, 82, 83, 85, 207, 208
laminar, 64, 71, 74, 81, 87, 88, 129, 162
lamination, 65, 71, 79
larva, 132
larynx, 199
latency, 226
left hemisphere, 187
lens, 96, 150
lesions, 18, 21, 53, 57, 117, 122, 138, 147, 182, 241, 264
leucine, 54
ligand, 138
light cycle, 123
limbic system, 2, 13, 14, 19, 33, 86, 143, 166
limitation, 35, 135, 230
line, x, 68, 69, 70, 75, 77, 108, 110, 111, 112, 145, 161, 233
lipids, 80
lithium, 25
lithotripsy, 50
localization, 24, 40, 41, 44, 47, 56, 69, 87, 89, 130, 135, 136, 138, 180, 227
locomotor, 132
locus, viii, 2, 3, 13, 16, 18, 22, 34, 110, 115, 126, 132, 134, 137
lordosis, 21
LTD, 114
luteinizing hormone, 139, 141

M

magnesium, vii, 1, 26, 35, 38
magnetic resonance imaging (MRI), 22, 24, 34, 39, 47, 49, 57, 83, 90, 91
maltreatment, 201, 204
mammal, 61, 86, 166, 211
mammalian brain, 122
mapping, 78, 82, 83, 85, 88, 90, 97, 227, 263
marital conflict, 200
mast cells, 29
matrix, 124, 192
maturation, 86, 94, 108, 111, 119, 202
measurement, 38, 206, 226, 246, 247, 248
measures, 242, 243, 244
median, 12, 130, 131, 227, 255, 260, 261, 262
mediation, 15, 196
medulla, 2, 3, 4, 7, 8, 14, 16, 17, 19, 20, 21, 22, 30, 31, 33, 35, 41, 42, 46, 52, 55, 56, 57, 129
medulla oblongata, 7, 30, 31, 46, 55
MEK, 114
melanin, 136, 137, 138
membranes, 97, 210
memory, 15, 172, 178, 204
memory formation, 172, 178
meninges, 2, 29
meningitis, vii, 1
mental state, 50
mental states, 50
mentor, 166
meridian, 155
mesencephalon, 6, 11, 133, 134, 142
mesenteric vessels, 11
messengers, 44, 56
metabolic syndrome, 205
metabolism, vii, 1, 26, 38, 48, 70, 130
methanol, 97
micrometer, 97
microscope, 69, 70, 82, 98, 125
microscopy, 70
microstructure, 79, 90
midbrain, 2, 3, 5, 6, 16, 21, 24, 34, 38, 39, 127, 133, 142
migraine headache, 2, 12, 22, 26, 28, 29, 37, 43, 45, 46, 53
MIP, 147, 151
mitochondria, 74
mobility, 209
modeling, 212, 214, 239, 241

models, xii, 27, 29, 36, 40, 45, 47, 56, 58, 95, 112, 113, 147, 152, 153, 199, 207, 208, 214, 215, 216, 217, 218, 224, 225, 238, 239, 240, 241, 245, 249, 252, 258

modulations, 16

modules, x, 67, 82, 145, 150, 151, 152, 153, 161, 163

mole, 61, 63, 86, 87

molecular biology, 75, 82, 85, 208

molecules, 29, 43, 75, 86, 88, 91, 94, 239, 263

monoclonal antibody, 97

mood, 16, 20, 200

morphine, 54

morphology, viii, 45, 59, 60, 69, 76, 79, 129, 136, 143, 184, 185, 188, 212, 214

morphometric, xii, 90, 207, 208, 209, 212, 214, 226, 239, 259

mosaic, 159, 230, 264

motion, x, 63, 145, 148, 152, 161, 205

motor fiber, 219, 220, 221, 222, 229, 233, 238, 259

motor neurons, 16, 212, 239, 262

motor system, 238, 239

movement, 25, 132, 162

mRNA, ix, 9, 44, 94, 99, 100, 101, 103, 104, 107, 108, 111, 112, 113, 115, 116, 117, 118, 132, 142

mtDNA, 188

mucosa, 58, 172, 174

muscles, vii, 1, 2, 5, 6, 52, 133, 221, 227, 228, 238, 259, 263

mutant, 132, 257

mutation, 107, 109, 113, 139, 140

myelin, 60, 66, 70, 72, 78, 80, 84, 210, 211, 230, 256

myocardium, 198

N

Na$^+$, vii, 2, 27, 40, 56

narcolepsy, 122, 139, 140, 143

natural selection, 192

nausea, 25, 26

negative influences, 201

neocortex, viii, 59, 60, 61, 62, 64, 67, 69, 70, 73, 75, 78, 79, 80, 86, 88, 91, 264

neonates, 200

nerve fibers, vii, xii, 8, 9, 11, 12, 13, 29, 41, 42, 50, 55, 56, 207, 208, 209, 210, 211, 216, 218, 220, 226, 227, 228, 230, 236, 238, 250, 255, 256, 257, 262, 264

nerve growth factor, 10, 32, 117

nervous system, viii, 6, 15, 51, 89, 93, 94, 114, 117, 119, 142, 166, 195, 205, 208, 245

network, ix, x, 21, 28, 31, 61, 62, 94, 107, 145, 149, 159, 160, 161, 162

neural development, 87, 88, 95, 111

neural function, 67

neural network, 160

neuralgia, 4, 46

neurobiology, 50, 163, 166, 180, 182, 206

neuroblasts, viii, 93, 94, 108, 179, 182

neurodegenerative diseases, xi, 171

neurodegenerative disorders, 172, 180, 241

neurofibrillary tangles, 172, 177, 178, 179, 265

neurogenesis, 111, 115, 264

neuroimaging, 24, 39, 72, 83, 198

neurokinin, 8, 9, 29, 35, 42, 43, 45, 53

neuromotor, 130

neuronal apoptosis, 117

neuronal cells, 31, 90, 94

neuronal systems, 132, 140

neuropathic pain, 52, 258

neuropathy, 255

neuropeptides, viii, ix, 2, 8, 9, 10, 23, 26, 29, 31, 32, 33, 44, 45, 53, 121, 122, 129, 141

neurophysiology, 53, 199

neuroprotection, 114, 115

neuroscience, vii, 88, 169, 181

neurosecretory, ix, 121, 130, 140

neuroses, 199

neurosurgery, 180

neurotoxicity, 258

neurotransmitter, 2, 5, 9, 11, 12, 13, 16, 17, 19, 25, 31, 32, 33, 50, 52

neurotrophic factors, viii, 32, 93, 94, 107, 109, 113, 117

nitric oxide, viii, 2, 10, 13, 30, 33, 43, 50, 51, 55, 56

nitric oxide synthase, 10

NMR, 90

nodes, x, 146, 149, 159, 160, 210

norepinephrine, 41, 199

normal development, 108, 118, 239

nuclei, 2, 3, 4, 6, 7, 13, 14, 16, 17, 18, 20, 21, 33, 35, 38, 58, 70, 73, 76, 94, 98, 99, 102, 106, 134, 136, 141, 184, 198, 200, 238, 239

nucleic acid, 70

nucleus tractus solitarius, 13, 15, 18, 19, 22, 35, 48, 57

null hypothesis, 244

Index

275

O

obligate, 190
observations, 48, 67, 69, 70, 73, 135, 227, 247
occipital cortex, 27, 57, 64, 71, 79, 147
occipital lobe, 163
oculomotor, 227, 262
oculomotor nerve, 262
olfaction, 182
omission, 125
opiates, 11
opioids, 20
optic chiasm, 173
optic nerve, ix, 93, 95, 108, 113, 116
oral cavity, 44
order, 5, 6, 9, 13, 14, 29, 63, 79, 80, 88, 98, 124, 130, 185, 199, 201, 209, 230, 244
organ, 127, 196, 211, 227
organism, 15, 73
ovaries, 142
ovulation, 142
oxygen, 25

P

pain, 1, 2, 3, 5, 7, 8, 9, 10, 11, 12, 13, 14, 16, 17, 18, 20, 21, 22, 23, 24, 25, 28, 29, 30, 31, 32, 33, 34, 35, 36, 37, 39, 40, 41, 42, 43, 44, 45, 46, 48, 49, 50, 52, 53, 54, 55, 56, 57, 58, 258, 261
palate, 199
pancreas, 198
panic disorder, 200, 204
parallel processing, 67, 147, 148, 155
parameter, 215, 216, 217, 220, 234, 240, 241, 244, 246, 249
parameters, 81, 90, 214, 215, 217, 224, 225, 240
parasympathetic nervous system, 198
parenchyma, 29
parietal cortex, 91, 147, 161, 162
paroxetine, 37
partition, 230, 233, 238, 244
parvalbumin, 10, 75, 76, 86
pathogenesis, viii, 2, 12, 26, 27, 28, 180, 241, 264
pathology, x, 44, 165, 179, 180, 181, 182
pathophysiology, 3, 18, 22, 25, 26, 34, 43, 44, 54, 55
pathways, 2, 3, 13, 15, 16, 17, 19, 34, 35, 37, 38, 52, 55, 57, 86, 90, 109, 148, 152, 162, 163, 201, 202
PCR, 96, 100, 101, 103, 104, 108, 112
PEP, 10

peptides, 8, 11, 22, 31, 39, 41, 42, 45, 46, 50, 55, 58, 132, 134, 136, 137, 138, 140
percentile, 233
periodicity, 24
peripheral nervous system, 241
permeability, 29
permit, 15, 199
personal communication, 84
personality, 199, 200, 202, 203
personality disorder, 200, 202
personality traits, 199
PET, 24, 26, 34, 49, 91
pH, 96, 97, 99
phantom limb pain, 4
pharmacogenetics, 51
pharmacology, 41, 56
pharynx, 199
phenotype, 141
phosphorylation, 26, 35
photophobia, 25, 26
photosensitivity, 137
phrenology, 69
physical activity, 26
physical health, 203
physical treatments, 23
physiology, 40, 44, 135, 162, 203, 208
plasma, 8, 11, 12, 23, 24, 28, 29, 39, 41, 42, 49
plasma levels, 23
plasma membrane, 28
plasticity, 10, 32, 44, 45, 118, 201
plexus, 261
polymerase, 96
polymorphism, xi, 184, 187, 188, 193, 206
polypeptide, 9, 36, 44, 47, 55, 137, 140
pons, viii, 2, 3, 5, 6, 14, 19, 26, 34, 46
population density, 74, 78, 81
porosity, 264
positron, 24, 26, 34, 35
positron emission tomography, 24
potassium, 28, 70
power, 204, 211, 246
precipitation, 75
predictors, 205
prefrontal cortex, 89, 198
prematurity, 202
preschool children, 203
pressure, 4, 5, 14, 62, 85, 211
prevention, 25
primary cells, 6

Index

primary visual cortex, viii, 59, 67, 74, 77, 78, 82, 83, 86, 89, 162

primate, 63, 74, 86, 87, 88, 89, 90, 146, 162, 163, 164, 195, 206

probability, 217, 242, 244, 246, 247, 248, 250, 251

probability density function, 217, 250

probability distribution, 244, 247, 251

probe, 112

problem drinking, 203

processing pathways, 33, 147

prodrome, 26

production, 29, 30, 33

program, 187, 193, 228, 233

programming, 203, 204

prolactin, 139

proliferation, 98

promoter, 10

propagation, 28

prophylactic, 25, 54

prophylaxis, 55

prostaglandins, 10, 29

prostheses, xii, 207, 226, 238

prosthesis, 252, 255

protein synthesis, 70

proteins, xi, 32, 70, 87, 94, 115, 130, 171

protocol, 124, 239

proto-oncogene, 118

psychiatric disorders, 201

psychopathology, 201, 202

psychosomatic, 199

puberty, 143

pupil, 150

purification, 75

purity, 98

pyramidal cells, 61, 62, 66, 67, 70, 75, 76, 77

Q

quality of life, 3

quinolinic acid, 21

R

radiation, xi, 177, 178, 183, 190

radius, 243, 251

rain, 35, 36, 48, 260, 261

Ramadan, 8, 31, 52

range, 5, 9, 13, 60, 61, 66, 78, 80, 84, 166, 194, 198, 201, 210, 217, 220, 221, 222, 223, 226, 238, 240

rapid eye movement sleep, 142

reactivity, 58, 199, 200, 203, 204, 206

receptive field, 29, 87, 162

receptor sites, 18

receptors, viii, ix, 2, 4, 6, 9, 10, 11, 17, 29, 30, 32, 33, 35, 40, 41, 43, 44, 45, 48, 55, 56, 58, 59, 78, 91, 93, 94, 95, 107, 109, 110, 113, 115, 116, 117, 118, 119, 122, 130, 131, 134, 135, 136, 141, 142, 172, 211, 259

recognition, 87, 146, 147

reconcile, 82, 83, 85

reconstruction, 81, 84, 187, 243

recovery, 200, 206, 257

recurrence, 57

redevelopment, 193, 195

reductionism, 155

redundancy, 193

reflexes, 6, 257

regenerate, 238

regeneration, xii, 208, 213, 214, 226, 239, 241, 258, 262, 264

region, x, 2, 3, 16, 18, 21, 24, 29, 34, 36, 38, 61, 68, 75, 81, 82, 83, 85, 87, 91, 97, 126, 131, 136, 151, 155, 165, 167, 175, 176, 178, 186, 187, 230, 251

regression, 65, 214

regulation, 11, 13, 18, 30, 33, 38, 50, 111, 112, 114, 115, 118, 131, 132, 134, 136, 142, 193, 198, 199, 200, 203, 204, 205, 206

relationship, x, 14, 44, 63, 65, 81, 84, 89, 121, 142, 151, 152, 158, 162, 210, 211, 212, 213

relaxation, 13, 29

relevance, 36, 43, 47, 78, 172, 255

reliability, 72, 80, 83, 85

relief, 12, 16, 26, 34, 45, 54

REM, 122, 133, 143, 182

reproduction, ix, 121, 122, 129, 130

reptile, 122, 166

resistance, 209

resolution, 3, 22, 69, 83

resources, 201

respiration, 18, 20, 150, 200

respiratory, 200, 203, 205

respiratory rate, 201

responsiveness, xii, 40, 114, 197, 201

retina, ix, 86, 91, 94, 95, 96, 99, 100, 102, 105, 106, 107, 108, 109, 110, 111, 112, 114, 115, 116, 117, 118, 119, 146, 241, 264

retinol, 74

reverse transcriptase, 96

rheumatoid arthritis, 54, 55

Index

rhino, 180
rhinorrhea, 23
rhythm, 118
riboflavin, 54
ribose, 70
rice, 172, 173, 175, 177, 178
right hemisphere, 146, 147, 148, 150, 151, 159, 187
risk, 39, 139, 174, 181, 201
risk factors, 39
RNA, 96

S

sampling, 200, 214, 241, 264
saturation, 162
scanning electron microscopy, 255
secrete, 114, 133
secretion, 10, 141
segregation, 61, 67, 147, 148, 150, 152, 153, 162, 163
selective serotonin reuptake inhibitor, 23
selectivity, 89, 130, 162, 208, 226, 255
selenium, 86
sensation, 4, 7, 9, 14, 16, 33, 39, 49, 54
sensations, 14, 19
sensitivity, 20, 23, 25, 44, 82, 85, 130, 201, 228
sensitization, 8, 18, 28, 31, 35
sensory experience, 108
sensory modalities, 172
sensory modality, 261
sensory projection, 51, 260
septum, 126, 127, 128, 133, 185
serotonin, vii, 1, 12, 26, 30, 44, 47, 142
serum, viii, 2, 24, 97, 124
serum albumin, 97
sex differences, 135
sex hormones, 11, 44
sexual behavior, 140
shape, 6, 81, 148, 159, 184, 210
sheep, 70, 129, 135, 136, 141
shyness, 200, 203, 204, 205, 206
signal transduction, 94, 118
signaling pathway, 10, 119
signalling, ix, 9, 16, 38, 94, 95, 111, 117, 118
signals, 22, 60, 94, 110, 111, 115, 201
signal-to-noise ratio, 84
signs, 24
silver, 70, 86, 181
simulation, 243
sinoatrial node, 198, 199

sinus, 9, 24, 29, 30, 32, 38, 39, 46, 58, 200, 203, 204, 205
sinus arrhythmia, 200, 203, 204, 205
sinuses, vii, 1, 5, 29, 30
skeletal muscle, 259, 260, 264
skills, 200
skin, 2, 4, 6, 7, 8, 9, 19, 23, 33, 41, 52, 222, 223, 259, 261
smooth muscle, 29
SMS, 12, 46
SNS, 198, 199
sociability, 200, 205
social phobia, 206
social policy, 167
social stress, 143, 206
social withdrawal, 200
sodium, 2, 27, 32, 40, 75, 97, 124, 149, 202
soleus, 259
somata, 10, 142
somatomotor, 6
space, 14, 28, 51, 147, 148, 159, 199, 203, 230, 238, 242, 243, 244, 245
spatial information, 61
specialization, vii, 64, 67, 73, 130, 131, 135, 160
speciation, 189, 193
species, ix, xi, 40, 60, 62, 63, 64, 65, 66, 67, 72, 74, 78, 80, 81, 82, 83, 85, 88, 121, 129, 130, 131, 132, 134, 135, 149, 166, 172, 183, 184, 185, 187, 188, 189, 190, 191, 192, 193, 202, 211, 212, 213, 226, 259
spectroscopy, 24, 48
speech, 69
spinal cord, 2, 4, 5, 8, 11, 12, 13, 16, 17, 19, 21, 31, 34, 36, 37, 38, 39, 44, 45, 46, 48, 49, 50, 52, 54, 55, 57, 58, 137, 143, 199, 238, 239, 260, 262, 263
spindle, 70, 211, 221, 259
standard deviation, 240
statistics, xii, 203, 207
stimulus, 4, 14, 31, 44, 130, 149, 150, 155, 226
stochastic model, 239
strategies, 23, 25, 205
stress, ix, xii, 20, 23, 121, 122, 138, 197, 198, 199, 200, 201, 204, 205, 206
stressors, 200
striae, 173
striatum, 126, 127, 133, 143, 185
stroke, 12, 57
structural changes, 24, 73
subcutaneous injection, 24
subjectivity, viii, 59

substrates, vii, viii, 1, 2, 3, 111, 205
sucrose, 96, 123, 124
suprachiasmatic nucleus, 125, 136
survival, viii, 32, 61, 93, 94, 95, 102, 105, 106, 107, 108, 109, 110, 111, 112, 113, 114, 115, 116, 117, 118, 119, 228
susceptibility, 27, 56
swelling, 29, 44
symmetry, 219, 258
sympathectomy, 41
sympathetic nervous system, 198
symptoms, xi, 12, 23, 24, 26, 27, 28, 55, 122, 171, 172, 179
synapse, 4, 6, 14, 174, 263
synaptic strength, 35
synaptic vesicles, 75
syndrome, 23, 43, 49
synergistic effect, 10
synovial fluid, 55
synovial tissue, 11, 54, 55
synthesis, 10, 11, 29, 43, 55, 108

T

targets, 18, 75, 109, 179, 208, 226, 239
task conditions, 203
task demands, 162
tau, xi, 171, 172, 176, 177, 178
taurocholic acid, 46
taxonomy, 189, 193, 194
telencephalon, ix, xi, 121, 127, 129, 134, 141, 142, 179, 183, 184, 185, 186, 187, 191, 192, 193, 194
temperament, 203, 204, 205, 206
temperature, 4, 9, 39, 123, 150, 226
temporal lobe, 69, 173
tension, 1, 22, 23, 36, 37, 38, 47, 51, 55, 209
tension headache, 1, 23
terminals, 7, 8, 11, 16, 22, 30, 31, 36, 46, 56, 58, 76, 86, 89, 159
territory, 9, 31
tetrapod, 125
thalamus, 5, 13, 14, 24, 33, 62, 76, 88, 126, 127, 128, 129, 132, 133, 134, 139
therapeutics, 43, 52
therapy, 36, 40, 49, 56, 138
three-dimensional reconstruction, 84
three-dimensional space, 163
tissue, 1, 3, 4, 5, 20, 21, 23, 26, 28, 30, 54, 56, 60, 69, 70, 75, 79, 81, 84, 94, 96, 99, 111, 124, 125,

137, 140, 142, 143, 209, 233, 242, 243, 244, 245, 265
tonic, vii, xii, 48, 197
topology, 243, 260
torus, 127, 128, 129, 132, 133
toxicology, xii, 208
tracking, 91, 202
trajectory, 159
transcatheter, 37
transcription, 32
transducer, 9
transduction, 4
transection, 95
transformations, 63
transforming growth factor, 115
transition, 68, 73
translation, 198, 242
transmission, 2, 16, 17, 20, 21, 22, 30, 31, 32, 33, 55, 58, 182, 255, 257
transport, 1, 19, 26, 28, 29, 44, 52, 55, 260
transverse section, 184, 186
trapezius, 23
trauma, 201
triceps, 257
tricyclic antidepressant, 23
tricyclic antidepressants, 23
trigeminal nerve, 2, 5, 6, 7, 8, 9, 25, 28, 29, 31, 33, 51
triggers, 46
trypsin, 99
tumors, 5, 54
tyrosine hydroxylase, 142, 143, 180, 182

U

underlying mechanisms, 53
urinary bladder, 52

V

vagus, vii, 1, 5, 7, 198, 199
vagus nerve, 7
variability, 62, 66, 67, 78, 80, 85, 200, 202, 203, 204, 205, 206
variance, 80, 81, 214, 246
vasculature, 8, 55
vasoactive intestinal peptide, viii, 2, 9, 43, 58
vasoconstriction, 13
vasodilation, 8, 9, 11, 13, 28, 29, 30, 33

vasodilator, 10, 25, 29, 33, 38
vasomotor, 33, 41, 45, 52
vasopressin, 9, 139
vasospasm, 12
vector, 247, 248, 249
vein, 23, 24
velocity, 4, 25, 28, 38, 198, 210, 211, 212, 216, 219, 256, 257, 259
ventilation, 15
ventricle, 125, 126, 127, 131, 174
venules, 29
vertebrates, vii, ix, x, 121, 122, 126, 129, 130, 131, 133, 134, 135
vesicle, 73
vessels, 5, 6, 9, 10, 11, 12, 13, 25, 29, 32, 33, 35, 40, 41, 44, 50, 55
viscera, 4, 18, 198
vision, x, 64, 145, 146, 147, 148, 152, 160, 162, 163, 173
visual area, x, 62, 63, 89, 145, 146, 147, 149, 150, 151, 152, 153, 154, 155, 156, 157, 159, 160, 161, 162, 163, 164
visual field, 89, 154, 156, 163, 241
visual impression, 230
visual processing, 148, 149
visual stimuli, 148, 150, 154, 155
visual system, 64, 87, 91, 108, 116, 118, 119, 146, 149, 159, 163, 164
visualization, 70, 80, 81, 83, 242
vomiting, 25, 26
vulnerability, xii, 197, 198, 199, 201, 204, 205

W

wavelengths, 164
wavelet, 201
white matter, 84, 149, 184

Y

young adults, 204, 206

Z

zinc, 75, 86, 89, 90, 91